Second Edition

Current

PSYCHOTHERAPEUTIC

Drugs

Second Edition

Current

PSYCHOTHERAPEUTIC

Drugs

Frederic M. Quitkin, MD
David C. Adams, MD
Charles L. Bowden, MD
Eric J. Heyer, MD, PhD
Arthur Rifkin, MD
Edward M. Sellers, MD, PhD, FRCPC
Rajiv Tandon, MD
Bonnie P. Taylor, MA

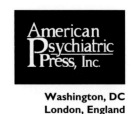

American Psychiatric Press, Inc.

Washington, DC
London, England

DEVELOPED BY CURRENT MEDICINE, INC., PHILADELPHIA

Current Medicine, Inc.
400 Market Street
Suite 700
Philadelphia, PA 19106

Director of Product Development: *Lori J. Bainbridge*
Developmental Editor: *Danielle Shaw*
Assistant Editor: *Jennifer Schafhauser*
Art Director: *Paul Fennessy*
Designers: *Christine Keller-Quirk, Robert LeBrun, Ryan Walsh,
 and Patrick Ward*
Illustration Director: *Ann Saydlowski*
Illustrator: *Beth Starkey*
Production Manager: *Lori Holland*
Production and Marketing Assistant: *Amy Watts*
Drug Company Liaison: *Robin Garstkiewicz*
Indexer: *Lawrence Meyer*

Although every effort has been made to ensure that drug doses and other information are presented accurately in this publication, the ultimate responsibility rests with the prescribing physician. Neither the publishers nor the authors can be held responsible for errors or for any consequences arising from the use of information contained herein. Products mentioned in this publication should be used in accordance with the prescribing information prepared by the manufacturers. No claims or endorsements are made for any drug or compound at present under clinical investigation.

Distributed by American Psychiatric Press, Inc.,
1400 K Street, N.W., Washington, DC 20005

ISBN: 0-88048-994-4
ISSN: 1083-9410
Printed in the United States by Edwards Brothers on acid-free paper
5 4 3 2 1

CONTRIBUTORS

David C. Adams, MD
Assistant Professor
Department of Anesthesiology
College of Physicians and Surgeons of Columbia University;
Assistant Attending Physician
Columbia-Presbyterian Medical Center
New York City, New York

Charles L. Bowden, MD
Professor and Chairman
Department of Psychiatry;
Professor of Pharmacology
University of Texas Health Science Center at San Antonio
San Antonio, Texas

Eric J. Heyer, MD, PhD
Assistant Attending Physician
Herbert Irving Assistant Professor of Anesthesiology
Assistant Professor of Neurology
College of Physicians and Surgeons of Columbia University
New York City, New York

Frederic M. Quitkin, MD
Professor
Department of Psychiatry;
Director, Depression Evaluation Service
College of Physicians and Surgeons of Columbia University
New York City, New York

Arthur Rifkin, MD
Professor of Psychiatry
Albert Einstein College of Medicine
Bronx, New York;
Director
MRIDD Service
Hillside Hospital Division
Long Island Jewish Medical Center
Glen Oaks, New York

Edward M. Sellers, MD, PhD, FRCPC
Professor
Department of Pharmacology, Medicine, and Psychiatry
Centre for Research in Women's Health
Women's College Hospital
University of Toronto
Toronto, Ontario, Canada

Rajiv Tandon, MD
Associate Professor of Psychiatry
University of Michigan Medical School;
Director
Hospital Services Division;
Director
Schizophrenia Program
University of Michigan Medical Center
Ann Arbor, Michigan

Bonnie P. Taylor, MA
Assistant Research Scientist
New York State Psychiatric Institute
New York City, New York

CONTENTS

Stimulants

Arthur Rifkin

■ AMPHETAMINES

This class consists of amphetamine sulfate (the racemic form of amphetamine); its dextro isomer, dextroamphetamine, which has more central nervous system (CNS) effect and less cardiovascular effect than does the racemic form and has largely replaced it; methamphetamine; methylphenidate, the most commonly prescribed member of this class; and pemoline, which works more slowly. A recent addition is a combination of the neutral sulfate salts of dextroamphetamine and amphetamine with the dextro isomer of amphetamine saccharate and d,1-amphetamine aspartate.

EFFICACY AND USE

Few drug treatments of a mental disorder have been as well-documented as stimulants for attention-deficit hyperactivity disorder (ADHD). Hundreds of studies have compared stimulants with placebo and have shown that stimulants alleviate symptoms of short-attention span, hyperactivity, and impulsivity [1]. Systematic laboratory tests also have shown that they improve the performance of repetitive tasks [2].

Systematic observations in the classroom have shown improvements in arithmetic, graphing, and attention [3] as well as motor movements, noncompliance, and overall hyperactivity [4]. However, the effect of treatment on actual school achievement is uncertain. Some studies have shown a lack of improvement [5], yet recent studies have shown otherwise [6].

Overall, about 75% of children with ADHD show moderate to marked improvement in the defining symptoms [7]. Methylphenidate is the most widely used stimulant, followed by dextroamphetamine and pemoline. Initially it seemed paradoxical that drugs that cause overstimulation in adults also could calm hyperactive children. However, moderate acute doses improve attention, concentration, and cognitive functioning in adults and normal children [8]. Children with ADHD slow down and become calmer with stimulants, but the apparent calmness may be due in part to enhanced attention and concentration.

Stimulants also are used for narcolepsy, especially methylphenidate, dextroamphetamine, and pemoline.

MODE OF ACTION

These drugs have sympathomimetic activity centrally and peripherally. The most common explanation for the mechanism of the disorder and of the effect of stimulant treatment involves theories of overarousal and underarousal.

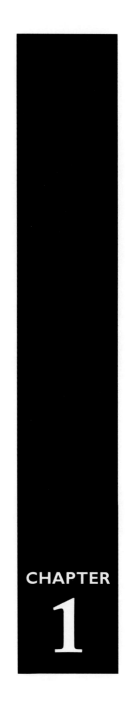

CHAPTER

1

The underarousal theory [9] asserts that children with ADHD are underaroused and seek excessive outside stimulation. A stimulant, therefore, would correct this problem. The overarousal theory posits the presence of excessive neurotransmitters, such as norepinephrine, which stimulants correct by downregulation of the receptor [10]. Tests of arousal, however, such as skin conductance, cortical evoked potentials, and electroencephalography (EEG), have not shown consistent differences between normal children and those with ADHD nor have studies shown differences in peripheral measures of neurotransmitters.

Stimulants affect a wide range of neurotransmitters. Specific agents that stimulate or block the dopamine receptor—L-dopa and haloperidol—have little effect on ADHD, and the evidence is unclear that responders change catecholamine metabolites more than do nonresponders [11].

PHARMACOKINETICS

These drugs are absorbed readily from the gastrointestinal (GI) tract and widely distributed. See descriptions of the individual drugs for details. For dextroamphetamine, the plasma half-life is 7 to 8 hours, (longer when urine is more alkaline), and the drug is metabolized in the liver. Methylphenidate has a plasma half-life of 4 to 5 hours and is metabolized by the liver, and alkalinization of the urine increases the drug's half-life. Pemoline has a plasma half-life of about 12 hours and is metabolized by the liver.

INDICATIONS

These drugs should be used to treat ADHD in children and possibly in adolescents and adults. They should not be used as an appetite suppressant. These amphetamines also are used to treat narcolepsy.

SPECIAL GROUPS

Race: Generally effective regardless of race.
Children: Indicated for children with ADHD and narcolepsy.
Adolescents and adults: Symptoms of ADHD may persist past puberty, and treatment with stimulants may continue to be helpful. Used also in this group for narcolepsy.
Renal impairment: Renal impairment will impair excretion, and stimulants should be used cautiously in such instances.
Hepatic impairment: Hepatic impairment will decrease metabolism and extend the plasma half-life.
Pregnancy: Safety for use during pregnancy has not been established. Cardiac abnormalities and biliary atresia have been associated with stimulant use.
Breast-feeding: Stimulants are excreted in breast milk; do not breast-feed.

PATIENT INFORMATION

Stimulants, by causing stimulation, may mask a decrease in performance due to fatigue and may cause insomnia, poor appetite, nervousness, restlessness, dry mouth, nausea, dizziness, irritability, and GI disturbances. They may elevate blood pressure and cause a rapid heart rate. If any of these effects become pronounced, notify a physician immediately. Follow-up medical examinations and laboratory studies to check blood pressure (adults and children) and growth charts (children) and to reassess the need for continued treatment are necessary. Stimulant users should be monitored closely by a physician, should not chew or crush sustained-release or long-acting tablets, and should not take more than is prescribed.

SPECIAL PRECAUTIONS

Users of amphetamines can develop extensive abuse and dependence, manifested by tolerance, withdrawal symptoms, and the taking of larger amounts than prescribed; persistent unsuccessful efforts to stop or cut down use; impairment of important social occupational, or recreational activities; persistent use despite the causing of physical or psychological problems; and use in physically hazardous situations, such as when driving an automobile. Abuse and dependence are not problems, however, in children receiving amphetamines for ADHD nor in adults under medical supervision.

Amphetamines may mask fatigue and, in large doses, cause psychosis and delirium during intoxication. They may exacerbate some mental disorders, such as schizophrenia, thyroid disease, and cardiovascular disease.

Pills that contain tartrazine may cause an allergic reaction.

CONTRAINDICATIONS

Amphetamines should not be used in people for whom noradrenergic stimulation would pose a risk, such as those with heart disease (including hypertension), hyperthyroidism, glaucoma, or mental agitation; those who are vulnerable to drug abuse; and especially, those taking monoamine oxidase (MAO) inhibitors. In all cases, the value of the drug should be balanced against the risk. These contraindications rarely apply for children with ADHD.

INTERACTIONS

Because of noradrenergic stimulation, amphetamines have been thought to interact dangerously with MAO inhibitors, but I do not believe this is an absolute contraindication. Use of the combination, however, should be left to experts.

ADVERSE REACTIONS

The most common side effects are loss of appetite, weight loss, insomnia, headaches, irritability, and emotional lability. These adverse reactions are dose related, and tolerance often develops. Growth suppression is of most concern; it may occur at a rate of up to 3 cm/y in children receiving more than 20 mg/d of methylphenidate for at least 3 years. Growth appears to rebound when the children stop taking the drug [12]. When followed through adulthood, children with ADHD treated with methylphenidate were as tall as a control group of nontreated adults without ADHD who were matched for socioeconomic status, age, and ethnicity [12].

Persistent tics may be a side effect. Some authors express concern that stimulants may worsen tics in children predisposed to Tourette disorder [13], whereas others doubt the connection and assert that stimulants, with haloperidol, may help control tics in that disorder [14]. No experimental studies have been done to resolve this disagreement.

OVERDOSAGE AND ACCIDENTAL POISONING

Overdosage exacerbates the usual adverse reactions: excitement, agitation, hypertension, tachycardia, mydriasis, ataxia, tremor, tachypnea, fever, headache, and psychosis (usually with persecutory delusions and auditory hallucinations). Psychosis usually does not occur with acute overdosage but chronic overdosage. At higher doses, overdosage causes fever, heart failure, convulsions, and coma. Treatment consists of close monitoring, lavage, and sedative use.

ANALEPTICS

Two drugs constitute the analeptic class: caffeine and doxapram. These drugs increase arousal and stimulate ventilation.

EFFICACY AND USE

These drugs are used for the primary apnea of prematurity [15,16], such as the absence of respiratory effort lasting more than 20 seconds, often with cyanosis and bradycardia. Caffeine also is used to lower the seizure threshold during electroconvulsive therapy.

MODE OF ACTION

The presumed mode of action is CNS stimulation causing increased sensitivity of the carbon dioxide sensors in the medulla, which increases alveolar ventilation and decreases $PaCO_2$ [17].

SPECIAL GROUPS

Children: Used for premature infants with primary apnea.
Elderly: Caffeine may be used as an adjuvant for electroconvulsive therapy to help induce seizures.

SPECIAL PRECAUTIONS

Excessive dosage causes CNS overstimulation, such as tachypnea, tachycardia, and vomiting.

ANOREXIANTS

The anorexiants consist of catecholamine agonists, including benzphetamine, diethylpropion, mazindol, phendimetrazine, phenmetrazine, phentermine, and phenylpranolamine. These drugs are sympathomimetic-like amphetamines that also suppress appetite, but anorexiants have fewer adverse effects of overstimulation than do amphetamines. The serotonin agonists fenfluramine and dexfenfluramine were marketed as anorexiants but were withdrawn because of the risk of causing pulmonary hypertension and heart valve abnormalities [18,19].

EFFICACY AND USE

Several studies demonstrated that brief dosing in normal volunteers reduces appetite [20–22], and the decrease in food intake accounts for weight loss [23,24]. Despite the hope of separating the anorexic and stimulant properties, the catecholamine agonists that suppress appetite have stimulant properties. For example, phenmetrazine causes excitement and euphoria and has been abused [25]. As with amphetamines, phenmetrazine in large doses causes persecutory delusions [26].

How effective are these drugs in reducing weight beyond the clear effects on short-term appetite? A comprehensive review by the United States Food and Drug Administration [27] of 160 double-blind, controlled studies involved 7725 subjects. In 90% of these studies the drug was superior to placebo, but in only 40% was this difference statistically significant. The mean weight loss on the drug was 0.2 kg/wk; however, the drop-out rate was about 50%, and most of the studies were short-term (ie, < 12 wk).

Silverstone [28] summarized the results of six double-blind, placebo-controlled studies of at least 12 weeks' duration and found that all drugs showed similar results: the drug was superior to placebo, no drug seemed superior to others, mean weight loss on the drug ranged from 0.2 to 0.6 kg/wk, and weight loss tended to reach a plateau after 8 weeks.

How persistent is the weight loss? All studies assessing short-term effects in crossover studies of anorexic drug and placebo show that subjects who lost weight during initial treatment with an anorexiant regained it during a subsequent placebo period [29–32]. Similarly, follow-up studies after long-term treatment with anorexiants show rebound weight gain [33,34]. Studies conducted for 9 months [35–39] found no further weight loss after 6 months but no weight gain during the remainder of the study. One double-blind, placebo-controlled study [38] assessed the combination of fenfluramine (60 mg/d) plus phentermine (15 mg/d) in 121 obese subjects for 34 weeks, along with behavior modification, caloric restriction, and exercise. Those on active treatment lost an average of 14.2 kg (15.9% of initial weight) versus 4.6 kg (0.9% of initial weight) in those given placebo, a statistically significant difference. Side effects were mild. During open-label treatment for an additional 70 weeks, most of those who remained on active treatment regained some weight but were, on average, 11.6 kg lighter at the end of 104 weeks of treatment [39].

MODE OF ACTION

The noradrenergic anorexiants appear to act by inducing satiety through increasing the action of norepinephrine and dopamine and decreasing parasympathetic stimulation [40]. Fenfluramine releases serotonin and inhibits its intake, which appears to induce satiety.

PHARMACOKINETICS

Phentermine's blood levels peaks at 4 to 8 hours; the other anorexiants peak at 1 to 2 hours. The half-life, except for delayed release preparations, range from 8 to 20 hours. The catecholamine agonists are excreted unchanged in acid urine. Benzphetamine gets metabolized to amphetamine and methamphetamine.

INDICATIONS

Anorexiants may be useful for weight loss when combined with efforts to reduce calories by behavior therapy, nutritional counseling, and exercise.

SPECIAL GROUPS

Elderly: Recommended only for adults or adolescents; elderly patients are particularly vulnerable to their adverse effects; administer with caution.
Renal or hepatic impairment: Impaired metabolism; administer with caution.
Pregnancy and breast-feeding: These drugs have not been proven safe and should be avoided.

PATIENT INFORMATION

These drugs may cause overstimulation, euphoria, abuse, rapid heart beat, elevated blood pressure, agitation, nervousness, and in large amounts, a severe mental disorder.

SPECIAL PRECAUTIONS

Aside from fenfluramine, these drugs may be abused and lead to dependence. Large doses may cause psychosis, usually manifested by persecutory delusions and auditory hallucinations. They may worsen hypertension and other forms of cardiovascular disease. Using these drugs to combat fatigue may give the erroneous impression that fatigue has not interfered with performance, such as driving. Some agents contain tartrazine, which may cause an allergic reaction.

CONTRAINDICATIONS

Anorexiants should be avoided in patients with heart disease, hyperthyroidism, hypersensitivity to such compounds, glaucoma, history of substance abuse, pregnancy, lactation, and in those taking monoamine oxidase (MAO) inhibitors.

INTERACTIONS

The noradrenergic anorexiants may cause a hypertensive reaction if given with MAO inhibitors and increase the risk of arrhythmia if given with thyroid hormones.

ADVERSE REACTIONS

The noradrenergic anorexiants produce central nervous system (CNS) stimulation and may cause nervousness, irritability, insomnia, decreased sense of fatigue, initial increase in alertness, and euphoria (with subsequent rebound depression and fatigue). They also cause dry mouth, blurred vision, dizziness, tachycardia, cardiac arrhythmia, hypertension, and nausea.

OVERDOSAGE AND ACCIDENTAL POISONING

Overdosage of noradrenergic anorexiants causes excitement, agitation, hypertension, tachycardia, arrhythmia, mydriasis, tremor, hyperreflexia, fever, headache, confusion, aggressivenesss, and psychosis (with symptoms of persecutory delusions and auditory hallucinations). With larger overdoses, fever, rhabdomyolysis, chest pain, cardiovascular collapse, convulsions, and coma may occur.

REFERENCES

1. Solanto MV: Neuropharmacological basis of stimulant drug action in deficit disorder with hyperactivity: a review and synthesis. *Psychol Bull* 1984, 95:387–409.

2. Rapport MD, Murphy HA, Bailey S: Ritalin vs. response cost in the control of hyperactive children: a within-subject comparison. *J Appl Behav Anal* 1982, 15:205–216.

3. Whalen CK, Alkus SR, Adams D, *et al.*: Behavior observations of hyperactive children and methylphenidate (Ritalin) effects in systematically structured classroom environments: now you see them, now you don't. *J Pediatr Psychol* 1978, 3:177–184.

4. Abikoff H, Gittelman R: The normalizing effects of methylphenidate on the classroom behavior of ADHD children. *J Abnorm Child Psychol* 1985, 13:33–44.

5. Cunningham CE, Barkley RA: The role of academic failure in hyperactive behavior. *J Learning Disabilities* 1978, 11:15–21.

6. Klein RG, Bessler AW: Stimulant side effects in children. In *Adverse Effects of Psychotropic Drugs.* Edited by Kane JM, Lieberman JA. New York: Guilford Press; 1992:470–496.

7. Dulcan MK: Using psychostimulants to treat behavioral disorders of children and adolescents. *J Child Adolesc Psychopharmacol* 1990, 1:7–20.

8. Rapoport JL, Buchsbaum M, Zahn TP, *et al.*: Dextroamphetamine: cognitive and behavioral effects in normal prepubertal boys. *Science* 1978, 199:560–562.

9. Zentall SS, Zentall TR: Optimal stimulation: a model of disorderd activity and performance in normal and deviant children. *Psychol Bull* 1983, 94:446–471.

10. Kornetsky C: Psychoactive drugs in the immature organism. *Psychopharmacologia* 1970, 17:105–136.

11. Zametkin AJ, Rapoport JL: Neurobiology of attention deficit disorder with hyperactivity: where have we come in 50 years? *J Am Acad Child Adolesc Psychiatry* 1987, 26:676–686.

12. Gittelman-Klein R, Mannuzza S: Hyperactive boys almost grown up: III. Methylphenidate effects on ultimate height. *Arch Gen Psychiatry* 1988, 45:1131–1134.

13. Golden GS: The effect of central nervous system stimulants on Tourette syndrome. *Ann Neurol* 1977, 2:69–70.

14. Comings DE, Comings BG: A controlled study of Tourette syndrome: I. Attention-deficit disorder, learning disorders and school problems. *Am J Hum Genet* 1987, 41:701–741.

15. Higbee MD, Bosso JA: Apnea of prematurity. *Drug Intell Clin Pharm* 1979, 13:24–29.

16. Aranda JV, *et al.*: Ontogeny of human caffeine and theophylline metabolism. *Dev Pharmacol Ther* 1984, 7(suppl 1):18–25.

17. Davi MJ, *et al.*: Physiologic changes induced by theophylline in treatment of apnea in preterm infants. *J Pediatr* 1978, 92:91–95.

18. Mark EJ, Patalas ED, Change HT, *et al.*: Fatal pulmonary hypertension associated with short-term use of fenfluramine and phentermine. *N Engl J Med* 1997, 337:602–606.

19. Connolly HM, Crary JL, McGoon MD, *et al.*: Valvular heart Disease associated with fenfluramine-phentermine. *N Engl J Med* 1997, 337:581–588.

20. Bahnsen P, Jacobsen E, Thesleff H: The subjective effect of beta-phenylisopropylaminsulfate on normal adults. *Acta Med Scand* 1938, 97:89–131.

21. Jacobsen E, Wollstein A: Studies on the subjective effects of the cephalotropic amines in man I. β-penylisopropylamine sulphate. *Acta Med Scand* 1939, 100:159–202.

22. Dimascio A, Buie DH: Psychopharmacology of chlorphentermine and D-amphetamine. *Clin Pathol Ther* 1964, 5:174–184.

23. Harris SC, Ivy AC, Searle CM: The mechanism of amphetamine-induced loss of weight. *JAMA* 1947, 134:1468–1475.

24. Silverstone T, Stunkard A: The anorectic effect of dexamphetamine sulphate. *Br J Pharmacol Chemother* 1968, 33:513–522.

25. Martin WK, Sloan JW, Sapira JD, *et al.*: Physiologic, subjective, and behavioral effects of amphetamine, methamphetamine, ephedrine, phenmetrazine, and methylphenidate in man. *Clin Pharmacol Ther* 1971, 12:245–258.

26. Evans J: Psychosis and addiction to phenmetrazine (Preludin). *Lancet* 1959, 2:152–155.

27. Scoville BA: Review of amphetamine-like drugs by the Food and Drug Administration: clinical data and value judgements. In *Obesity in Perspective DHEW*, Pub No (NIH 75-708). Edited by Bray GA. Washington DC: US Government Printing Office, 1975, 441–443.

28. Silverstone T: Clinical use of appetite suppressants. *Drug and Alcohol Dependence* 1986, 17:151–167.

29. Haugen HN: Double blind cross-over study of a new appetite suppressant AN 448. *Eur J Clin Pharmacol* 1975, 8:71–74.

30. Lawson AAH, Roscoe P, Strong JA, *et al.*: Comparison of fenfluramine and metformin in treatment of obesity. *Lancet* 1970, 1:437–441.

31. Miach PJ, Thomson W, Doyle AE, *et al.*: Double-blind cross-over evaluation of maxindol in the treatment of obese hypertensive patients. *Med J Aust* 1976, 2:378–380.

32. Brightwell DR, Naylor CS: Effects of a combined behavioral and pharmacologic program on weight loss. *Int J Obesity* 1979, 3:141–148.

33. Langlois KJ, Forbes JA, Bell GW, *et al.*: A double-blind clinical evaluation of the safety and efficacy of phentermine hydrochloride (Fastin) in the treatment of exogenous obesity. *Curr Ther Res* 1974, 16:289–296.

34. Vernace BJ: Controlled comparative investigation of mazindol, d-amphetamine, and placebo. *Obesity/Bariatric Med* 1974, 3:124–129.

35. Silverstone T, Solomon T: The long-term management of obesity in general obesity in general practice. *Br J Clin Pract* 1965, 19:395–398.

36. Munro JF, MacCuish AC, Wilsom EM, *et al.*: Comparison of continuous and intermittent anorectic therapy in obesity. *Br Med J* 1968, 1:352—354.

37. Steel JM, Munro JF, Duncan LJP: A comparative trial of different regimens of fenfluramine and phentermine in obesity. *Practitioner* 1973, 211:232–236.

38. Weintraub M, Sundaresan PR, Madan M, *et al.*: Long-term weight control study. I (weeks 0 to 34). The enhancement of behavior modification, caloric restriction, and exercise by fenfluramine plus phentermine versus placebo. *Clin Pharmacol Ther* 1992, 51:586–594.

39. Weintraub M, Sundaresan PR, Schuster B, *et al.*: Long-term weight control study. II (weeks 34 to 104). An open-label study of continuous fenfluramine plus phentermine versus targeted intermittent medication as adjuncts to behavior modification, caloric restriction, and exercise. *Clin Pharmacol Ther* 1992, 51:595–601.

40. Bray GA: Approach to control of food intake in humans. *Med Clin North Am* 1989, 73:29–45.

AMPHETAMINE SULFATE

Amphetamine sulfate is a sympathomimetic amine that stimulates CNS activity by releasing norepinephrine and, at high doses, dopamine. This drug is a racemic preparation and shares pharmacologic properties with other stimulants. The major indication is for the treatment of ADHD. Dosing for this indication varies widely and should be titrated clinically, raising the dose for persistent symptoms until adverse effects (eg, overstimulation, restlessness, insomnia, anorexia) appear. The short half-life usually requires a divided dosage. This form of amphetamine has not been used frequently.

SPECIAL GROUPS

Children: Not recommended to treat attention deficit disorders in children younger than 3 years old.
Elderly: Not indicated for use.
Pregnancy: Category C drug. Safety for use during pregnancy has not been established. Congenital defects associated with amphetamine sulfate include cardiac abnormalities and biliary atresia.
Breast-feeding: Amphetamine sulfate is excreted in breast milk; discontinue nursing or avoid drug use.

DOSAGE

Adults: 5 to 20 mg, one to three times daily; start with 10 mg daily, raising in increments of 10 mg/d at weekly intervals and reducing if adverse reactions occur. Long-acting forms can be used for once-a-day dosage; with tablets or elixir give first dose on awakening and additional one to two doses every 4 to 6 hours.
Children: 3 to 5 years old, 2.5 mg daily, increasing in increments of 2.5 mg/d at weekly intervals until optimum response is obtained (usual range, 0.1–0.5 mg/kg/dose every morning); children at least 6 years of age, 5 mg one or two times daily, increasing in increments of 5 mg/d (usual range 0.1–0.5 mg/kg/dose every morning); long-acting forms can be used as a once-a-day dose; first dose of tablets or elixir can be given on awakening, with additional one or two doses at intervals of 4 to 6 hours.

In Brief

INDICATIONS
ADHD narcolepsy, obesity

CONTRAINDICATIONS
Advanced arteriosclerosis, symptomatic cardiovascular disease, hypertension, hyperthyroidism, glaucoma, hypersensitivity to sympathomimetric amines

INTERACTIONS
Guanethidine, MAO inhibitors, TCAs, urinary alkalinizers, general anesthetics, carbonic anhydrase inhibitors, β-adrenergic blockers, doxazosin, furazolidine, haloperidol, nabilone, phenothiazines, prazosin
Drug/laboratory test interactions: Plasma corticosteroid levels may increase; urinary steroid determinations may be altered

ADVERSE EFFECTS
Palpitations, tremor, tachycardia, headache, elevated blood pressure, changes in libido, reflex decrease in heart rate, arrhythmia, exacerbated motor and phonic tics in Tourette disorder, overstimulation, dry mouth, restlessness, unpleasant taste, dizziness, diarrhea, insomnia, constipation, dyskinesia, anorexia, euphoria, urticaria, dysphoria, impotence, reversible elevations in serum thyroxine levels

PHARMACOKINETICS AND PHARMACODYNAMICS
Onset of action: response is individualized and varies
Peak plasma level: 5–10 μg/dL (4–24 h)
Plasma half-life: 7–8 h for urinary acidification to pH < 5.6; alkalinization increases half-life (range, 18.6–33.6 h); every 1 unit of increase in urinary pH yields average 7-h increase in plasma half-life
Bioavailability: readily absorbed from GI tract and widely distributed throughout most tissue, with highest concentrations in the brain and cerebrospinal fluid.
Metabolism: metabolized in the liver by aromatic hydroxylation, N-dealkylation, and deamination; accumulated hydroxylated metabolites have been implicated in development of amphetamine psychosis
Excretion: excretion through kidneys
Effect of food: none expected
Renal impairment: excreted slowly (5–7 d); cumulative effects may occur with continued administration
Hepatic impairment: cumulative effects may occur with continued administration

PROLONGED USE
Prolonged treatment is usually required. Abuse or dependence has not been a problem in children. Adolescents and adults should be monitored carefully.

OVERDOSAGE
Restlessness, irritability, insomnia, tremor, hyperreflexia, rhabdomyolysis, rapid respiration, hyperpyrexia, assaultiveness, hallucinations, panic states, diaphoresis, mydriasis, flushing, hyperactivity, confusion, hypertension or hypotension, extrasystoles, tachypnea, fever, delirium, self-injury, arrhythmia, convulsions, coma, circulatory collapse, attempted suicide. Nausea, vomiting, diarrhea, and abdominal cramps may occur; fatigue and depression usually follow the central stimulation.
Treatment is largely symptomatic and included gastric evaluation followed by administration of activated charcoal (1 g/kg) and saline cathartic.

AVAILABILITY
Tablets—5 and 10 mg in 1000s (without tartrazine)

DEXTROAMPHETAMINE SULFATE

This D-stereoisomer of amphetamine is about twice as potent as racemic amphetamine. There is not clear evidence that one form of amphetamine is more clinically useful than the other. Despite the potential for abuse, amphetamines do not cause abuse or dependence in children treated for ADHD. The adverse effect of most concern is reduced growth. It is not clear if the sustained-release form is more or less effective than the regular form (ie, whether it eliminates the need for divided doses).

SPECIAL PRECAUTIONS

Dextroamphetamine sulfate is a Schedule II–controlled substance.

SPECIAL GROUPS

Children: Children should be monitored for growth retardation. Dextroamphetamine is not recommended to treat attention deficit disorders in children younger than 3 years of age.

Renal and hepatic impairment: The drug and its metabolites may accumulate. Use caution in dosing.

Pregnancy: Category C drug. No adequate and well-controlled studies in pregnant women. Safety for use during pregnancy has not been established. Congenital defects associated with the drug include cardiac abnormalities and biliary atresia. Infants born to mothers dependent on dextroamphetamine have an increased risk for premature delivery and low birth weight. Also, these children may experience symptoms of withdrawal by dysphoria, including agitation and significant lassitude. Use during pregnancy only if potential benefit justifies potential risk to the fetus.

Breast-feeding: Excreted in breast milk; mothers taking this drug should be advised to refrain from nursing.

DOSAGE

Adults: When prescribing for ADHD, begin with 5 mg/d and increase weekly by 5 mg/d or slower to a maximum dose of 20 mg/d. For ADHD and narcolepsy; 5 to 20 mg/d, divided according to individual needs of the patient. Long-acting forms can be used to reduce the need for divided doses.

Children: 3 to 5 years old 2.5 mg daily, increasing in increments of 2.5 mg/d at weekly intervals until optimum response is obtained (usual range, 0.1–0.5 mg/kg/dose every morning); children at least 6 years of age; 5 mg once or twice daily, increasing in increments of 5 mg/d (usual range, 0.1–0.5 mg/kg/dose every morning); long-acting forms can be used as a once-daily dose; first dose of tablets or elixir can be given on awakening, with additional one or two doses at intervals of 4 to 6 hours.

Impaired renal function: The drug and its metabolites may accumulate. Use caution in dosing.

(Continued on next page)

In Brief

INDICATIONS
ADHD and narcolepsy

CONTRAINDICATIONS
Advanced arteriosclerosis, symptomatic cardiovascular disease, hypertensions, hyperthyroidism, glaucoma, hypersensitivity to sympathomimetic amines

INTERACTIONS
Guanethidine, MAO inhibitors, TCAs, urinary alkalinizers, general anesthetics, carbonic anhydrase inhibitors, β-adreneragic blockers, doxazosin, furazolidine, haloperidol, nabilone, phenothiazines, prazosin, antihistamines, antihypertensives, chlorpromazine, ethosuximide, lithium carbonate, meperidine, methenamine, norepinephrine, phenobarbital, phenytoin, propoxyphene, veratrum alkaloids
Drug/laboratory test interactions: Plasma corticosteroid levels may increase; urinary steroid determinations may be altered.

ADVERSE EFFECTS
Palpitations, tachycardia, elevation of blood pressure, cardiomyopathy, psychotic episodes at recommended doses, overstimulation, restlessness, dizziness, insomnia, euphoria, dyskinesia, dysphoria, tremor, headache, exacerbation of motor and phonic tics in Tourette syndrome, dryness of the mouth, unpleasant taste, diarrhea, constipation, anorexia, weight loss, urticaria, impotence, changes in libido

PHARMACOKINETICS AND PHARMACODYNAMICS
Onset of action: response is individualized and varies
Peak plasma levels: 5–10 μg/dL (4–24 h)
Plasma half-life: 7–8 h for urinary acidification to pH < 5.6; alkalinization increases half-life (range, 18.6–33.6 h); every 1 unit of increase in urinary pH yields average 7-h increase in plasma half-life
Bioavailability: readily absorbed from GI tract and widely distributed throughout most tissue, with highest concentrations in the brain and cerebrospinal fluid
Metabolism: metabolized in the liver by aromatic hydroxylation, N-dealkylation, and deamination; accumulated hydroxylated metabolites have been implicated in development of amphetamine psychosis
Excretion: excreted through kidneys
Effect of food: none expected
Renal impairment: excreted slowly (5–7 d); cumulative effects may occur with continued administration
Hepatic impairment: cumulative effects may occur with continued administration

PROLONGED USE
Prolonged use usually is indicated for ADHD and narcolepsy. Abuse or dependence has not been a problem in children. Adolescents and adults should be monitored carefully.

OVERDOSAGE
Symptoms of acute overdose include restlessness, irritability, insomnia, tremor, hyperreflexia, rhabdomyolysis, rapid respiration, hyperpyrexia, assaultiveness, hallucinations, panic states, diaphoresis, mydriasis, flushing, hyperactivity, confusion, hypertension or hypotension, extrasystoles, tachypnea, fever, delirium, self-injury, arrhythmia, convulsions, coma, circulatory collapse, and attempted suicide. Nausea, vomiting, diarrhea, and abdominal cramps may occur; fatigue and depression usually follow the central stimulation.

(Continued on next page)

DEXTROAMPHETAMINE SULFATE (CONTINUED)

OVERDOSAGE (CONTINUED)

Treatment is largely symptomatic and includes gastric lavage and sedation with a barbiturate. Experience with hemodialysis or peritoneal dialysis is inadquate to permit recommendation. Acidification of the urine increases excretion of the drug. If acute severe hypertension complicates overdosage, administration of IV phentolamine has been suggested; however, a gradual drop in blood pressure usually results when sufficient sedation has been achieved. Chlorpromazine antagonizes the central stimulant effects and can be used to treat intoxication from this drug.

PATIENT INFORMATION

This drug may cause insomnia. Avoid taking it near bedtime. Use caution when driving or performing other activities that require especial alertness because this drug could mask the subjective feeling of fatigue without affecting the diminished performance from fatigue. It may cause nervousness, agitation, difficulty sleeping, diminished appetite, dizziness, and drug mouth. Discuss these with your physician, should they occur.

AVAILABILITY

Tablets—5 mg with or without tartrazine in 500s and 1000s; 10 mg without tartrazine in 100s, 500s, and 1000s
Capsules (sustained-release)—5 mg with tartrazine in 50s; 10 mg with tartrazine in 50s and 500s; 15 mg without tartrazine in 250s and 1000s and with tartrazine in 50s and 500s
Elixir—5 mg/5 mL with tartrazine, 10% alcohol, in 480 mL

DEXTROAMPHETAMINE SULFATE, AMPHETAMINE SULFATE, D-AMPHETAMINE SACCHARATE, and D,1-AMPHETAMINE ASPARTATE

(Adderall)

This drug is the combination of several amphetamine salts. There are no studies indicating its superiority to other amphetamines. As with other amphetamines, it is a sympathomimetic amine with CNS stimulant activity. Its indication is for ADHD and narcolepsy. It remains to be seen if this combination is preferable to old preparations of amphetamines.

SPECIAL PRECAUTIONS

Amphetamine is a schedule II controlled substance. It should be given cautiously to patients with a history of drug dependence or alcoholism because such patients may increase the dose on their own initiative. Chronically abusive use can lead to tolerance and dependence. Persecutory delusions can occur with large doses. Use cautiously in patients with hypertension.

SPECIAL GROUPS

Children: It may exacerbate psychotic symptoms in psychotic children. Safety and efficacy have not been established in children younger than 3 years old.
Renal and hepatic impairment: This drug and its metabolites may accumulate. Use cautiously in such patients.
Pregnancy: Safe use during pregnancy has not been established.
Breast-feeding: Amphetamine is excreted in human breast milk. Mothers taking amphetamine should avoid nursing.

(Continued on next page)

In Brief

INDICATIONS

Attention deficit disorders (children > 3 y), narcolepsy

CONTRAINDICATIONS

Symptomatic cardiovascular disease, hypertension, hyperthyroidism, glaucoma, hypersensitivity to sympathomimetic amines

INTERACTIONS

Guanethidine, MAO inhibitors, TCAs, urinary alkalinizers, general anesthetics, carbonic anhydrase inhibitors, ß-adrenergic blockers, doxazosin, furazolidone, haloperidol, nabilone, phenothiazines, prazosin, antihistamines, antihypertensives, chlorpromazine, ethosuximide, lithium carbonate, meperidine, methenamine, norepinephrine, phenobarbital, phenytoin, propoxyphene, veratrum alkaloids
Drug/laboratory test interactions: Plasma corticosteroid levels may increase; urinary steroid determinations may be altered

ADVERSE EFFECTS

Palpitations, tachycardia, elevation of blood pressure, cardiomyopathy, psychotic episodes at recommended doses, overstimulation, restlessness, dizziness, insomnia, euphoria, dyskinesia, dysphoria, tremor, headache, exacerbation of motor and phonic tics in Tourette syndrome, dryness of the mouth, unpleasant taste, diarrhea, constipation, anorexia, weight loss, urticaria, impotence, changes in libido.

PHARMACOKINETICS AND PHARMACODYNAMICS

Peak action: mean time to peak plasma concentration, 2.9 h (range, 1.5–8.0 h)
Plasma half-life: 11.1 h (range, 7.35–15.36 h)

PROLONGED USE

Prolonged use usually is indicated for ADHD and narcolepsy. Abuse and dependence have not been problems in children. Adolescents and adults should be monitored carefully.

DOSAGE

Adults: Start dosage at 5 mg once or twice daily; increase by 5 mg/wk if necessary. The usual maximum dose is 40 mg/d. Avoid dosing after 6 PM if the drug causes insomnia.

Elderly: Same as adult dosage.

Children: Not recommended for children younger than 3 years of age. Before age 6, start with 2.5 mg/d, increasing by 2.5 mg/d at weekly intervals until optimal result. In older children, use adult dosage.

Renal impairment: The drug and its metabolites may accumulate. Use cautiously.

OVERDOSAGE

Symptoms of overdose are restlessness, tremor, hyperreflexia, tachypnea, cognitive impairment, aggressiveness, hallucinations, panic, persecutory delusions, hyperpyrexia, rhabdomyolysis, arrhythmias, hypertension, circulatory collapse, nausea, vomiting, diarrhea, cramps, convulsions, and coma. Treatment is largely symptomatic and includes gastric lavage, activated charcoal, sedation, and cathartics. Experience with hemodialysis or peritoneal dialysis is inadequate to permit recommendation. Acidification of the urine increases excretion. If acute severe hypertension complicates overdosage, administration of IV phentolamine has been suggested; however, a gradual drop in blood pressure usually results when sufficient sedation has been achieved. Chlorpromazine antagonizes the central stimulant effects and can be used to treat intoxication from this drug.

PATIENT INFORMATION

This drug may cause insomnia. Avoid taking it near bedtime. It may mask the feeling of fatigue without affecting the diminished performance from fatigue, so use caution when driving or performing other activities that require special alertness. It may cause nervousness, agitation, diminished appetite, dizziness, and dry moth. Discuss these with your physician if they occur.

AVAILABILITY

Tablets—10 mg and 20 mg in 100s

METHYLPHENIDATE HYDROCHLORIDE
(Ritalin)

Pharmacologically this drug acts like an amphetamine, although chemically it is a piperidine. The dosage for ADHD varies widely and should be titrated clinically. Children with ADHD often require doses far in excess, per pound, of those that adults tolerate. The most common adverse effects are restlessness, overstimulation, insomnia, and anorexia. Methylphenidate, and amphetamines in general, should not be used for weight reduction. Growth retardation may be the most serious side effect.

SPECIAL PRECAUTIONS

There is some clinical evidence that methylphenidate may lower the convulsive threshold in patients with a prior history of seizures, prior EEG abnormalities in the absence of seizures, and no prior EEG evidence of seizures.

Methylphenidate should be given cautiously to emotionally unstable patients, such as those with a history of drug dependence or alcoholism, because these patients may increase the dose on their own initiative. Chronically abusive use can lead to marked tolerance and psychic dependence, with varying degrees of abnormal behavior. Frank psychotic episodes can occur. Careful supervision is required during drug withdrawal because severe depression and the effects of chronic overactivity can be unmasked. Long-term follow-up may be required because of the patient's basic personality disturbances.

In Brief

INDICATIONS

Attention deficit disorders (children > 6 y), narcolepsy

CONTRAINDICATIONS

Marked anxiety, tension, agitation; known hypersensitivity to methylphenidate; patients with glaucoma; patients with motor tics or with family history or diagnosis of Tourette syndrome

INTERACTIONS

Guanethidine, MAO inhibitors, warfarin, anticonvulsants, TCAs

Drug/laboratory test interactions: Increase urinary excretion of epinephrine

ADVERSE EFFECTS

Nervousness, insomnia, skin rash, urticaria, fever, arthralgia, exfoliative dermatitis, erythema multiforme, anorexia, nausea, dizziness, palpitations, headache, dyskinesia, drowsiness, blood pressure and pulse changes, tachyardia, angina, cardiac arrhythmia, abdominal pain, weight loss during prolonged therapy, cerebral arteritis and occlusion, leukopenia, anemia, transient depressed mood, hair loss

PHARMACOKINETICS AND PHARMACODYNAMICS

Peak plasma levels: 1.9 h for tablets and 4.7 h for sustained-release tablets

Plasma half-life: 1–3 h, but concentrations in the brain exceed those in plasma

Bioavailability: readily absorbed; 105% in children and 101% in adults

Metabolism: metabolized in liver; major metabolite is de-esterified product, ritalinic acid

(Continued on next page)

(Continued on next page)

METHYLPHENIDATE HYDROCHLORIDE (CONTINUED)

SPECIAL PRECAUTIONS (CONTINUED)

Use cautiously in patients with hypertension. Blood pressure should be monitored at appropriate intervals in all patients taking the drug.

Symptoms of visual disturbances have been encountered; difficulties with accommodation and blurring of vision have been reported.

SPECIAL GROUPS

Children: Methylphenidate should not be used in children younger than 6 years of age because safety and efficacy in this age group have not been established. Long-term effects of the drug on children have not been well-established.

Renal and hepatic impairment: The drug and its metabolites may accumulate. Use caution in dosing.

Pregnancy: Safe use during pregnancy has not been established; do not prescribe to women of childbearing age unless, in the opinion of the physician, potental benefits outweigh possible risks.

Breast-feeding: It is unknown whether methylphenidate is excreted in human breast milk; use with caution in lactating women.

DOSAGE

Adults: *Tablet*—Administer in divided doses two or three times daily, preferably 30 to 45 minutes before meals. Average dose is 20 to 30 mg daily. Some patients may require 40 to 60 mg daily; 10 to 15 mg daily is adequate for other patients. Patients who are unable to sleep if drug is taken late in the day should take the last dose before 6 PM. *Sustained-release tablets*—Use in place of tablets when 8-hour dose of sustained-release tablet corresponds to titrated 8-hour dose of tablets. Do not crush or chew tablets. Administer one to three times daily every 8 hours, preferably on an empty stomach.

Elderly: Same as adult doses.

Children: Not recommended younger than 6 years old. *Attention deficit disorders*—Initiate in small doses with gradual weekly increments. Daily doses over 60 mg are not recommended. If improvement is not observed after appropriate dose adjustment over a 1-month period, discontinue drug use. Periodically discontinue drug therapy to assess child's condition. Drug treatment should not and need not be indefinite and usually can be discontinued after puberty. Start with 5 mg twice daily (before breakfast and lunch), with gradual increments of 5 to 10 mg weekly. *Narcolepsy*—20 mg, one to three times daily. Do not crush or chew sustained-release tablets.

Renal impairment: The drug and its metabolites may accumulate. Use caution in dosing.

PHARMACOKINETICS AND PHARMACODYNAMICS (CONTINUED)

Excretion: eliminated in kidneys and excreted in urine; ritalinic acid accounts for 80% of dose excreted; average of 67% of sustained-release dose excreted in children compared with 86% in adults

Effect of food: none expected

Renal and hepatic impairment: the drug and its metabolites may accumulate; use caution in dosing.

PROLONGED USE

Prolonged treatment usually is required. Abuse or dependence has not been a problem in children. Adolescents and adults should be monitored carefully.

OVERDOSAGE

Symptoms of acute overdose include vomiting, agitation, tremors, hyperreflexia, muscle twitching, convulsions (may be followed by coma), euphoria, confusion, hallucinations, delirium, sweating, flushing, headache, hyperplexia, tachycardia, palpitations, cardiac arrhythmias, hypertension, mydriasis, and dryness of mucous membranes.

Treatment consists of appropriate supportive measures. Patients must be protected against self-injury and external stimuli that would aggravate overstimulation already present. If symptoms are not too severe and the patient is conscious, gastric contents can be evacuated by induction of emesis or gastric lavage. In the presence of severe intoxication, use a carefully titrated dose of a *short-acting* barbiturate *before* performing gastric lavage. Intensive care must be provided to maintain adequate circulation and respiratory exchange; external cooling procedures may be required for hyperpyrexia. Efficacy of peritoneal dialysis or extracorporeal hemodialysis has not been established.

PATIENT INFORMATION

Use caution when driving or operating hazardous machinery. Patients or their parents should record the patient's weight two times a week and report any significant loss. Any changes in mood should be reported to the physician, as should any evidence of skin rashes, fever, or pain in the joints. The sustained-release tablets should not be crushed or chewed.

AVAILABILITY

Tablets—5 and 10 mg in 100s
Tablets (sustained-release)—20 mg in 100s

PEMOLINE
(Cylert)

Pemoline has a chemical structure different from that of amphetamine but a similar pharmacologic action. Its adverse effects are the same as those for amphetamines; however, it has a slower onset and a longer half-life, and for this reason, and perhaps its less intense effect, it has not been associated with abuse. It would seem to be the preferred drug for ADHD except for the usual impression that it is less effective. Abuse has not been a problem in using other stimulants in children with ADHD.

SPECIAL PRECAUTIONS

Decrements in predicted growth rate (ie, weight gain, height) have been reported with long-term use of pemoline. Patients requiring long-term therapy should be carefully monitored.

Pemoline is a Schedule IV controlled substance. Psychologic and physical dependence might occur. There have been isolated reports of transient psychotic symptoms occurring in adults after long-term misuse of excessive doses of pemoline.

Mild adverse reactions appearing early during the course of treatment often remit with continuing therapy. If adverse reactions are of a significant or protracted nature, the dose should be reduced or drug therapy discontinued.

SPECIAL GROUPS

Children: Safety and efficacy in children younger than 6 years old have not been established. Long-term effects have not been established. Suppression of growth also has been reported. Pemoline has been reported to precipitate motor and phonic tics and Tourette syndrome in children. Clinical evaluation for tics and Tourette syndrome in children and their families should precede use of this drug.
Renal impairment: Administer with caution to patients with significantly impaired renal function.
Hepatic impairment: Use with caution in patients with impaired hepatic function. In all patients, liver function tests should be performed before and periodically during therapy. Drug therapy should be discontinued if abnormalities are revealed and confirmed with follow-up tests.
Pregnancy: Category B drug. No adequate and well-controlled studies in pregnant women; this drug should be used during pregnancy only if clearly needed.
Breast-feeding: It is unknown whether pemoline is excreted in human breast milk; caution should be exercised when administered to a nursing woman.

DOSAGE

Adults: *Narcolepsy and ADHD*—50–200 mg/d in two divided doses.
Elderly: Same as for adults.
Children: Not recommended for patients younger than 6 years of age. *Attention deficit disorder*—Administer as single oral dose each morning. Recommended starting dose is 37.5 mg/d gradually increased by 18.75 mg at 1-week intervals until desired clinical response is obtained. Effective daily dose ranges from 56.25 to 75 mg. Maximum recommended daily dose is 112.5 mg. When using recommended schedule of dose titration, significant benefit may not be evident until third or fourth week of drug administration.

In Brief

INDICATIONS

Narcolepsy in adults; attention deficit disorders in children > 6 years of age

CONTRAINDICATIONS

Patients with impaired hepatic function; known hypersensitivity or idiosyncratic reaction to pemoline

INTERACTIONS

Have not been studied in humans; patients who are receiving pemoline concurrently with other drugs, especially drugs with CNS activity, should be monitored carefully. Do not use with MAO inhibitors. **Drug/laboratory test interactions:** Increased AST, ALT, and serum LDH

ADVERSE EFFECTS

Hepatic-related fatalities, hepatitis, jaundice, aplastic anemia, convulsive seizures, Tourette syndrome, hallucinations, dyskinetic movements, abnormal oculomotor function, mild depression, dizziness, increased irritability, headache, drowsiness, insomnia, anorexia, weight loss, nausea, stomach ache, growth suppression, skin rash

PHARMACOKINETICS AND PHARMACODYNAMICS

Onset of action: gradual; requires 2–3 wk or more for significant clinical benefits
Peak plasma levels: 2–4 h
Plasma half-life: about 12 h
Bioavailability: rapidly absorbed from GI tract
Metabolism: metabolized by liver; metabolites include pemoline conjugate, pemoline dione, mandelic acid, and unidentified polar compounds
Excretion: eliminated primarily by kidneys with about 50% excreted in urine unchanged and only minor fractions present as metabolites
Protein binding: about 50% plasma protein bound
Renal impairment: the drug and its metabolites may accumulate; use caution in dosing
Hepatic impairment: elevated liver enzyme levels occur regularly; these reactions appear to be reversible on drug therapy discontinuance; most patients with elevated liver enzyme levels are asymptomatic

PROLONGED USE

When possible, drug administration should be interrupted occasionally to determine whether there is recurrence of behavioral symptoms sufficient to require continued therapy.

OVERDOSAGE

Symptoms of acute overdose include vomiting, agitation, tremors, hyperreflexia, muscle twitching, convulsions (may be followed by coma), euphoria, confusion, hallucinations, delirium, sweating, flushing, headache, hyperpyrexia, tachycardia, palpitations, cardiac arrhythmias, hypertension, mydriasis, and dryness of mucous membranes.
Treatment consists of appropriate supportive measures. Patients must be protected against self-injury and external stimuli that would aggravate overstimulation already present. If symptoms are not too severe and the patient is conscious, gastric contents can be evacuated by induction of emesis or gastric lavage. Chlorpromazine has been reported to be useful in decreasing CNS stimulation and sympathomimetic effects. Efficacy of peritoneal dialysis or extracorporeal hemodialysis has not been established.

(Continued on next page)

PEMOLINE (CONTINUED)

PATIENT INFORMATION
A printed list of drug effects should be provided to the patient or patient's family. Physician should be notified immediately if agitation, restlessness, hallucinations, or tachycardia develop. The importance of periodic liver function tests should be emphasized. Patient or patient's family should be advised of the gradual onset of action and that the benefits of the drug will not be notice-able for several weeks. Parents of patients taking pemoline should measure the child's height every month and weigh the child twice a week; all measurements should be recorded on a graph and presented during each follow-up medical visit to the physician.

AVAILABILITY
Tablets—18.75, 37.5, and 75 mg in 100s
Tablets (chewable)—37.5 mg in 100s

CAFFEINE
(Cafergot)

Caffeine is a xanthine, present in many beverages, that pharmacologically acts as a stimulant. Its therapeutic uses are limited to an unlabeled use in neonatal apnea and as an adjuvant agent during electroconvulsive therapy to lower the seizure threshold in patients who do not have seizures from the usual doses of electricity. People should be aware it is a drug with many adverse reactions and not merely a harmless addition to popular drinks. Despite popular belief, caffeine is not indicated for neutralization of the effects of intoxication with alcohol or other CNS depressants.

SPECIAL PRECAUTIONS
Analeptic use is strongly discouraged by most clinicians.

Too-vigorous treatment with parenteral caffeine can produce further depression in already depressed patients; therefore, do not exceed 1 g as a single dose of caffeine and sodium benzoate.

Large quantities of caffeine-containing products may reactivate duodenal ulcers.

Higher blood glucose levels may result from caffeine.

High doses can elicit tremor, insomnia, and hyperalgesia.

As with other xanthines, caffeine can readily produce grand mal seizures; patients with asthma should be monitored carefully.

SPECIAL GROUPS
Children: Used for neonatal apnea.
Elderly: May be more sensitive to the effects. Use caution in dosing.
Renal impairment: Use with caution in patients with compromised kidney function. Some increase in renal blood flow and glomerular filtration rate occurs.
Hepatic impairment: Use with caution in patients with alcoholic liver disease.
Pregnancy: Category C drug. Safety for use in pregnancy has not been established. Pregnant women should consume sparingly or avoid caffeine-containing drugs. Excessive caffeine intake has been weakly associated with increased fetal loss, low birth weight, and premature deliveries.
Breast-feeding: Caffeine use is not recommended because caffeine appears in the breast milk of nursing mothers; about 1.5 to 3.1 mg of caffeine is ingested by a nursing infant whose mother consumes 1 cup of coffee.

(Continued on next page)

In Brief

INDICATIONS
Off-label: For neonatal apnea and as an adjuvant agent to lower the seizure threshold during electroconvulsive therapy

CONTRAINDICATIONS
History of duodenal ulcers; pregnancy or lactation

INTERACTIONS
Cimetidine, oral contraceptives, disulfiram, fluoroquinolones (ciprofloxacin, enoxacin), phenylpropanolamine, tobacco
Drub/laboratory test interactions: False-positive elevations of serum urate levels as measured by the Bittner method; in urine levels, slight increases in vanillymandelic acid (VMA), catecholamines, and 5-hydroxyindoleacetic acid; high urine levels of VMA or catecholamines may result in false-positive diagnosis of pheochromocytoma or neuroblastoma; avoid caffeine intake during tests for these disorders

ADVERSE EFFECTS
Anxiety disorder: Large doses of caffeine may produce symptoms of anxiety neurosis (eg, tremulousness, muscle twitching, sensory disturbances, irritability, flushing, tachypnea, palpitations, arrhythmias, GI disturbances, diureses).
Withdrawal: Headache, anxiety, lethargy, and muscle tension may occur after abrupt cessation from regular consumption.
General: Insomnia, nausea, restlessness, vomiting, excitement, diarrhea, nervousness, stomach pain, tinnitus, tachycardia, scintillating scotoma, extrasystoles, muscular tremor, palpitations, headaches, diuresis, lightheadedness

PHARMACOKINETICS AND PHARMACODYNAMICS
Excretion: 0.5%–3.5% excreted unchanged in urine; in neonates, almost entirely eliminated unchanged in urine; almost completely absorbed with peak plasma levels appearing in about 30 min; it readily enters the CNS and crosses the placenta
Renal impairment: some increases in renal blood flow and glomerular filtration; major portion of diuretic action probably involves inhibition of renal tubular reabsorption of sodium
Hepatic impairment: clearance decreased in patients with alcoholic liver disease

PROLONGED USE
Tolerance and withdrawal symptoms may appear, but the evidence is not definite that these symptoms are clinically significant.

DOSAGE

Adults: *Parenteral*—Sodium benzoate increases caffeine's solubility in aqueous solutions; administered 500 mg (250 mg caffeine) IM (or slow IV injection in emergency respiratory failure) or maximum single dose of 1 g (500 mg of caffeine). Usual dose is 500 mg.
Elderly: Same as for adults; monitor patient for arrhythmia and hyperglycemia.
Children: Not recommended for use.

OVERDOSAGE
Treatment should be symptomatic and supportive.

PATIENT INFORMATION
Used for difficult breathing in newborns and to facilitate electroconvulsive treatment for mental disorders. It should be used only in the presence of a physician.

AVAILABILITY
Injection—250 mg/mL (equal parts caffeine and sodium benzoate) in 2-mL ampules

DOXAPRAM HYDROCHLORIDE
(Dopram)

Doxapram has similar properties to caffeine. Its only indication seems to be for off-label use in neonatal apnea. It probably has no clear indication as a respiratory stimulant in other causes of respiratory embarrassment. The drug is used by anesthesiologists.

SPECIAL PRECAUTIONS
Use only in neonates.

Doxapram HCl is no longer considered the drug of choice in the treatment of CNS depression caused by severe overdose of sedatives and hypnotics.

Administer doxapram in a closely monitored environment.

Ensure patient airway; administer oxygen along with doxapram HCl in patients with chronic pulmonary insufficiency.

Have short-acting barbiturates, oxygen, and resuscitative equipment available in case of overdose from excessive CNS stimulation.

Avoid extravasation or use of single injection site for extended period; thrombophlebitis or local skin irritation may occur. Rapid infusion may result in hemodialysis.

Monitor blood pressure and deep tendon reflexes to prevent overdose.

SPECIAL GROUPS
Used only in neonates.

DOSAGE
Children: Neonates—0.5–1.0 mg/kg.

In Brief

INDICATIONS
Off-label: Neonatal apnea

CONTRAINDICATIONS
None

INTERACTIONS
Sympathomimetics, MAO inhibitors, halothane, cyclopropane, enflurane, muscle relaxants; increased likelihood of adverse reactions to dexaprom
Drug/laboratory test interactions: Hemoglobin, hematocrits, RBCs, BUN, proteinuria

ADVERSE EFFECTS
Headache, bronchospasm, dizziness, hiccoughs, apprehension, rebound hypoventilation, disorientation, phlebitis, pupillary dilation, variations in cardiac rate, hyperactivity, lowered T waves, convulsions, arrhythmia, bilateral Babinski, chest pain, involuntary movements, tightness in chest, muscle spasticity, increase in blood pressure, increase deep tension reflexes, nausea, clonus, vomiting, pyrexia, diarrhea, flushing, desire to defecate, sweating, urinary retention, pruritus and paresthesia, spontaneous voiding, cough, proteinuria, dyspnea, tachypnea, laryngospasm, decreased hemoglobin, decreased hematocrit, decreased RBC count, further WBC decrease in presence of preexisting leukopenia, elevation in BUN

PHARMACOKINETICS AND PHARMACODYNAMICS
Metabolism: rapid; metabolizes in the liver
Excretion: metabolites excreted in urine

PROLONGED USE
Not designed for prolonged use; doxapram is a habit-forming agent.

OVERDOSAGE
Early symptoms include excessive pressor effect, tachycardia, skeletal muscle hyperactivity, and enhanced deep tendon reflexes. Monitor blood pressure, pulse rate, and deep tendon reflexes periodically. Treatment is supportive because there is no specific antidote and no evidence that doxapram is dialyzable.

AVAILABILITY
Injection—20 mg/mL in 20-mL vials

BENZPHETAMINE HYDROCHLORIDE

(Didrex)

This drug has the properties of other noradrenergic anorexiants: it helps short-term weight loss of modest proportions, which reaches a plateau after 1 to 2 months. Following discontinuation of therapy, the user tends to regain the lost weight. Although less likely to cause stimulant adverse reactions than amphetamine, it *can* cause these effects, which limits its use. It may cause dependence and abuse.

SPECIAL PRECAUTIONS

Benzphetamine is a Schedule II–controlled substance. Abuse may be associated with intense psychologic dependence and severe social dysfunction. The most severe manifestation of chronic intoxication is psychosis, often clinically indistinguishable from schizophrenia.

Insulin requirements may be altered in association with drug and concomitant dietary restrictions.

Benzphetamine may produce dizziness, extreme fatigue, and depression after abrupt cessation of therapy; patients should use caution when driving or performing any task that requires alertness.

Use with caution and monitor blood pressure in patients with mild hypertension; benzphetamine is not recommended for use in patients with symptomatic cardiovascular disease, including arrhythmias.

Tolerance to the anorectic effects may develop within a few weeks; cross-tolerances are almost universal.

If agent contains tartrazine, monitor patient for allergic reactions, including bronchial asthma.

SPECIAL GROUPS

Children: Not recommended for children younger than 12 years of age.
Elderly: Use with caution, especially in patients suffering from hypertension, hyperexcitability, or debilitated states.
Renal and hepatic impairment: Clearance of active drug reduced.
Pregnancy: Category X drug; contraindicated during pregnancy.
Breast-feeding: Benzphetamine is excreted in breast milk; advise patients to refrain from nursing.

DOSAGE

Adults: Initial dosage of 25 to 50 mg once daily; increase according to patient response. Dosage generally ranges from 25 to 50 mg, one to three times daily.
Elderly: Same as for adults; use with caution.
Children: Not recommended for children < 12 years of age.
Impaired renal function: Clearance of active drug reduced.

In Brief

INDICATIONS
Obesity

CONTRAINDICATIONS
Advanced arteriosclerosis, symptomatic cardiovascular disease, moderate to severe hypertension, hyperthyroidism, known hypersensitivity or idiosyncratic reaction to sympathomimetic amines, glaucoma, agitated states, history of drug abuse, administration of MAO inhibitors during or within 14 d, pregnancy, lactation

INTERACTIONS
MAO inhibitors CNS stimulants, antihypertensives, urinary alkalinizing agents, urinary acidifying agents
Drug/laboratory test interactions: Increase in urinary catecholamine levels, increase in plasma corticosteroid levels

ADVERSE EFFECTS
Palpitations, tachycardia, elevation of blood pressure, cardiomyopahy, overstimulation, restlessness, dizziness, insomnia, tremor, sweating, headache, psychotic episodes, depression following withdrawal of drug therapy, dry mouth, unpleasant taste, nausea, diarrhea, urticaria and other allergic reactions involving the skin, changes in libido

PHARMACOKINETICS AND PHARMACODYNAMICS
Onset of action: within 1–2 h
Metabolism: benzphetamine is metabolized to methamphetamine
Excretion: most of the drug and its metabolites excreted through kidneys
Effect of food: drug should be taken on an empty stomach; effectiveness dependent on caloric intake and patient's eating habits
Renal and hepatic Impairment: cumulative effects may occur with continued administration

PROLONGED USE
Tolerance, withdrawal symptoms, abuse, or dependence may occur if used excessively.

OVERDOSAGE
Acute overdose may result in restlessness, tremor, tachypnea, confusion, assaultiveness, and panic states. Fatigue and depression usually follow the central stimulation. Cardiovascular effects include arrhythmia, hypertension or hypotension, and stimulatory collapse. GI symptoms include nausea, vomiting, diarrhea, and abdominal cramps. Hyperpyrexia and rhabdomyolsis have been reported and can lead to a number of associated complications. Fatal poisoning is usually manifested by convulsions and coma.
Overdose with benzphetamine HCl is extremely limited. Management of acute intoxication is primarily symptomatic and includes sedation with a barbiturate. If hypertension is marked, use of a nitric or rapidly action α-receptor blocker should be considered. Experience with hemodialysis or peritoneal dialysis is inadequate to permit recommendation. Acidification of the urine increase excretion.

PATIENT INFORMATION
Insomnia may occur; avoid taking drug late in the day. Weight reduction requires strict adherence to dietary restriction. Do not take more frequently than prescribed. Notify physician if palpitations, nervousness, or dizziness occurs. Also notify physician if dry mouth and constipation become pronounced. Observe caution driving or cease driving: dizziness and blurred vision may occur. Take drug on an empty stomach.

AVAILABILITY
Tablets—25 mg with tartrazine in 100s; 50 mg in 100s and 500s

DIETHYLPROPION HYDROCHLORIDE

(Tenuate, Tepanil)

This drug, as with other noradrenergic anorexiants, has pharmacologic properties similar to amphetamines, but has less intense adverse reactions. It usually causes modest weight loss during short-term treatment and maintains that loss during long-term treatment. Its adverse effects necessitate careful monitoring in people with heart disease and a vulnerability to psychoactive substance abuse.

SPECIAL PRECAUTIONS

If tolerance develops, the recommended dose should not be exceeded in an attempt to increase the effect; therapy should be discontinued.

When prescribed, consideration must be given to the possibility of adverse interactions with alcohol.

Diethylpropion is a Schedule IV–controlled substance, and there have been reports of patients becoming psychologically dependent on it. The possibility of abuse should be kept in mind when evaluating the desirability of including this drug as part of a weight-reduction program.

Exercise caution when dispensing drug to patients with hypertension or symptomatic cardiovascular disease; monitor blood pressure. Do not prescribe to patients with severe hypertension.

Convulsions may increase in some epileptics; dose titration or drug therapy discontinuance may be necessary.

The least amount should be prescribed or dispensed at one time to minimize the possibility of overdose.

SPECIAL GROUPS

Children: Not recommended for children younger than 12 years of age.

Elderly: Use with caution, especially in patients suffering from hypertension, hyperexcitability, or debilitated states.

Renal impairment: Clearance of drug may be reduced; dose reduction usually is required.

Hepatic impairment: Transformation to inactive metabolites may be reduced; dose reduction may be required.

Pregnancy: Category B drug. No adequate and well-controlled studies in pregnant women. Safe use during pregnancy has not been established. Use in women who may become pregnant only when clearly needed and when potential benefits outweigh potential hazards to the fetus.

Breast-feeding: Diethylpropion and its metabolites are excreted in milk; advise patient to avoid nursing while taking drug.

In Brief

INDICATIONS

Appetite suppression for obesity

CONTRAINDICATIONS

Advanced arteriosclerosis, symptomatic cardiovascular disease, moderate to severe hypertension, hyperthyroidism, known hypersensitivity or idiosyncratic reaction to sympathomimetic amines, glaucoma, agitated states, history of drug abuse, administration of MAO inhibitors during or within 14 d

INTERACTIONS

Insulin, general anesthetics, antihypertensive agents

ADVERSE EFFECTS

Precordial pain, arrhythmia, ECG changes, tachycardia, elevation of blood pressure, palpitation, convulsive episodes, psychotic episodes, dyskinesia, blurred vision, overstimulation, nervousness, restlessness, dizziness, jitters, insomnia, anxiety, euphoria, depression, dysphoria, tremor, mydriasis, drowsiness, malaise, headache, vomiting, diarrhea, abdominal discomfort, dryness of the mouth, unpleasant taste, nausea, constipation, urticaria, rash, ecchymosis, erythema, impotence, changes in libido, gynecomastia, menstrual upset, bone marrow depression, agranulocytosis, leukopenia, dysuria, dyspnea, hair loss, muscle pain, increased sweating, polyuria

PHARMACOKINETICS AND PHARMACODYNAMICS

Onset of action: immediate

Plasma half-life: 4–6 h

Bioavailability: rapidly absorbed through the GI tract; active metabolites believed to cross blood–brain barrier and placenta

Metabolism: metabolized extensively through complex pathway of biotransformation involving dealkylation and reduction; many of the metabolites are biologically active and may participate in therapeutic action of drug; circulating levels of the metabolites are affected by urinary pH

Excretion: most of the drug and its metabolites are excreted through kidneys; between 75% and 106% of the dose is recovered in the urine within 48 h after dosing

Effect of food: drug should be taken on an empty stomach; effectiveness dependent on caloric intake and patient's eating habits

Renal and hepatic impairment: cumulative effects may occur with continued administration

PROLONGED USE

Tolerance, withdrawal symptoms, abuse, or dependence may occur if used excessively.

OVERDOSAGE

Acute overdose manifested by restlessness, tremor, hyperreflexia, rapid respiration, confusion, assaultiveness, hallucinations, and panic attacks. Cardiovascular symptoms include arrhythmia, hypertension or hypotension, and circulatory collapse. GI symptoms include nausea, vomiting, diarrhea, and abdominal cramps. Overdose may result in convulsions, coma, and death.

Management of acute diethylpropion intoxication is largely symptomatic and includes lavage and sedation with a barbiturate.

Experience with hemodialysis or peritoneal dialysis is inadequate to permit recommendation. IV phentolamine has been suggested on pharmacologic grounds for possible acute severe hypertension if this complicates overdose.

(Continued on next page)

DIETHYLPROPION HYDROCHLORIDE *(CONTINUED)*

DOSAGE

Adult: *Tablets*—25 mg three times daily 1 hour before meals and in the evening if needed to overcome night hunger. *Sustained-release tablets*—75 mg once daily in midmorning.
Elderly: Same as for adult; use with extreme caution.
Children: Not recommended for children younger than 12 years of age.
Impaired renal function: Clearance of drug reduced.

PATIENT INFORMATION

Patient advised not to consume alcohol while taking drug. Insomnia may occur. Weight reduction requires strict adherence to dietary restriction. Do not take more frequently than prescribed. Notify physician if palpitations, nervousness, or dizziness occurs.

AVAILABILITY

Tablets—25 mg in 100s, 500s, 1000s
Tablets (sustained release)—75 mg in 30s, 100s, 250s, 500s, 1000s

MAZINDOL

(Mazanor, Sanorex)

This drug is an analogue of amphetamine and shares the indications and adverse effects of other noradrenergic anorexiants. It leads to short-term weight loss with rebound weight gain. Prominent adverse effects are similar to those caused by amphetamines, but less intense. Its efficacy and adverse reactions do not differ from those of other noradrenergic anorexiants.

SPECIAL PRECAUTIONS

Not recommended for severely hypertensive patients or for patients with symptomatic cardiovascular disease, including arrhythmias.

Mazindol is a Schedule IV–controlled substance. In widespread clinical use, however, there have been no reports of physical or psychologic dependence, drug tolerance, habituation, chronic abuse, or symptoms of withdrawal or abstinence.

May impair ability of patients to engage in potentially hazardous activities; patients should be cautioned accordingly.

Can decrease the hypotensive effect of guanethidine and similar substances; patients should be monitored accordingly.

Can markedly potentiate the pressor effect of exogenous catecholamines. If a pressor amine agent must be given to a patient who has recently been taking mazindol, extreme care should be taken in monitoring blood pressure at frequent intervals and initiating pressor therapy with a low initial dose and careful titration.

Can potentiate blood pressure increases in patients taking sympathomimetic drugs.

Moderately lowers blood glucose levels independent of apppetite suppressant effects by increasing glucose uptake in human muscle.

SPECIAL GROUPS

Children: Not recommended for children younger than 12 years of age.
Elderly: Use with caution, especially in patients suffering from hypertension, hyperexcitability, or debilitated states.
Pregnancy: Category C drug. Safe use during pregnancy has not been established. Use in women who may become pregnant only when clearly needed and when potential benefits outweigh potential hazards to fetus; animal studies report an increase in neonatal mortality and incidence of rib anomalies.
Breast-feeding: The extent to which mazindol may be transferred to breast milk is unknown; mothers who are nursing should not receive this drug.

(Continued on next page)

In Brief

INDICATIONS

Appetite suppression for obesity

CONTRAINDICATIONS

Advanced arteriosclerosis, symptomatic cardiovascular disease, moderate to severe hypertension, hyperthyroidism, known hypersensitivity or idiosyncratic reaction to sympathomimetic amines, glaucoma, agitated states, history of drug abuse, administration of MAO inhibitors during or within 14 d, lactation

INTERACTIONS

Guanethidine, catecholamines, sympathomimetic drugs, pressor amine agents, MAO inhibitors

ADVERSE EFFECTS

Most common: Dry mouth, tachycardia, constipation, nervousness, insomnia
Others: Palpitation, edema, overstimulation, restlessness, dizziness, insomnia, dysphoria, tremor, headache, depression, drowsiness, weakness, dryness of mouth, unpleasant taste, diarrhea, constipation, nausea, vomiting, abdominal discomfort, rash, excessive sweating, clamminess, impotence, changes in libido (rare), blurred vision, fainting sensation, hot or cold flashes, hyperdipsia, paresthesia, dysuria, pollakiuria

PHARMACOKINETICS AND PHARMACODYNAMICS

Onset of action: 30–60 min
Peak plasma level: 0.003–0.012 mg/mL (no time specified)
Excretion: excreted in urine partially unchanged
Effect of food: none expected
Renal and hepatic impairment: cumulative effects may occur with continued administration

PROLONGED USE

Tolerance, withdrawal symptoms; abuse or dependency may occur if used excessively.

OVERDOSAGE

Approximately 50% overdose cases have involved children 1–4 y of age; reported doses ingested were 4–40 mg. All patients recovered. In general, overdose symptoms include irritability, agitation, hyperactivity, tachycardia, arrhythmia (premature ventricular contractions), and tachypnea.

(Continued on next page)

DOSAGE

Adults: 1 mg three times daily 1 hour before meals or 2 mg once daily 1 hour before lunch; initiate therapy at 1 mg once daily and adjust to patient response; take with meals to avoid GI discomfort.
Elderly: Same as for adults; use with caution.
Children: Not recommended for children younger than 12 years of age.
Impaired renal function: Clearance of drug may be reduced; dose reduction usually is required.

OVERDOSAGE (CONTINUED)

Symptomatic treatment includes emesis (if patient is conscious), inducing vomiting with ipecac syrup (15–30 mL). In unconscious patients, gastric lavage should not be attempted unless cuffed endotracheal intubation has been done. Sedate patient with chlorpromazine. Forced acid diuresis may be necessary. Data on hemodialysis or peritoneal dialysis are unavailable; however, mazindol is soluble only in acid, so dialysis with base or neutral solvents would not remove the drug.

PATIENT INFORMATION

Insomnia may occur; avoid taking drug late in day. Weight reduction requires strict adherence to dietary restriction. Do not take more frequently than prescribed. Notify physician if palpitations, nervousness, or dizziness occurs. Also notify physician if dry mouth and constipation become pronounced. Use caution when driving or cease driving; dizziness and blurred vision may occur. To minimize GI irritation, take drug with meals.

AVAILABILITY

Tablets—1 mg in 30s and 100s; 2 mg in 100s

PHENDIMETRAZINE TARTRATE

(Adipost, Bontril PDM, Melfiat-105, Plegine, Prelu-2, Statobex)

This drug, as a phenethylamine, acts like an amphetamine but has fewer adverse effects at therapeutically equivalent doses for the induction of weight loss. It shares this property with other noradrenergic anorexiants. It causes short-term weight loss by suppressing appetite, and rebound weight gain occurs when the drug therapy is stopped. Common adverse effects are sympathomimetic, such as palpitations, hypertension, overstimulation, agitation, insomnia, dry mouth, and in large doses, psychosis and abuse.

SPECIAL PRECAUTIONS

Use of phendimetrazine within 14 days after administration of MAO inhibitors may result in a hypertensive crisis.

Abrupt cessation of administration after prolonged high doses results in extreme fatigue and depression. Because of the effect on the CNS, phendimetrazine can impair the ability of patients to engage in potentially hazardous activities.

Phendimetrazine is a Schedule III–controlled substance. Abuse may be associated with intense psychologic dependence and severe social dysfunction.

Caution should be exercised in using phendimetrazine for patients with even *mild* hypertension; monitor blood pressure.

Insulin requirements in diabetes mellitus may be altered in association with the use of this agent and a concomitant dietary regimen.

May decrease the hypotensive effect of guanethidine.

The least amount feasible should be prescribed or dispensed at one time to minimize the possibility of overdose.

Not recommended for use in patients with symptomatic cardiovascular disease, including arrhythmias.

In Brief

INDICATIONS

Appetite suppression for obesity

CONTRAINDICATIONS

Advanced arteriosclerosis, symptomatic cardiovascular disease, moderate to severe hypertension, hyperthyroidism, known hypersensitivity or idiosyncratic reaction to sympathomimetic amines, glaucoma, agitated states, history of drug abuse, administration of MAO inhibitors during or within 14 d

INTERACTIONS

Guanethidine, insulin and sulfonylurease, MAO inhibitors, TCAs, thiazide diuretics
Drug/laboratory test interactions: Increase in urinary catecholamines increase in plasma corticosteroid levels

ADVERSE EFFECTS

Palpitations, tachycardia, elevation of blood pressure, overstimulation, restlessness, dizziness, insomnia, tremor, headache, psychotic episodes, agitation, flushing, sweating, blurred vision, dryness of the mouth, diarrhea, constipation, nausea, stomach pain, changes in libido, urinary frequency, dysuria

PHARMACOKINETICS AND PHARMACODYNAMICS

Onset of action: immediate
Plasma half-life: 1.9–9.8 h, with average of 3.7 h for both timed and untimed forms
Metabolism: some of the drug is metabolized to phenmetrazine and phendimetrazine-*N*-oxide.
Excretion: most of the drug and its metabolites are excreted through kidneys
Effects of food: drug should be taken on an empty stomach; effectiveness dependent on caloric intake and patient's eating habits
Renal and hepatic impairment: cumulative effects may occur with continued administration

(*Continued on next page*)

PHENDIMETRAZINE TARTRATE
(CONTINUED)

SPECIAL GROUPS

Children: Not recommended for children younger than
12 years of age.
Elderly: Use with caution, especially in patients suffering from mild
hypertension, hyperexcitability, or debilitated states.
Pregnancy: Category C drug. Safe use during pregnancy has not
been established. Use in women who may become pregnant only
when clearly needed and when potential benefits outweigh potential hazards to fetus.
Breast-feeding: Safety for use in nursing mother has not been
established.

DOSAGE

Adults: *Tablets and capsules*—35 mg two or three times daily
1 hour before meals. *Sustained-release capsules*—105 mg once daily in
the morning before breakfast.
Elderly: Same as for adults; use with extreme caution.
Children: Not recommended for children younger than 12 years of age.
Renal Impairment: Clearance of drug may be reduced; dose
reduction usually is required.

PROLONGED USE
Tolerance, withdrawal symptoms; abuse or dependence may occur if
used excessively.

OVERDOSAGE
Manifestations of acute overdose include restlessness, tremor, hyperreflexia, rapid respiration, confusion, assaultiveness, hallucinations, and
panic states. Fatigue and depression usually follow the central stimulation. Cardiovascular symptoms include arrhythmia, hypertension or
hypotension, and circulatory collapse. GI symptoms include nausea,
vomiting, diarrhea, and abdominal cramps. Fatal poisoning usually
terminates in convulsions and coma.
Treatment of acute intoxication is largely symptomatic and includes
lavage and sedation with a barbiturate. Experience with hemodialysis
or peritoneal dialysis is inadequate to recommend as treatment
measure.

PATIENT INFORMATION
Insomnia may occur; avoid taking drug late in day. If taking timed-
release form, limit dose to one capsule in the morning. Weight
reduction requires strict adherence to dietary restriction. Do not
take more frequently than prescribed. Notify physician if palpitations, nervousness, or dizziness occurs. Also notify physician if dry
mouth and constipation become pronounced. Use caution when
driving or cease driving; dizziness and blurred vision may occur.
Take drug on an empty stomach.

AVAILABILITY
Tablets—35 mg without tartrazine in 100s, 500s, 1000s; 35 mg with
tartrazine in 100s and 1000s
Capsules—35 mg in 100s and 1000s
Capsules (sustained-release)—105 mg in 100s, 250s, 500s, 1000s

PHENMETRAZINE HYDROCHLORIDE
(Preludin)

This drug mechanism of action is similar to that of other noradrenergic anorexiants. It causes short-term weight loss with rebound
weight gain upon discontinuation of treatment. Adverse effects are
mainly a result of its sympathomimetic action and include palpitations, hypertension, overstimulation, agitation, insomnia, dry mouth,
and nausea. In large doses it may cause psychosis and dependence.

SPECIAL PRECAUTIONS

May produce dizziness, extreme fatigue, and depression after abrupt
cessation of therapy; patients should observe caution when driving or
performing any task that requires alertness.

Use with caution and monitor blood pressure in patients with mild
hypertension; phenmetrazine is not recommended for use in patients
with symptomatic cardiovascular disease, including arrhythmias.

There is a potential for drug abuse and dependency, especially in
patients with a history of alcohol or drug intoxication.

Contains tartrazine; patients should be monitored closely for allergic reactions, including bronchial asthma.

In Brief

INDICATIONS
Appetite suppression for obesity

CONTRAINDICATIONS
Advanced arteriosclerosis, symptomatic cardiovascular disease,
moderate to severe hypertension, hyperthyroidism, known hypersensitivity or idiosyncratic reaction to sympathomimetic amines,
glaucoma, agitated states, history of drug abuse, administration of
MAO inhibitors during or within
14 d, pregnancy, lactation

INTERACTIONS
Guanethidine, insulin, MAO inhibitors, TCAs, thiazide diuretics
Drug/laboratory test interactions: Increase in urinary cate-
cholamines, increase in plasma corticosteroid levels

ADVERSE EFFECTS
Palpitations, tachycardia, arrhythmia, hypertension or hypotension,
fainting, precordial pain, pulmonary hypertension, overstimulation,
nervousness, restlessness, dizziness, insomnia, weakness or fatigue,
malaise, anxiety, tension, euphoria, elevated mood, drowsiness,
depression, agitation, dysphoria, tremor, dyskinesia, dysarthria,
confusion, incoordination, headache, change in libido, dry mouth,
unpleasant taste, nausea, vomiting, abdominal discomfort, diarrhea,
constipation, urticaria, burning sensation, mydriasis, eye irritation,
urinary frequency, impotence, menstrual upset, muscle pain, chest
pain, excessive sweating, fever, psychotic episodes

(Continued on next page)

SPECIAL GROUPS
Children: Not recommended for children younger than 12 years of age.
Elderly: Use with caution, especially in patients suffering from hyperexcitability or debilitated states.
Pregnancy: Category C drug. Safe use during pregnancy has not been established. Animal (dog) studies show adversely affected conception rate; survival and body weight of pups also affected. Congenital malformations are associated with phenmetrazine use, but a causal relationship has not been proven.
Breast-feeding: Safety for use in nursing mothers has not been established.

DOSAGE
Adults: Maximum dose of 75 mg once daily; provides appetite suppression for about 12 hours; determine administration time by period of day anorectic effect is desired.
Elderly: Same as for adults; use with caution.
Children: Not recommended for children younger than 12 years of age.

PHARMACOKINETICS AND PHARMACODYNAMICS
Onset of action: immediate
Excretion: most of the drug and its metabolites is excreted through the kidneys
Effects of food: drug should be taken on an empty stomach; effectiveness dependent on caloric intake and patient's eating habits
Renal and hepatic binding: cumulative effects may occur with continued administration

PROLONGED USE
Tolerance, withdrawal symptoms; abuse or dependence may occur if used excessively.

OVERDOSAGE
Symptoms of the CNS include restlessness, tremor, hyperreflexia, rapid respiration, hyperpyrexia, tachypnea, dizziness, confusion, belligerence, assaultivensss, hallucinations, and panic states; depression and fatigue usually follow central stimulation. Cardiovascular symptoms are arrhythmia (tachycardia), hypertension or hypotension, and circulatory collapse. Nausea, vomiting, diarrhea, and abdominal cramps also can occur. Convulsions, coma, and death may result. Doses less than 5 mg/kg are toxic; 5–10 mg/kg may produce coma and convulsions. Most deaths result from respiratory failure and cardiac arrest. Toxic effects occur within 30–60 min and progress rapidly.
Treatment includes symptomatic and supportive therapy. Sedate patient with a barbiturate and monitor respiratory exchange and cardiac function. Chlorpromazine may antagonize CNS effects. Experience with hemodialysis or peritoneal dialysis is inadequate to recommend as therapy.

PATIENT INFORMATION
Weight reduction requires strick adherence to dietary restriction. Avoid taking drug late in day, because insomnia can occur. Do not take more frequently than prescribed. Notify physician if palpitations, nervousness, or dizziness occurs. Also notify physician if dry mouth and constipation become pronounced. Do not drive unless absolutely necessary, because dizziness and blurred vision can occur. Take drug on an empty stomach.

AVAILABILITY
Tablets (sustained release)—75 mg with tartrazine in 100s

PHENTERMINE HYDROCHLORIDE

(Ionamin)

This drug is a noradrenergic anorexiant similar in its effect and adverse reactions to other members of this class. Therapy with this drug causes short-term weight loss with rebound weight gain following its discontinuation. Its adverse effects are amphetamine-like, although usually less intense than those produced by amphetamine use, such as palpitations, hypertension, dry mouth, nausea, and, in high dose, psychosis and dependence.

SPECIAL PRECAUTIONS

Concomitant use of alcohol with phentermine HCl may result in an adverse drug reaction.

Phentermine is a Schedule IV–controlled substance. The possibility of abuse should be kept in mind, evaluating the desirability of including this drug as part of a weight-reduction program.

May produce dizziness, extreme fatigue, and depression after abrupt cessation of therapy; patients should use caution when driving or performing any task that requires alertness.

Use with caution and monitor blood pressure in patients with mild hypertension; not recommended for use in patients with symptomatic cardiovascular disease, including arrhythmias.

SPECIAL GROUPS

Children: Not recommended for children younger than 12 years of age.
Elderly: Use with caution, especially in patients suffering from hyperexcitability or debilitated states.
Renal impairment: Clearance of drug may be reduced; dose reduction usually is required.
Hepatic impairment: Transformation to inactive metabolites may be reduced; dose reduction may be required.
Pregnancy: Category C drug. Safe use during pregnancy has not been established. Use by women who are or may become pregnant and by those in the first trimester of pregnancy necessitates that potential benefit of the drug be weighed against the possible hazard to the mother and infant.
Breast-feeding: Safety for use in nursing mothers has not been established.

DOSAGE

Adults: 8 mg three times daily 0.5 hours before meals or 15 to 37.5 mg as a single daily dose before breakfast or 10 to 14 hours before retiring.
Elderly: Same as for adults.
Children: Not recommended for children younger than 12 years of age.
Impaired renal function: Clearance of drug may be reduced; dose reduction usually is necessary.

In Brief

INDICATIONS
Appetite suppression for obesity

CONTRAINDICATIONS
Advanced arteriosclerosis, symptomatic cardiovascular disease, moderate to severe hypertension, hyperthyroidism, known hypersensitivity or idiosyncratic reaction to sympathomimetic amines, glaucoma, agitated states, history of drug abuse, administration of MAO inhibitors within 14 d, pregnancy, lactation

INTERACTIONS
Guanethidine, insulin, MAO inhibitors, TCAs, thiazide diuretics
Drug/laboratory test: Increase in urinary catecholamines, increase in plasma corticosteroid levels

ADVERSE EFFECTS
Palpitations, tachycardia, elevation of blood pressure, overstimulatio
Renal and hepatic impairment: cumulative effects may occur with continued administration

PHARMACOKINETICS AND PHARMACODYNAMICS
Onset of action: immediate
Excretion: most of the drug and its metabolites are excreted through the kidneys
Effect of food: drug should be taken on an empty stomach; effectiveness dependent on caloric intake and patient's eating habits

PROLONGED USE
Tolerance, withdrawal symptoms, abuse, or dependence may occur.

OVERDOSAGE
Symptoms of the CNS include restlessness, tremor, hyperreflexia, rapid respiration, hyperpyrexia, tachypnea, dizziness, confusion, belligerence, assaultiveness, hallucinations, and panic states; depression and fatigue usually follow central stimulation. Cardiovascular symptoms are arrhythmia (tachycardial), hypertension or hypotension, and circulatory collapse. Nausea, vomiting, diarrhea, and abdominal cramps also can occur. Convulsions, coma, and death may result. Doses < 5 mg/kg are toxic; 5–10 mg/kg may produce coma and convulsions. Most deaths result from respiratory failure and cardiac arrest. Toxic effects occur within 30–60 min and progress rapidly.
Treatment includes symptomatic and supportive therapy. Sedate patient with a barbiturate and monitor respiratory exchange and cardiac function. Chlorpromazine may antagonize CNS effects. Experience with hemodialysis or peritoneal dialysis is inadequate to recommend as therapy.

PATIENT INFORMATION
Avoid taking drug late in day because insomnia may occur. Weight reduction requires strict adherence to dietary restriction. Do not take more frequently than prescribed. Notify physician if palpitations, nervousness, or dizziness occurs. Also notify physician if dry mouth and constipation become pronounced. Use caution when driving or cease driving because dizziness and blurred vision can occur. Take drug on an empty stomach.

AVAILABILITY
Tablets—8 mg (equivalent to 6.4-mg base) in 100s and 1000s; 30 mg (equivalent to 24-mg base) in 100s and 1000s; 37.5 mg (equivalent to 30-mg base) in 30s, 100s, 500s, 1000s
Capsules—15 mg (equivalent to 12-mg base) in 100s and 1000s; 18.75 mg (equivalent to 15-mg base) in 100s, 500s, and 1000s; 30 mg (equivalent to 24-mg base) in 7s, 30s, 100s, 150s, 450s, 1000s; 37.5 mg (equivalent to 30-mg base) in 100s, 500s, 1000s; 15 mg (as resin complex) in 100s and 400s; 30 mg (as resin complex) in 100s and 400s

PHENYLPROPANOLAMINE HYDROCHLORIDE AND PHENYLPROPANOLAMINE COMBINATIONS

(Phenoxine, Dextrim Pre-Meal, Prolamine, Maximum Strength Dex-A-Diet Caplets, Phenyldrine, Control Maximum Strength Dex-A-Diet, Maximum Strength Dexatrim, Unitrol, Acutrim 16 Hour, Acutrim Late Day, Acutrim II-Max, Stay Trim)

Unlike other noradrenergic anorexiants, this drug is available over the counter and is used mainly as a decongestant. It is also effective, however, in causing weight loss in the short-term, with rebound weight gain occurring upon discontinuation of therapy. Its over-the-counter status comes from the likelihood of causing less amphetamine-like adverse effects at recommended doses, although this is probably a matter of dose and not a qualitative difference. It should be considered as effective and toxic as are other noradrenergic anorexiants.

SPECIAL PRECAUTIONS

Do not use in patients with high blood pressure or diabetes.

Do not use if patients have taken any MAO inhibitors within the past 2 weeks.

Do not use if patients have taken digitalis preparations within the past 7 days.

Do not use concomitant with other over-the-counter medications.

SPECIAL GROUPS

Children: Safety and efficacy for use in children have not been established; not recommended as an anorexiant for children younger than 12 years of age; anorexiant dose must be individualized for children 12 to 18 years of age.

Elderly: Monitor blood pressure frequently; adults older than 60 years of age are more likely to develop high blood pressure, heart-rhythm disturbances, and angina.

Renal impairment: Hypertensive crisis and possible kidney failure.

Hepatic impairment: Transformation to inactive metabolites may be reduced; dose reduction may be required.

Pregnancy: Safety and efficacy during pregnancy have not been established; use is not recommended.

Breast-feeding: Safety and efficacy during lactation have not been established; avoid nursing.

In Brief

INDICATIONS

Nasal congestion resulting from colds, hay fever, and allergies. Short-term treatment of exogenous obesity in conjunction with weight-reduction program that includes reduced caloric intake, exercise, and behavior modification.

CONTRAINDICATIONS

Arteriosclerosis, cardiovascular disease, hypertension, hyperthyroidism, kidney disease, diabetes, hypersensitivity or idiosyncratic reaction to sympathomimetic amines, glaucoma, depression, during or within 14 d after administration of MAO inhibitors

INTERACTIONS

Furazolidone, guanethidine, MAO inhibitors, indomethacin, general anesthetics, antihypertensives, β-adrenergic blockers, digitalis preparations, epinephrine, ergot preparations, methyldopa, phenothiazines, rauwolfia, tarazoain, alcohol, caffeinated beverages

ADVERSE EFFECTS

Serious CNS effects attributable to abuse of drug—Agitation, tremor, increased motor activity, hallucinations, seizures, and stroke; death can occur; hypertension may be severe and can lead to a crisis
Common—Palpitation, tremor, tachycardia, increased motor activity, blood pressure elevation, agitation, severe hypertension, hallucinations, hypertensive crisis, seizures, possible renal failure, stroke, restlessness, dry mouth, dizziness, nasal dryness, insomnia, nausea, headache, dysuria, bizarre behavior

PHARMACOKINETICS AND PHARMACODYNAMICS

Onset of action: 30–60 min (anorexiant); 15–30 min (decongestant)
Peak plasma levels: 60–200 ng/mL; average, 100 ng in 1–2 h
Plasma half-life: 3–4 h
Bioavailability: rapidly absorbed through gastrointestinal tract
Metabolism: small amounts metabolized in the liver to active hydroxylated metabolites
Excretion: 80%–90% excreted unchanged in urine
Renal impairment: clearance of drug may be reduced; dose reduction usually is required.
Hepatic impairment: transformation to inactive metabolites may be reduced; dose reduction may be required

PROLONGED USE

Tolerance, withdrawal symptoms, abuse, or dependence may occur if used excessively.

(Continued on next page)

PHENYLPROPANOLAMINE HYDROCHLORIDE AND PHENYLPROPANOLAMINE COMBINATIONS (CONTINUED)

DOSAGE

Adults: *Decongestant*—25 mg every 4 hours or 50 mg every 6 to 8 hours; maximum dose, 150 mg/d. *Anorexiant*—Immediate-release tablets, 25 mg three times daily 0.5 hour before meals; timed-release tablets and capsules, 75 mg once daily in the morning; precision-release tablets (16-hour duration), 75 mg after breakfast.

Elderly: Same as for adults; use with caution in patients older than 60 years of age.

Children: *Decongestant*—2 to 6 years of age, 6.25 mg every 4 hours not to exceed 37.5 mg in 24 hours; 6 to 12 years of age, 12.5 mg every 4 hours not to exceed 75 mg in 24 hours. *Anorexiant*—Not recommended for use in children younger than 12 years of age; dose must be individualized for children 12 to 18 years of age.

OVERDOSAGE

Overdose symptoms of the CNS include restlessness, tremor, hyper-reflexia, tachypnea, confusion, assaultive behavior, and hallucinations. Cardiovascular symptoms include arrhythmia and hypertension; GI symptoms are nausea and vomiting.

Treatment is symptomatic. Gastric lavage, activated charcoal, seizure control, cardiac monitoring, and acidification of urine are recommended.

PATIENT INFORMATION

Do not exceed recommended dosage. Use only in conjunction with a calorie-restrictive diet. Use cautiously, if at all, with alcohol. Do not use other over-the-counter drugs with similar actions. Discontinue use if rapid pulse, dizziness, nervousness, insomnia, or palpitations occur. Older men are cautioned to report to physicians any difficulty in voiding, because they are more susceptible to drug-induced urinary retention.

AVAILABILITY

Phenylpropanolamine HCl: *Tablets*—25 mg in 1000s; *Tablets (timed release)*—75 mg in 24s and 100s; *Tablets (precision release)*—75 mg in 20s and 40s; *Capsules*—37.5 mg in 20s; *Capsules (timed release*—75 mg in 3s, 10s, 14s, 20s, 28s, and 40s (*Note*: also available as gum [8.33 mg in 20s] and mints [12.5 mg in 36s].)

Phenypropanolamine HCl combinations: *Tablets*—25 mg in 30s; *chewable*:12.5 mg in 42s and 90s; *capsules (timed release)*—75 mg (with grapefruit extract) in 4s and 24s and in 10s and 20s; 75 mg (with 180 mg vitamin C) in 20s; 30 mg (with grapefruit extract, tartrazine) in 20s and 50s

Antidepressants

Frederic M. Quitkin
Bonnie P. Taylor

The development of psychopharmacologic approaches to treat affective disorders was a major advance. In the late 1950s, tricyclic antidepressants (TCAs) and monoamine oxidase (MAO) inhibitors were introduced for the treatment of depression. Pharmacologic agents have become the cornerstone for treating these disorders.

Depending on the method of categorization used, there are four or five classes of antidepressant compounds. These include the TCAs (also referred to as imipramine-like drugs or dibenzyl derivatives), the MAO inhibitors, the selective serotonin reuptake inhibitors (SSRIs), the tetracyclics, and a group of compounds referred to as second-generation drugs, which although chemically unrelated, have antidepressant properties.

These classes of drugs are discussed separately. Although there are a few exceptions, each drug within a class has a similar efficacy. The major difference between the drug classes is the side-effect profile. Some patients tolerate some classes of anti-depressants better than others. For example, TCAs tend to be more soporific than the SSRIs. Trial and error is involved when selecting a drug for a patient. Most outpatients tolerate the newer drugs, such as the SSRIs, bupropion, and venlafaxine, better than the other classes of drugs, although their efficacy is roughly equal.

Although not studied systematically, there is no evidence of long-term ill effects from prolonged use of these drugs.

PRESCRIPTION OF ANTIDEPRESSANTS

Several general principles apply to these drugs. The most frequent mistakes concerning their prescription have to do with the use of inappropriate dose and duration of a clinical trial before deciding a drug is ineffective.

Dosage

Several reports have suggested that these drugs should be used at their optimum dose [1–3]. If a drug is prescribed, every attempt should be made to increase slowly to the maximum dose suggested by the manufacturer before deciding that the drug is ineffective. There are surprisingly few dose-response studies, and a great deal is not known about the reasonable safe maximum dose. However, the few studies that exist clearly suggest that maximum doses are more effective than are doses in the middle range. For example, Simpson and coworkers [4] show that 300

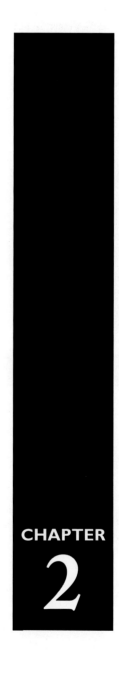

CHAPTER

2

mg of imipramine is superior to 150 mg, and Watt and coworkers [5] demonstrate that patients treated with 300 mg of desipramine are more likely to respond than those treated with 150 mg. Tyrer and coworkers [6] and Ravaris and coworkers [7] show that maximum doses of the MAO inhibitor phenelzine were superior to doses of 30 to 45 mg. Although dose-response curves have not shown that larger doses of SSRIs are superior to standard doses, anecdotal reports suggest that some patients who do not benefit from lower doses clearly benefit from maximum doses. Our experience in open trials suggests that roughly half of the patients who do not benefit from a 20-mg dose of fluoxetine benefit when the dose is raised to 40 to 80 mg. Dosage is an important issue when prescribing antidepressants.

Duration of Drug Trial

The other major mistake concerns duration of a drug trial before deciding the drug is ineffective. These drugs almost always take 1 to 2 weeks before they start to work. Only a minority of patients who eventually benefit show any improvement after 2 weeks of treatment [8]. The time it takes to go from a symptomatic state to a relatively symptom-free one can vary. Some patients show no improvement for 3 to 4 weeks and suddenly improve; others gradually get better over 2 weeks. Two studies demonstrate that patients taking a fixed dose of an antidepressant who have not improved at 4 weeks have a far greater chance of improving when the drug is extended to 6 weeks than do those taking placebo [9,10]. Therefore, patients should not be considered to be unresponsive until they have received a minimum of a 6-week trial of the antidepressant with a dose close to the maximum for at least 10 days.

Accommodating to Side Effects

Another mistake is that physicians stop raising the dose or terminate the drug trial if patients develop unpleasant side effects that have no serious consequence (ie, mild orthostatic hypotension). If unpleasant side effects occur, the correct procedure is to lower the dose slightly and wait until the patient accommodates to the drug. Most symptoms generally disappear and become tolerable within a few days to 1 week. The dose then can be raised gradually until the most effective dose is reached. This can take 4 or 5 weeks. If the

patients understand that these side effects, which are innocuous but unpleasant, can be controlled in this manner, the dose usually can be raised to the most effective level.

■ TRICYCLIC ANTIDEPRESSANTS

Imipramine, the first TCA, was developed in the search for antipsychotic agents of the phenothiazine type. The phenothiazine sulfur atom was replaced with a dimethyl bridge. Kuhn's [11] chance discovery, as a result of good clinical observation, was critical in recognizing the antidepressant effects of this class of compounds. TCAs available in the United States include amitriptyline, desipramine, doxepin, imipramine, amoxapine, nortriptyline, protriptyline, trimipramine, and clomipramine. All of these drugs have roughly equal therapeutic effect. The exception, clomipramine, has superior efficacy in obsessive-compulsive disorder [12].

CLASSIFICATION, MODE OF ACTION, AND SIDE EFFECTS

The side effects of this class of compounds vary considerably. Compounds with two methyl groups (eg, amitriptyline, imipramine) are tertiary amines and appear to block the reuptake of serotonin and norepinephrine [13]. TCAs that have one methyl group are referred to as secondary amines (desipramine, nortriptyline, protriptyline) and have a greater effect of blocking the reuptake of norepinephrine and relatively little effect on serotonin. TCAs exert their effect by increasing the availability of norepinephrine and serotonin in the synaptic cleft. Generally, TCAs that are tertiary amines are more soporific than secondary amines. Other than the particular efficacy of clomipramine in patients with obsessive-compulsive disorder, one drug in this class is not superior to another.

There is evidence that patients with cardiac conduction defects, particularly left bundle branch block, may develop heart block with TCAs [14]. Although the evidence is clearly indirect, caution is suggested when treating patients with ischemic heart disease with a TCA [15]. This stems from the increased mortality associated with flecainide, encainide, and moricizine in the collaborative cardiac

Table 2-1. Controlled Studies Comparing Tricyclics with Placebo for Treatment of Depression*

Drug studied	Inpatients		Outpatients		Mixed Group		Total (All Groups)	
	Superior to Placebo†	Not Superior	Superior to Placebo	Not Superior	Superior to Placebo	Not Superior	Superior to Placebo	Not Superior
Imipramine	23	15	6	4	1	1	30	20
Desipramine	3	2	1	0	0	0	4	2
Amitriptyline	7	4	7	2	0	0	14	6
Nortriptyline	4	3	1	0	0	0	5	3
Protriptyline	1	0	2	0	0	0	3	0
Doxepin	1	0	0	0	0	0	1	0
Amitriptyline, perphenazine	1	1	3	0	0	0	4	1
Totals	40	25	20	6	1	1	61	32

*Ninety-three treatment group comparisons in 85 studies.
†Superior in each column indicates significance at least at 0.05 level
Adapted from Morris and Beck [18].

arrhythmia suppression trial [16,17]. These drugs, called class I antiarrhythmics, also are sodium channel blockers. Direct evidence for a contraindication of TCAs in ischemic heart disease is lacking. However, TCAs share many of the characteristics of class I antiarrhythmics and are suspect in patients with anoxic heart disease. Many of the other antidepressants do not share this effect with the TCAs.

There is an additive anticholinergic effect with concomitant use of TCAs and other anticholinergic medicines, including antihistamines and antipsychotic agents. TCA drugs that have a sedative effect (ie, doxepin, amitriptyline, trimipramine, nortriptyline and imipramine) interact additively with alcohol and other central nervous system (CNS) depressants. In addition, TCAs may produce a seizure, especially in patients with a history of seizure disorder.

RELATIVE EFFICACY

In Table 2-1, trials of TCAs are compared with placebo [18]. Roughly 65% of the time, tricyclics are superior to placebo; 35% of the time there is no difference, and placebo is never superior to a TCA. These data clearly suggest that these drugs are effective for treating depressive illness. Trials contrasting different TCAs also are summarized in Table 2-2. In an overwhelming number of trials, there is no difference between the two active compounds that are contrasted. The logical conclusion is that all of these drugs have roughly equal efficacy.

Amoxapine is a derivative of the antipsychotic loxapine. It may be helpful in treating psychotic depression. It disadvantage is that it causes D2 blockade, which may lead to extrapyramidal and tardive dyskinesia.

DOSAGE AND TRIAL DURATION

It is not uncommon for TCAs to be mistakenly prescribed for a short duration [19] at subtherapeutic doses [19,20]. Imipramine, amitriptyline, desipramine, doxepin, trimipramine, and clomipramine can be given in doses up to 300 mg. The drug should be started at the lowest possible dose and slowly increased. Most of the drugs eventually can be given in a single dose at bedtime. This minimizes soporific effects during working hours. The possibility exists that there is a window in nortriptyline, and the dose is generally 50 to 150 mg/d with a serum level of 75 to 150 ng/d [21,22]. The dose of protriptyline is 10 to 60 mg.

These drugs should be prescribed for at least 5 to 6 weeks with 10 days at the maximum tolerated dose before determining that they are ineffective.

PATIENT INFORMATION

Patients should be told that these drugs cause orthostatic hypotension and anticholinergic side effects. Patients who experience dizziness when changing position should be cautioned to change position slowly or to have the dose temporarily lowered. Sugarless gum minimizes dry mouth, and stool softeners can be prescribed for constipation.

PROLONGED USE

Systematic studies have not been performed for all of the TCA compounds, but anecdotal experience collected over 30 years suggest that prolonged use of therapeutic doses is safe. Chronic use of TCAs may result in rapid cycling, recurrent periodic shifts in mood from depression to hypomania.

■ MONOAMINE OXIDASE INHIBITORS

The discovery of the antidepressant action of the MAO inhibitors was largely accidental. MAO is a widely distributed enzyme that oxidatively deaminizes tyramine, epinephrine, dopamine, and other biogenic amines to pharmacologically inactive acidic derivatives. Zeller and coworkers [23] found that MAO was inhibited by iproniazid, and Selikoff and coworkers [24] noticed the mood-elevating properties of iproniazine in tuberculosis patients. Crane [25] and Kline [26], working independently, found that MAO inhibitors were effective in depressed patients. Nonhydrazine MAO inhibitors were synthesized

Table 2-2. Drug Groups Showing Imipramine Superior, Inferior, or Equivalent to Other Tricyclics*

Comparison Drug	Inpatients			Outpatients			Mixed			Total		
	Superior	No Difference	Inferior	Superior	No Difference	Inferior	Superior	No Difference	Inferior	Superior	No Difference	Inferior
Desipramine	2	8	0	0	1	0	0	0	0	2	9	0
Amitriptyline	1	2	4	0	2	1	1	0	0	2	4	5
Nortriptyline	0	1	0	0	1	0	0	0	0	0	2	0
Protriptyline	0	0	0	0	2	0	0	0	0	0	2	0
Doxepin	0	3	0	0	0	0	0	0	0	0	3	0
Perphenazine, amitriptyline	0	0	1	0	0	0	0	0	0	0	0	1
Totals	3	14	5	0	6	1	1	0	0	4	20	6

*Thirty treatment group comparisons in 29 studies.
Adapted from Morris and Beck [18].

to avoid troublesome liver toxicity associated with the hydrazine MAO inhibitors. Tranylcypromine was the first of these developed. Other nonhydrazine MAO inhibitors have been shown to be effective.

CLASSIFICATION AND MODE OF ACTION

One classification for MAO inhibitors includes three groups: non-selective, including tranylcypromine (a nonhydrazine) and phenelzine (a hydrazine derivative); selective; and reversible inhibitors of MAO A. MAO exists in two forms, MAO A and MAO B. Selegiline is an example of selective MAO B inhibitor and is not approved as an antidepressant. There may be less toxicity associated with selective MAO inhibitors [27]. The third class includes drugs that are not marketed in the United States, including moclobemide [28]. MAO inhibitors are effective antidepressants and may have a superior effect in patients with atypical depression, those with reversed vegetative symptoms, such as overeating and oversleeping [29]. Atypical depression is a new parenthetical modifier in the *Diagnostic & Statistical Manual of Mental Disorders, 4th edition* (*DSM IV*). This is a major advantage of MAO inhibitors compared with the tricyclics, although preliminary observations suggest SSRIs may be as effective as MAO inhibitors in atypical depressive patients. The efficacy of SSRI in atypical depression requires validation.

For other diagnostic subtypes, the efficacy of MAO inhibitors is approximate to that of TCAs, but MAO inhibitors are considered second-line drugs because of their unfavorable side-effect profile. However, MAO inhibitors may be preferred for patients with seizure disorders because they do not lower the seizure threshold [30]. Concurrent administration of an MAO inhibitor with another antidepressant is not recommended; at least a 7-day delay after a tricyclic is discontinued and a 5-week delay after fluoxetine is discontinued are recommended before beginning a trial with an MAO inhibitor. Patients who cannot adhere to the dietary restrictions required when using an MAO inhibitor, as well as those who frequently drink alcohol, have pheochromocytoma, asthma, or severe cardiovascular, hepatic, or renal disease, should not take MAO inhibitors.

Monoamine oxidase inhibitors are effective antidepressants. MAO metabolizes a wide range of biogenic amines, including norepinephrine, serotonin, dopamine, phenylethylamine, and others. It generally is believed that inhibition of MAO increases the availability of the biogenic amines, which is responsible for their antidepressant effect.

CLASSIFICATION OF SIDE EFFECTS: HYPERTENSIVE CRISIS

The major disadvantage of MAO inhibitors is their complicated side-effect profile. The "cheese reaction," or hypertensive crisis, associated with the use of MAO inhibitors was first described by Ogilvie [31] in patients suffering from tuberculosis. Patients who have been taking an MAO inhibitor for a sufficient time and eat substances containing tyramine, dopamine, or sympathomimetics may develop a throbbing headache with a sudden onset, usually occipital, sometimes temporal. This often is preceded by cardiac palpitations, sudden rise in blood pressure, sweating, and chills. The syndrome represents a clinical picture similar to that seen with pheochromocytoma and can result in intracranial bleeding. This could be fatal. Patients must be cautioned when combining tyramine and dopamine. Sympathomimetics (*ie*, some cold medicines, amphetamines, cocaine, ephedrine, and methylphenidate) are markedly potentiated by MAO inhibitors. However, direct-acting sympathomimetics may be used in refractory patients if introduced slowly [32].

In general, the MAO inhibitors, although extremely effective in a variety of disorders, have become second-line drugs, and their use is recommended only in patients who have been refractory to at least two classes of other antidepressants.

■ TETRACYCLIC ANTIDEPRESSANTS

There are at least two tetracyclic antidepressants: mianserin, which is not approved for use in the United States, and maprotiline. Maprotiline's fourth ring is formed by a bridge across the central tricyclic ring. Thus, it has characteristics similar to TCAs. Maprotiline blocks the reuptake of norepinephrine and has anticholinergic effects and effects in the cardiovascular system.

Mianserin originally was developed to be used for allergic conditions. Itil and coworkers [33] suggested that using quantitative electroencephalogram (EEG), mianserin produced EEG changes typical of other antidepressants, referred to as "thymoleptic EEG reaction." This led to its being tested as an antidepressant. Mianserin does not block the reuptake of monoamines, such as norepinephrine, as the TCAs do. It has minimal if any effects on the autonomic nervous system and does not cause difficulty in accommodation or decreased salivary flow, which leads to dry mouth. Although these side effects clearly are not life threatening, some patients find them intolerable. Its other great advantage is its safety. Crome and Newman [34] were unable to find any evidence that it caused cardiac arrhythmia in overdose, a frequent cause of death with TCAs. Because death from overdosage of TCAs is common, it is a major advantage of mianserin. Mianserin is not available in the United States.

■ SELECTIVE SEROTONIN REUPTAKE INHIBITORS

MODE OF ACTION

Interest in developing drugs that selectively block the reuptake of serotonin stems from the possibility that serotonin may be involved in some forms of depressive illness. The major metabolite of serotonin, 5-hydroxyindoleacetic acid (5-HIAA), is at low levels in the brain tissue of deceased depressed patients [35]. In addition, 5-HIAA levels were reported to be low in the spinal fluid of some depressed patients [36]. Compounds that have specific effects on the reuptake of serotonin without effects on noradrenaline, dopamine, or acetylcholine would appear to be advantageous because they might be effective antidepressants without many of the unpleasant side effects associated with the older antidepressants [37].

SIDE EFFECTS AND METHOD OF PRESCRIPTION

Fluoxetine was the first of these drugs to be developed. It has far fewer anticholinergic effects and appears to be well tolerated in overdose, which is important because some depressed patients attempt to take their lives with the drugs prescribed to treat their depression. In general, SSRIs are well tolerated. However, they are more likely to cause nausea, nervousness, and insomnia when first prescribed. In general, these symptoms can be controlled by slowly introducing the drug in small doses. Some anxious depressive patients, especially those with a history of panic attacks, become agitated if started on too high a dose. Even anxious patients tolerate this class of drugs if the initial dose is low. Some patients eventually tolerate the SSRI if the starting dose is lower than the recommended starting dose.

EFFICACY AND USE

Fluoxetine has been shown to be effective [38]. In general, the drugs included in this class have a broad range of efficacy in depressive disorders. Their use in psychotic depression has not been studied.

They are effective in obsessive-compulsive and panic disorder. In addition to fluoxetine, three other SSRIs, sertraline, fluvoxemine, and paroxetine have been approved and have equal efficacy and similar side-effect profiles to that of fluoxetine.

SSRIs may be particularly useful in patients with coronary artery disease, hypertension, narrow-angle glaucoma, and prostate enlargement. They are also recommended for patients who can not tolerate the side effects of TCAs and MAO inhibitors and for elderly patients because they mediate little or no anticholinergic activity. They have also been useful in treating depressed patients with comorbid obsessive-compulsive disorder, panic disorder, eating disorders, and alcohol abuse.

DRUG INTERACTIONS

All members of this class of drugs have equivalent effects. Cytochrome P_{450} is a group of heme proteins found throughout the body with high concentration in the liver. One group of P_{450} proteins oxidizes drugs; another group of P_{450}s catalyzes the formation of fatty acids and steroid hormones [39]. Three of the SSRIs affect P_{450}, which metabolizes other drugs. It was originally thought that sertraline (Zoloft) had no effect on P_{450}. The manufacturer has stated that sertraline does have some effect but probably less than other SSRIs on P_{450} enzymes. Fluvoxamine inhibits CYPIA2, and paroxetine and fluoxetine inhibit CYP2D6. Table 2-3 indicates some drugs metabolized by the relevant isoenzymes. Caution is required when using these SSRIs and the relevant drugs of which the metabolism is inhibited.

Table 2-3. Drugs Metabolized by Specific Cytochrome P_{450} Enzymes

CYPIA2*	CYP2D6†
Amitriptyline HCl	Opiates
Clomipramine	Fluoxetine
Imipramine HCl	Citalopram
Propranolol HCl	Paroxetine HCl
	Tricyclics
	Neuroleptics
	β-Blockers

*Inhibited by fluvoxemine HCl
†Inhibited by fluoxetine HCl and paroxetine HCl
Adapted from Brosen [35].

CONTRAINDICATIONS

Toxic interactions between SSRIs and MAO inhibitors have been reported, and fatalities have resulted. At least 1 week should elapse between the elimination of an SSRI and its metabolites and the use of an MAO inhibitor. With fluoxetine this requires a 5-week wait.

PHARMACOKINETICS

After continuous administration of Prozac (Lilly, Indianapolis, Indiana), the half-life of fluoxetine is 4 to 6 days, and for its major metabolite, norfluoxetine, it may be as long as 16 days. Some metabolites may be present for at least 1 month following drug discontinuation. This is advantageous in patients who take drugs irregularly, but disadvantageous if the patient must switch to another drug class in which simultaneous use with an SSRI is hazardous (eg, MAO inhibitor). In contrast, the half-life of sertraline is approximately 24 hours, and paroxetine's half-life is approximately the same.

■ SECOND-GENERATION DRUGS

Tricyclics and MAO inhibitors are effective. TCAs frequently were characterized by anticholinergic and soporific effects, which many patients found intolerable. Patients receiving an MAO inhibitor had to follow a restricted diet. Many patients believed that these drugs limited their cognitive ability. As a result, new drugs were developed that had antidepressant properties but fewer anticholinergic and other unpleasant side effects. Included in the second-generation drugs are several unrelated compounds, such as trazodone, venlafaxine, mirtazapine, nefazodone, and bupropion. Bupropion is an effective drug that has several advantages, including little change in the electrocardiogram (ECG) and low anticholinergic effects, and it is relatively nonsedating. Its efficacy has been clearly established [40]. Trazodone, although it has minimal anticholinergic effects, is a sedating drug, which occasionally has been associated with priapism in men. Trazadone in low doses (25–75 mg) has been used as a sedating drug in patients using MAO inhibitors.

Venlafaxine is structurally unrelated to other antidepressants. Its mechanism of action is not understood, but it does block reuptake of serotonin and norepinephrine and is a weak inhibitor of dopamine uptake. There is some evidence that it is effective in patients refractory to other antidepressants. Nefazodone is well tolerated and has a low side-effect profile, including a low incidence of sexual dysfunction. REM sleep is increased, and nefazodone is recommended for patients with a sleep disturbance.

REFERENCES

1. Johnson DAP: A study in the use of antidepressant medication in general practice. *Br J Psychiatry* 1974, 125:1986–1992.
2. Ketai R: Family practitioners knowledge about treatment of depressive illness. *JAMA* 1976, 235:2600–2603.
3. Fauman MA: Tricyclic antidepressant description by general hospital physicians. *Am J Psychiatry* 1980, 137:490–491.
4. Simpson GM, Lee JH, Cuculica A, *et al.*: Two dosages of imipramine in hospitalized endogenous and neurotic depressives. *Arch Gen Psychiatry* 1976, 33:1093–1102.
5. Watt DC, Crammer JL, Elkes A: Metabolism, anticholinergic effects and therapeutic effects on outcome of desmethylimipramine in depressive illness. *Psychological Med* 1972, 2:397–405.
6. Tyrer P, Gardner M, Lambourn J, *et al.*: Clinical and pharmacokinetic factors affecting response to phenelzine. *Br J Psychiatry* 1980, 136:359–365.
7. Ravaris CL, Nies A, Robinson DS, *et al.*: A multiple-dose controlled study of phenelzine in depression-anxiety states. *Arch Gen Psychiatry* 1976, 33:347–350.
8. Qutikin FM, Rabkin JG, Markowitz JM: Use of pattern analysis to identify true drug response: a replication. *Arch Gen Psychiatry* 1987, 44:259–264.
9. Donovan SJ, Quitkin FM, Stewart JS, *et al.*: Duration of antidepressant trials: clinical and research implications. *J Clin Psychopharmacology* 1994, 14(1):64–66.
10. Quitkin FM, Rabkin JG, Ross, D, McGrath PJ: Duration of antidepressant drug treatment: what is an adequate trial? *Arch Gen Psych* 1984, 41(3):238–245.
11. Kuhn R: The treatment of depressive states with G-22355 (imipramine hydrochloride). *Am J Psychiatry* 1958, 115:459–464.
12. Rapoport JL: Recent advances in obsessive compulsive disorder. *Neuropsychopharmacology* 1991, 5:1–10.
13. Klein DF, Gittleman R, Quitkin FM, *et al.*: *Diagnosis and Drug Treatment of Psychiatric Disorders in Adults and Children.* Baltimore: Williams & Wilkins; 1980.
14. Glassman AH, Bigger JT Jr: Cardiovascular effects of therapeutic doses of tricyclic antidepressants: a review. *Arch Gen Psychiatry* 1981, 38:815–820.

15. Glassman AH, Roose SP, Bigger JT Jr: The safety of tricyclic antidepressants in cardiac patients: risk-benefit reconsidered. *JAMA* 1993, 26920:2673–2675.

16. The Cardiac Arrhythmia Suppression Trial (CAST) Investigators: Preliminary report: effect of encainide and flecainide on mortality in a randomized trial of arrhythmia suppression after myocardial infarction. *N Engl J Med* 1989, 321:406–412.

17. The Cardiac Arrhythmia Suppression Trial II Investigators: Effect of the antiarrhythmic agent moricizine on survival after myocardial infarction. *N Engl J Med* 1992, 327:227–233.

18. Morris JB, Beck AT: The efficacy of antidepressant drugs. *Arch Gen Psychiatry* 1974, 30:667–674.

19. MacDonald TM, McMahon AD, Reid IC, *et al.*: Antidepressant drug use in primary care: a record linkage study in Tayside, Scotland. *Br Med J* 1996, 313:860–861.

20. Donaghue JM, Tylee A: The treatment of depression: prescribing patterns of antidepressants in primary care in the UK. *Br J Psychiatry* 1996, 168:164–168.

21. Perry PJ, Pfohl BM, Holstads SG: The relationship between antidepressant response and tricyclic antidepressant plasma concentrations. *J Clin Pharmacokinet* 1987, 13:381–392.

22. Karagh-Sorensen T, Hansen C, Gaastrup T, *et al.*: Self inhibiting action of nortriptyline to antidepressant effects at high plasma levels. *Psychopharmacologia* 1976, 45:305–312.

23. Zeller EA, Barsky J, Fouts JR, *et al.*: Influence of isonicotinic and hydrazide (INH) and 1-isonicotinyl-2-isopropyl hydrazide (IIH) on bacterial and mammalian enzymes. *Experientia* 1952, 8:349–350.

24. Selikoff IJ, Robitzek EH, Ornstein GG: Toxicity of hydrazine derivatives of isonicotinic acid in the chemotherapy of human tuberculosis. *Q Bull SeaView Hosp* 1952, 13:17.

25. Crane GE: Iproniazid (Marsilid) phosphate, a therapeutic agent for mental disorders and debilitating disease. *Psychiatr Res Rep* 1957, 8:142–152.

26. Kline NS: Clinical experience with iproniazid (Marsilid). *J Clin Exp Psycopathol* 1958, 19(suppl 1):72–78.

27. Quitkin FM, Liebowitz MR, Stewart JW, *et al.*: L-Deprenyl in atypical depressives. *Arch Gen Psychiatry* 1984, 41:777–781.

28. Lecrubies Y, Guelfi JD: Efficacy of reversible inhibitors of monoamine oxidase A in various forms of depression. *Acta Psychiatr Scand* 1990, 360(suppl):18–23.

29. Quitkin FM, McGrath PJ, Stewart JW, *et al.*: Atypical depression, panic attacks, and response to imipramine and phenelzine. *Arch Gen Psychiatry* 1990, 47:935–941.

30. Richardson WJ, Richelson E: Antidepressants: a clinical update for medical practitioners. *Mayo Clin Proc* 1984, 59:330–337.

31. Ogilvie C: The treatment of pulmonary tuberculosis with iproniazid and isoniazid. *Q J Med* 1955, 24:175–189.

32. Feighner JP, Herbstein J, Damlouji N: Combined MAOI, TCA, and direct stimulant therapy of treatment-resistant depression. *J Clin Psychiatr* 1985, 46:206–209.

33. Itil TM, Polvan N, Hsu W: Clinical and EEG effects of GB-94, a "tetracyclic" antidepressant. *Curr Ther Res* 1972, 14:395–413.

34. Crome P, Newman G: Poisoning with maprotiline and mianserin [letter]. *Br Med J* 1977, 2:260.

35. Beskow J, Gottfries CG, Roos BE, *et al.*: Determination of monoamine metabolites in the human brain, postmortem studies in a group of suicides in a control group. *Acta Psychiatr Scand* 1976, 53:7–20.

36. Asberg M, Thoren T, Traskman L, *et al.*: Serotonin depression: a biochemical subgroup within the affective disorders? *Science* 1976, 191:478–180.

37. Anderson IM, Tomenson BM: Treatment discontinuation with selective serotonin reuptake inhibitors compared with tricyclic antidepressants: a meta-analysis. *Br Med J* 1995, 310:1433–1438.

38. Stark P, Hardison CD: A review of multi-center controlled studies of fluoxetine vs imipramine and placebo in outpatients with major depressive disorder. *J Clin Psychiatr* 1985, 46:53–58.

39. Brosen K: Isozyme specific drug oxidation: genetic polymorphism and drug-drug interactions. *Nord J Psychiatry* 1993, 47(suppl 30):21–26.

40. Soroko FE, Mehta NB, Maxwell RA, *et al.*: Buprorion hydrochloride: a novel antidepressant agent. *J Pharm Pharmacol* 1977, 29:767–770.

AMITRIPTYLINE HYDROCHLORIDE

(Elavil, Endep, Etrafon, Limbitrol)

Amitriptyline hydrochloride (HCl) is a TCA with significant anticholinergic and sedative effects; it may cause orthostatic hypotension.

SPECIAL PRECAUTIONS

Use with caution in patients with a history of seizures and, because of its atropine-like action, patients with a history of urinary retention, angle-closure glaucoma, or increased intraocular pressure. In patients with angle-closure glaucoma, even average doses may precipitate an attack.

Patients with cardiovascular disorders should be watched closely, particularly those with conduction defects or heart disease. Amitriptyline has been reported to produce arrhythmias, sinus tachycardia, and prolongation of conduction time.

It may block the antihypertensive action of guanethidine or similarly acting compounds.

Close supervision is required when amitriptyline is given to hyperthyroid patients or patients receiving thyroid medication.

Elevated and lowered blood sugar have been reported with the use of amitriptyline.

SPECIAL GROUPS

Children: Safety and efficacy in children younger than age 12 years have not been established.

Elderly: Lower doses are recommended for elderly patients.

Hepatic impairment: Amitriptyline should be used with caution in patients with impaired liver function.

Pregnancy: Category C drug. No adequate and well-controlled studies have been conducted in pregnant women. Amitriptyline should be used during pregnancy only if potential benefit justifies potential risk to fetus.

Breast-feeding: Amitriptyline and its metabolite, nortriptyline, are excreted in breast milk. A decision should be made whether to discontinue nursing or discontinue the drug, taking into account the importance of the drug to the mother.

In Brief

INDICATIONS
Relief of symptoms of depression; endogenous depression is more likely to be alleviated than other depressive status; useful in patients with insomnia if given at bedtime

CONTRAINDICATIONS
Contraindicated during acute recovery phase following myocardial infarction

INTERACTIONS
Alcohol, anticholinergic agents or sympathomimetic drugs, barbiturates and other CNS depressants, cimetidine, ethchlorvynol, guanethidine or similarly acting compounds, MAO inhibitors, thyroid medications

ADVERSE EFFECTS
Most are rare. Observed in patients taking amitriptyline but often causality is not established. Hypotension, hypertension, tachycardia, palpitation, myocardial infarction, arrhythmias, heart block, stroke, confusional states, disturbed concentration, disorientation, delusions, hallucinations, excitement, anxiety, restlessness, insomnia, nightmares, numbness, tingling and parethesias of the extremities, peripheral neuropathy, loss of coordination, ataxia, tremor, seizures, alteration in EEG patterns, extrapyramidal symptoms, tinnitus, dry mouth, blurred vision, disturbance of accommodation, increased intraocular pressure, constipation, paralytic ileus, urinary retention, dilation of urinary tract, skin rash, urticaria, photosensitization, edema of face and tongue, bone marrow depression, nausea, epigastric distress, vomiting, anorexia, stomatitis, peculiar taste, diarrhea, parotid swelling, black tongue, hepatitis, testicular swelling and gynecomastia in the male, breast enlargement and galactorrhea in the female, increased or decreased libido, elevation and lowering of blood sugar levels, syndrome of inappropriate antidiuretic hormone secretion, dizziness, weakness, fatigue, headache, weight gain or loss, edema, increased perspiration, urinary frequency, mydriasis, drowsiness, alopecia

PHARMACOKINETICS AND PHARMACODYNAMICS
Onset of action: drug effectiveness may require up to 42 d

Peak plasma levels: 4 h for parent drug (amitriptyline); 10 h for metabolite (nortriptyline)

Plasma half-life: 31–46 h

Bioavailability: about 50% (both parent drug and metabolite)

Metabolism: metabolized in liver; amitriptyline mainly demethylated to nortriptyline; both undergo preferential oxidation at the 10 position; 10-hydroxy metabolites may have some biologic activity; conjugation of hydroxylated metabolites with glucuronic acid extinguishes any remaining biologic activity; metabolism slower in elderly and adolescents

Excretion: inactivation and elimination occur over several days; secreted into hepatobiliary circulation and stomach and reabsorbed; less than 2% excreted in the urine

Protein binding: about 96% plasma protein bound

Hepatic impairment: distribution and metabolism prolonged; accumulation of parent drug and major metabolite

PROLONGED USE
Use > 4 consecutive mo has not been studied, but drug has been available for 30 y with no evidence of long-term toxicity.

(Continued on next page)

AMITRIPTYLINE HYDROCHLORIDE (CONTINUED)

DOSAGE

Adults: *Oral for outpatients*—Start with 25 mg/d and gradually increase to 75 mg/d. Can increase to 150 mg/d. Make increases preferably in late afternoon or at bedtime. A sedative effect may be apparent before the antidepressant effect is noted. An adequate therapeutic effect may take as long as 30 days to develop. Alternatively, initiate therapy with 25 to 50 mg at bedtime. Increase by 25 to 50 mg as necessary to a total of 200 to 300 mg if necessary and tolerated. Total daily dose can be given in a single dose, preferably at bedtime. When patient has satisfactorily improved, reduce dose to lowest effective amount. Continue 3 to 6 months or longer to lessen possibility of relapse. *IM*—Do not administer IV. Initially, 20 to 30 mg four times per day. When used for initial therapy in patients unable or unwilling to take tablets, the tablets should replace the injection as soon as possible.

Elderly: Start with 10 mg/d. Can cause orthostatic hypotension. In elderly patients who cannot tolerate higher doses, 10 mg three times per day with 20 mg at bedtime may be satisfactory.

Child: Not recommended for children younger than 12 years. For adolescents aged 12 to 18 years, 10 mg three times per day may be satisfactory for those who cannot tolerate higher doses.

Impaired renal function: Given in low doses, 10 to 25 mg/d; slowly increase as tolerated (increase 10–25 mg every 3–4 days).

OVERDOSAGE

High doses may cause temporary confusion, disturbed concentration, or transient visual hallucinations. Overdose may cause drowsiness, hypothermia, tachycardia and other arrhythmic abnormalities, evidence of impaired conduction, congestive heart failure, dilated pupils, disorders of ocular motility, convulsions, severe hypotension, stupor, and coma. Other symptoms include agitation, hyperactive reflexes, muscle rigidity, vomiting, hyperpyresia, or any of those listed under Adverse Effects.

All patients suspected of having taken an overdose should be admitted to the hospital as soon as possible. Treatment is symptomatic and supportive. Empty the stomach by emesis followed by gastric lavage on arrival at the hospital. After gastric lavage, activated charcoal can be administered. IV administration of physostigmine salicylate has reportedly reversed the symptoms of overdose. Because physostigmine may be toxic, it is not recommended for routine use. Standard measures should be used to manage circulatory shock and metabolic acidosis. Cardiac arrhythmia may be treated with neostigmine, pyridostigmine, or propranolol. Anticonvulsants can be given to control convulsions. Dialysis is of no value. Because overdose is often deliberate, patients may attempt suicide by other means during the recovery phase.

AVAILABILITY

Tablets—10 mg in 30s, 40s, 50s, 100s, 250s, 1000s, UD 32s, and UD 100s; 25 mg in 15s, 21s, 30s, 60s, 90s, 100s, 250s, 500s, 1000s, UD 32s, and UD 100s; 75 mg in 30s, 36s, 100s, 250s, 500s, 1000s, UD 32s, and UD 100s; 100 mg in 100s, 250s, 500s, 1000s, UD 32s, and UD 100s; 150 mg in 30s, 100s, 250s, 500s, 1000s, and UD 100s
Injection—10 mg/mL in 10-mL vials with and without dextrose and parabens

AMOXAPINE

(Asendin)

Amoxapine is a TCA with a sedative component to its action. The mechanism of clinical action is not well understood, but it is believed that amoxapine reduces the uptake of norepinephrine and serotonin and blocks the response of dopamine receptors to dopamine.

SPECIAL PRECAUTIONS

Tardive dyskinesia, a syndrome of potentially irreversible, involuntary dyskinetic movements, may develop in patients. The risk of developing the syndrome and likelihood that it will become irreversible increase as duration of treatment and total cumulative dose of the drug administered to the patient increase.

A potentially fatal symptom complex sometimes referred to as neuroleptic malignant syndrome has been reported.

Should be used with caution in patients with a history of urinary retention, angle-closure glaucoma, or increased intraocular pressure. Patients with cardiovascular disorders also should be watched closely.

Extreme caution should be used when treating patients with a history of convulsive disorder or those with overt or latent seizure disorders.

In Brief

INDICATIONS

Effective in endogenous and psychotic depressions; outcome in other groups not well studied

CONTRAINDICATIONS

Contraindicated during acute recovery phase following myocardial infarction

INTERACTIONS

Anticholinergics, barbiturates, cimetidine, MAO inhibitors, and other CNS depressants

ADVERSE EFFECTS

Most are rare. Observed in patients taking amoxapine, but causal link not established.

(Continued on next page)

(Continued on next page)

SPECIAL GROUPS

Children: Safety and efficacy in children younger than age 16 years have not been established.

Elderly: In general, lower doses are recommended for these patients. The prevalence of tardive dyskinesia is highest among the elderly, especially elderly women.

Pregnancy: Category C drug. No adequate and well-controlled studies in pregnant women. Amoxapine should be used during pregnancy only if potential benefit justifies potential risk to fetus.

Breast-feeding: Amoxapine is excreted in human breast milk. Because effects of the drug on infants are unknown, caution should be exercised when administered to nursing women.

DOSAGE

Adults: Initially 25 to 50 mg daily. Depending on tolerance, increase dose to 100 mg two times daily by the end of the first week. Increase above 300 mg/d only if 300 mg/d has been ineffective for at least 2 weeks. Once an effective dose is established, the drug can be given in a single bedtime dose (not to exceed 300 mg). If total daily dose exceeds 300 mg, give in divided doses. Adequate trial period is unclear but is probably 4 to 6 weeks. If no response is seen at 300 mg, increase dose to 400 mg/d. Patients refractory to antidepressant therapy and who have no history of convulsive seizures may have dose cautiously increased to 600 mg/d in divided doses. Maintenance dose is lowest dose that will maintain remission. If symptoms reappear, increase dose to the earlier level until they are controlled.

Elderly: Initially, 25 mg daily. If tolerated, dose can be increased to 50 mg two or three times daily at the end of the week. Although 100 to 150 mg/d may be adequate, some may require higher doses; carefully increase up to 300 mg/d.

Children: Not recommended for children younger than age 16 years.

ADVERSE EFFECTS *(CONTINUED)*

Drowsiness, dry mouth, constipation, blurred vision, anxiety, insomnia, restlessness, nervousness, palpitations, tremor, confusion, excitement, nightmares, ataxia, alterations in EEG patterns, edema, skin rash, elevation of prolactin levels, nausea, dizziness, headache, fatigue, weakness, excessive appetite, increased perspiration, anticholinergic symptoms, hypotension, hypertension, syncope, tachycardia, drug fever, urticaria, photosensitization, pruritus, vasculitis, hepatitis, tingling, paresthesias of extremities, tinnitus, disorientation, seizures, hypomania, numbness, loss of coordination, disturbed concentration, hyperthermia, extrapyramidal symptoms (including tardive dyskinesia), neuroleptic malignant syndrome, leukopenia, agranulocytosis, epigastric distress, vomiting, flatulence, abdominal pain, peculiar taste, diarrhea, increased or decreased libido, impotence, menstrual irregularity, breast enlargement and galactorrhea in the female, lacrimation, weight gain or loss, altered liver function, painful ejaculation, paralytic ileus, atrial arrhythmias, myocardial infarction, stroke, heart block, hallucinations, thrombocytopenia, eosinophilia, purpura, petechiae, parotid swelling, change in blood glucose levels, pancreatitis, hepatitis, jaundice, urinary frequency, testicular swelling, anorexia, alopecia

PHARMACOKINETICS AND PHARMACODYNAMICS

Onset of action: not clearly established; a minimum of 1–2 wk
Peak plasma levels: 90 min
Plasma half-life: 8 h for amoxapine; 30 h for major metabolite (8-hydroxy)
Bioavailability: well absorbed from GI tract
Metabolism: relatively little information has been published on the metabolism of this drug; primarily converted in the liver to major active metabolite 8-hydroxyamoxapine but also to active metabolite 7-hydroxyamoxapine
Excretion: excreted in the urine
Effect of food: none anticipated
Protein binding: highly plasma protein bound

OVERDOSAGE

Toxic symptoms of overdose differ significantly from those of other tricyclic antidepressants. CNS effects, particularly grand mal seizures, occur frequently, and treatment should be directed toward prevention or control of seizures. Status epilepticus may develop and constitutes a neurologic emergency. Coma and acidosis are other serious complications. Renal failure may develop 2–5 d after toxic overdose in patients who may appear otherwise recovered. Acute tubular necrosis with rhabdomyolysis and myoglobinuria is the most common renal complication.

Treatment should be symptomatic and supportive, with special attention to prevention of seizures. If the patient is conscious, induced emesis followed by gastric lavage with appropriate precautions to prevent pulmonary aspiration should be accomplished as soon as possible. Following lavage, activated charcoal can be administered. An adequate airway should be established in comatose patients and assisted ventilation instituted if necessary. Seizures may respond to standard anticonvulsant therapy. Convulsions typically begin within 12 h after ingestion. Treatment of renal impairment is the same as that for nondrug-induced renal dysfunction. Serious cardiovascular effects are rare.

PATIENT INFORMATION

Patients should be advised that some patients exposed chronically to this drug will develop tardive dyskinesia.

AVAILABILITY

Tablets—25 mg in 100s; 50 mg in 100s, 500s, and UD 100s; 100 mg in 100s and UD 100s; 150 mg in 30s and 100s

CLOMIPRAMINE HYDROCHLORIDE

(Anafranil)

Clomipramine HCl is a TCA with a high degree of anticholinergic and sedative effects and moderate orthostatic hypotension. Clomipramine is believed to influence obsessive and compulsive behaviors through its effects on serotoninergic neuronal transmission. The actual neurochemical mechanism is unknown, but the drug's capacity to inhibit the reuptake of serotonin is important.

SPECIAL PRECAUTIONS

During premarketing evaluation, seizure was identified as the most significant risk of clomipramine. Caution should be used when administering the drug to patients with a history of seizures or other predisposing factors and concomitant use with other drugs that lower the seizure threshold. Fatalities in association with seizures have been reported by foreign postmarketing surveillance but not in United States clinical trials.

Modest orthostatic decreases in blood pressure and modest tachycardia were seen in about 20% of patients taking clomipramine in clinical trials. Caution is necessary when treating patients with cardiovascular disease, and gradual dose titration is recommended.

Postmarketing reports have shown leukopenia, agranulocytosis, thrombocytopenia, anemia, and pancytopenia in association with clomipramine use. Leukocyte and differential blood counts should be obtained in patients who develop fever and sore throat during treatment.

Before elective surgery with general anesthetics, clomipramine therapy should be discontinued for as long as clinically feasible, and the anesthetist should be informed of when therapy ceased.

Clomipramine should be used with caution in patients with increased intraocular pressure, history of narrow-angle glaucoma, or urinary retention (because of anticholinergic properties of the drug).

Many withdrawal symptoms have been reported in association with abrupt discontinuation of this drug. Although the withdrawal effects have not been systematically evaluated in controlled trials, it is recommended that the dose be tapered gradually and the patient monitored carefully during discontinuation.

(Continued on next page)

In Brief

INDICATIONS

Treatment of obsessions and compulsions in patients with obsessive-compulsive disorder that causes distress, is time consuming, or significantly interfere with social or occupational functioning

CONTRAINDICATIONS

Heart disease with left bundle branch block

INTERACTIONS

The risks of using clomipramine in combination with other drugs have not been systematically evaluated. Given the primary CNS effects of the drug, caution is advised when using it concomitantly with other CNS-active drugs. Clomipramine should not be used with MAO inhibitors.

ADVERSE EFFECTS

Most are rare. Observed in patients taking clomipramine, but causal link not always clearly established. Somnolence, nausea and vomiting, general edema, increased susceptibility to infection, malaise, dependent edema, withdrawal syndrome, abnormal ECG, arrhythmia, bradycardia, cardiac arrest, extrasystoles, pallor, aneurysm, atrial flutter, bundle branch block, cardiac failure, cerebral hemorrhage, heart block, myocardial infarction, myocardial ischemia, peripheral ischemia, thrombophlebitis, vasospasm, ventricular tachycardia, abnormal hepatic function, blood in stool, colitis, duodenitis, gastric ulcer gastritis, gastroesophageal reflux, gingivitis, glossitis, hemorrhoids, hepatitis, increased saliva, irritable bowel syndrome, peptic ulcer, rectal hemorrhage, tongue ulceration, tooth caries, cheilitis, chronic enteritis, discolored feces, gastric dilation, gingival bleeding, hiccups, intestinal obstruction, oral or pharyngeal edema, paralytic ileus, salivary gland enlargement, hypothyroidism, goiter, gynecomastia, hyperthyroidism, lymphadenopathy, leukemoid reaction, lymphoma-like disorder, bone marrow depression, dehydration, diabetes mellitus, gout, hypercholesterolemia, hyperglycemia, hyperuricemia, hypokalemia, fat intolerance, glycosuria, arthrosis, dystonia, exostosis, lupus erythematosus rash, bruising, myopathy, myositis, polyarteritis nodosa, torticollis, abnormal thinking, vertigo, abnormal coordination, abnormal EEG, abnormal gait, apathy, ataxia, coma, convulsions, delirium, delusions, dyskinesia, dysphonia, encephalopathy, euphoria, extrapyramidal disorder, hallucinations, hostility, hyperkinesia, hypokinesia, leg cramps, manic reaction, neuralgia, paranoia, phobic disorder, psychosis, suicidal ideation, suicide attempt, suicide, bronchitis, hyperventilation, increased sputum, pneumonia, alopecia, cellulitis, erythematous rash, genital pruritus, abnormal accommodation, deafness, diplopia, earache, eye pain, foreign body sensation, taste loss, endometriosis, hematuria, nocturia, oliguria, perineal pain, polyuria, renal calculus, renal pain, urethral disorder, urinary incontinence, uterine hemorrhage, vaginal hemorrhage, breast engorgement, premature ejaculation

PHARMACOKINETICS AND PHARMACODYNAMICS

Onset of action: 3–4 wk

Peak plasma levels: no pharmacokinetic information for doses ranging from 150–250 mg/d, the maximum recommended daily dose; after single 50-mg dose, peak levels occur within 2–6 h (mean, 4.7 h)

Plasma half-life: after 150-mg dose, half-life ranges from 19–37 h (mean, 32 h) for parent drug and 54–77 h (mean, 69 h) for major metabolite

Bioavailability: no data available; clomipramine distributes into cerebrospinal fluid and brain and into breast milk; major metabolite also distributes into cerebrospinal fluid

(Continued on next page)

SPECIAL GROUPS

Children: Safety and efficacy for use in children younger than 10 years have not been established.

Elderly: Clomipramine has not been systematically studied in older patients; however, 152 patients at least 60 years old participating in United States clinical trials received the drug for several months to several years. No unusual age-related adverse events have been identified in this population, but these data are insufficient to rule out possible age-related differences, particularly in elderly patients who have concomitant systemic illnesses or who are receiving other drugs concomitantly.

Renal impairment: Use with caution in patients with significantly impaired renal function.

Hepatic impairment: Extreme caution is indicated when treating patients with known liver disease, and periodic monitoring of hepatic enzyme levels is recommended in such patients.

Pregnancy: Category C drug. No adequate and well-controlled studies in pregnant women. Withdrawal symptoms, including jitters, tremor, and seizures, have been reported in neonates whose mothers had taken clomipramine until delivery. Use during pregnancy only if the potential benefit justifies potential risk to fetus.

Breast-feeding: Clomipramine has been found in human breast milk. Because of the potential for adverse reactions, a decision should be made whether to discontinue nursing or discontinue the drug, taking into account the importance of the drug to the mother.

DOSAGE

Adults: *Initial*—Initiate at 25 mg daily and gradually increase as tolerated to about 100 mg during the first 2 weeks. Administer in divided doses with meals to reduce GI side effects. Dose can be increased gradually over following weeks to a maximum of 250 mg/d. After titration, total daily dose can be given once at bedtime to minimize daytime sedation. *Maintenance*—Adjust dose to maintain patient on lowest effective dose, and periodically reassess patient to determine need for treatment.

Elderly: Same as adult dosage; monitor carefully.

Children: Not recommended for children younger than 10 years. For children older than 10 years and for adolescents, initiate at 25 mg daily and gradually increase during the first 2 weeks as tolerated to daily maximum of 3 mg/kg or 100 mg, whichever is smaller. Administer in divided doses with meals. Thereafter, the dose can be increased to a daily maximum of 3 mg/kg or 200 mg, whichever is smaller. After titration, total daily dose can be given once at bedtime to minimize daytime sedation. *See* Adult section for instructions on maintenance.

Renal impairment: Use continuously.

PHARMACOKINETICS AND PHARMACODYNAMICS
(CONTINUED)

Metabolism: extensively biotransformed in the liver into major active metabolite, desmethylclomipramine (DMI) and other metabolites and their glucuronide conjugates; DMI is pharmacologically active, but its effects on obsessive-compulsive disorder behaviors are unknown; clomipramine does not induce drug-metabolizing enzymes

Excretion: metabolites excreted in urine and feces following biliary elimination; combined urinary recoveries of clomipramine and DMI only about 0.8%–1% of administered dose

Effect of food: not significantly affected by food

Protein binding: about 97% protein bound, primarily to albumin, and independent of clomipramine concentration; interaction between clomipramine and other highly protein-bound drugs not fully evaluated but may be important

Renal impairment: effects of renal impairment on kinetic disposition of the drug not determined

Hepatic impairment: effects of hepatic impairment on kinetic disposition of the drug not determined

PROLONGED USE

Effectiveness for long-term use (*ie*, > 10 wk) has not been systematically evaluated; physician who elects to use for extended periods should periodically reevaluate long-term usefulness of the drug for individual patient.

OVERDOSAGE

In United States clinical trials, two deaths occurred in 12 reported cases of acute overdose with clomipramine either alone or in combination with other drugs. One death involved a patient suspected of ingesting 7000 mg; the other death involved a patient suspected of ingesting 5750 mg. The 10 nonfatal cases involved doses up to 5000 mg.

Symptoms vary depending on amount of drug absorbed, age of patient, and time elapsed since drug ingestion. First symptoms generally are severe anticholinergic reactions. CNS abnormalities include drowsiness, stupor, coma, ataxia, restlessness, agitation, delirium, severe perspiration, hyperactive reflexes, muscle rigidity, athetoid and choreiform movements, and convulsions. Cardiac abnormalities may include arrhythmia, tachycardia, ECG evidence of impaired conduction, signs of congestive heart failure, and in rare cases, cardiac arrest. Respiratory depression, cyanosis, hypotension, shock, vomiting, hyperpyrexia, mydriasis, oliguria or anuria, and diaphoresis may be present.

Because the recommended treatment for overdoses may change periodically, the physician should contact a Poison Control Center for current information on treatment.

PATIENT INFORMATION

Patients should be advised about the risk of seizure associated with this drug.

AVAILABILITY

Tablets—25, 50, and 75 mg in 100s and UD 100s

DESIPRAMINE HYDROCHLORIDE

(Norpramin, Pertofrane)

Desipramine HCl is a TCA thought to mediate its antidepressant effects by blocking the neuronal reuptake of serotonin and norepinephine. It may have greater activity in blocking norepinephrine reuptake.

SPECIAL PRECAUTIONS

Extreme caution should be used when this drug is given to patients with cardiovascular disease because of the possibility of conduction defects, arrhythmias, tachycardias, strokes, and acute myocardial infarction; patients with a history of urinary retention or glaucoma, because of the anticholinergic properties of the drug; patients with thyroid disease or those taking thyroid medication; and patients with a history of seizure disorder.

Desipramine is capable of blocking the antihypertensive effect of guanethidine and similarly acting compounds.

Close supervision and careful adjustment of dose are required when this drug is given concomitantly with anticholinergic or sympathomimetic drugs.

Concurrent administration of cimetidine psychostimulants or phenothiazines with desipramine can produce clinically significant increases in the plasma levels of the drug.

Concurrent use of barbiturates, alcohol, and tobacco reduces desipramine plasma levels.

Desipramine should be discontinued as soon as possible before elective surgery because of the possible cardiovascular effects.

Elevation and depression of blood sugar levels have been reported.

Leukocyte and differential counts should be performed in any patient who develops fever and sore throat during therapy; the drug should be discontinued if there is evidence of pathologic neutrophil depression.

SPECIAL GROUPS

Children: Safety and efficacy for use in children have not been established; use in adolescents only. Lower doses are recommended for adolescents.
Elderly: In general, lower doses are administered to older patients. The elderly are more susceptible to states of confusion when given this drug.
Pregnancy: Category C drug. Animal reproductive studies have been inconclusive. Safe use during pregnancy has not been established; therefore, if it is to be given to pregnant patients or women of childbearing age, possible benefits of drug must be weighed against possible hazards to mother and child.
Breast-feeding: Safe use in lactating women has not been established; weigh potential benefits of therapy against possible hazards to mother and child.

In Brief

INDICATIONS
Treatment of depression

CONTRAINDICATIONS
Contraindicated in patients during acute recovery period following myocardial infarction; concurrent use or use within 2 weeks of an MAO inhibitor

INTERACTIONS
Alcohol, barbiturates, cimetidine, MAO inhibitors, phenothiazines, psychostimulants, tobacco smoke, drugs metabolized by $P_{450}IID_6$

ADVERSE EFFECTS
Most are rare. Observed in patients taking TCAs including desipramine, but causal link not always established. Hypotension, hypertension, palpitations, heart block, myocardial infarction, stroke, arrhythmias, premature ventricular contractions, tachycardia, ventricular tachycardia, ventricular fibrillation, sudden death, confusional states (especially in the elderly) with hallucinations, disorientation, delusions, anxiety, restlessness, agitation, insomnia and nightmares, hypomania, exacerbation of psychosis, numbness, tingling, paresthesias of extremities, incoordination, ataxia, tremors, peripheral neuropathy, extrapyramidal symptoms, seizures, alteration in EEG patterns, tinnitus, dry mouth, blurred vision, disturbance of accommodation, mydriasis, increased intraocular pressure, constipation, paralytic ileus, urinary retention, delayed micturition, dilation of urinary tract, drug fever, petechiae, itching, skin rash, urticaria, photosensitization, bone marrow depression, anorexia, nausea and vomiting, peculiar taste, altered liver function, gynecomastia in the male, breast enlargement, and galactorrhea in the female, increased or decreased libido, impotence, painful ejaculation, elevation or depression of blood sugar levels, weight gain or loss, perspiration, flushing, urinary frequency, nocturia, drowsiness, dizziness, weakness and fatigue, headache, fever, alopecia, elevated alkaline phosphatase

PHARMACOKINETICS AND PHARMACODYNAMICS
Onset of action: at the earliest, 2–5 d; usually 2–3 wk
Bioavailability: rapidly absorbed from GI tract
Metabolism: metabolized in the liver; rate of metabolism varies widely from individual to individual; in general, elderly metabolize drug more slowly
Excretion: parent drug and metabolites excreted through gastric mucosa; reabsorbed from the GI; 70% is excreted in urine
Protein binding: 82% plasma protein bound
Renal impairment: amount bound to plasma proteins altered in patients with uremia

PROLONGED USE
Use beyond 4 consecutive mo is not recommended; however, if physician elects to do so, patient should undergo periodic physical examination once per year. Anecdotal observation suggests drug is safe over long periods.

(Continued on next page)

DOSAGE

Adults: Initial therapy can be given in divided doses or as single daily dose. Maintenance therapy can be given once daily. Usual adult dose is 100 to 200 mg/d. In more severely ill patients, dose may be gradually increased to 300 mg/d. Dosage should be administered at a lower level and titrated according to tolerance and clinical response.

Elderly: 25 to 100 mg/d. Doses higher than 150 mg are not recommended.

Children: Not recommended for children younger than 12 years. For adolescents aged 12 to 18 years, give 25 to 100 mg/d. Doses higher than 150 mg/d are not recommended.

OVERDOSAGE

Symptoms most often involved the cardiovascular system and CNS, including cardiac dysrhythmias, severe hypotension, convulsions, CNS depression, and changes in the ECG, particularly in QRS axis or width. Other signs include confusion, disturbed concentration, transient visual hallucinations, dilated pupils, agitation, hyperactive reflexes, stupor, drowsiness, muscle rigidity, vomiting, hypothermia, and hyperpyrexia.

There is no specific antidote for desipramine overdose. Because CNS involvement, respiratory depression, and cardiac arrhythmia can occur suddenly, hospitalization and close observation are generally advisable, even when the amount ingested is believed to be small or the initial degree of intoxication appears slight or moderate. Aggressive supportive therapy of cardiac, neurologic, or acid–base disturbance may be necessary. Forced diuresis, peritoneal dialysis, exchange transfusions, and hemodialysis are ineffective. Additional information regarding treatment of overdose is available from poison control centers.

AVAILABILITY

Tablets—10 mg in 100s and 1000s; 25, 50, and 75 mg in 30s, 100s, 500s, 1000s, and UD 100s; 100 mg in 100s and 500s; 150 mg in 50s and 100s

Capsules—25 and 50 mg in 100s

DOXEPIN HYDROCHLORIDE

(Adapin, Sinequan)

Doxepin HCl is in a class of psychotherapeutic agents known as dibenzoxepine TCAs. Chemically, doxepin is a dibenzoxepin derivative and is the first of a family of TCAs. The drug has antianxiety, anticholinergic, antiserotonin, sedative, antihistaminic, and hypotensive properties.

SPECIAL PRECAUTIONS

The once-a-day dose regimen for this drug in patients with concurrent illness or patients taking other medications should be adjusted carefully, especially if the other drugs have anticholinergic effects.

Withdrawal symptoms may develop on abrupt cessation of treatment after prolonged doxepin administration; these symptoms do not indicate addiction, and gradual withdrawal of medication should not cause these symptoms.

The once-a-day dose strength is intended for maintenance therapy only and is not recommended for initiation of treatment.

In Brief

INDICATIONS

Depression associated with alcoholism (not to be taken concomitantly with alcohol); depression associated with organic disease (possibility of drug interaction should be considered if patient is receiving other drugs concomitantly); psychotic depressive disorders associated with involutional depression and manic-depressive disorders

CONTRAINDICATIONS

Glaucoma or tendency for urinary retention

INTERACTIONS

Alcohol, anticholinergics, barbiturates, charcoal, cimetidine, clonidine, dicumarol, disulfiram, fluoxetine, guanethidine, haloperidol, levodopa, MAO inhibitors, phenothiazines, smoking

ADVERSE EFFECTS

Most are rare. Observed in patients taking doxepin, but causal link not always established. Dry mouth, blurred vision, constipation, urinary retention, drowsiness, confusion, disorientation, hallucinations, numbness, paresthesias, ataxia, extrapyramidal symptoms, seizures, hypotension, tachycardia (occasionally), skin rash, edema, photosensitization, pruritus, eosinophilia, agranulocytosis, leukopenia, thrombocytopenia, purpura, nausea, vomiting, indigestion, taste disturbances, diarrhea, anorexia, aphthous stomatitis, increased or decreased libido, testicular swelling, gynecomastia in males, enlargement of breasts and galactorrhea in females, increased or decreased blood sugar levels, inappropriate antidiuretic hormone secretion, dizziness, tinnitus, weight gain, sweating, chills, fatigue, weakness, flushing, jaundice, alopecia, headache

(Continued on next page)

DOXEPIN HYDROCHLORIDE
(CONTINUED)

SPECIAL GROUPS

Children: Because of a lack of clinical experience in children, doxepin is not recommended for use in children younger than 12 years.

Elderly: Clinical experience has shown that doxepin is safe and well tolerated in elderly patients; patients on the once-a-day dose regimen should be carefully observed.

Renal impairment: Use caution in patients with significant impaired renal function.

Hepatic impairment: Metabolism may be impaired, and drug accumulation may occur in patients with hepatic disease.

Pregnancy: Category C drug. Because there is no experience in pregnant women who have received this drug, safety in pregnancy has not been established.

Breast-feeding: Few data are available; however, apnea and drowsiness may occur in nursing infants whose mothers are taking doxepin.

DOSAGE

Adults: Total daily dose can be given on a divided or once-a-day dose. If the once-a-day capsule schedule is used, the maximum recommended dose is 150 mg/d. If the oral concentrate is used, dilute with 120 mL of liquid (eg, water, milk, and some fruit juices) just before administration. Do not mix with grape juice; some carbonated beverages are not compatible with concentrate. For patients on methadone maintenance, mix the concentrate with methadone and lemonade, orange juice, water, sugar water, or powdered fruit drink. *Depression*—Initially, 25 mg/d. Individualize dose. Usual optimum dose is 75 to 150 mg/d. Alternatively, total daily dose up to 150 mg can be given at bedtime. If necessary, gradually increase to 300 mg/d. Additional effectiveness is rarely obtained by exceeding 300 mg/d.

Elderly: Same as adult dosage.

Children: Not recommended for children younger than 12 years. For adolescents aged 12 to 18 years, same as adult dosage.

PHARMACOKINETICS AND PHARMACODYNAMICS

Onset of action: about 3–4 wk for antidepressant effect

Peak plasma levels: association between plasma levels and therapeutic effect has not been adequately defined

Plasma half-life: 8–24 h for parent drug and active metabolite desmethyldoxepin (nordoxepin)

Bioavailability: 27% ± 10%, assuming complete absorption, elimination only by liver, hepatic blood flow of 1500 mg/min, and equal partition between plasma and erythrocytes

Metabolism: metabolized in the liver to active metabolite, nordoxepin, by N-demethylation

Excretion: partially secreted into hepatobiliary circulation and stomach and reabsorbed and excreted in urine over several days

Effect of food: food does not alter absorption or bioavailability

Protein binding: strongly bound to plasma proteins

OVERDOSAGE

Symptoms of mild overdose include drowsiness, stupor, blurred vision, and excessive dryness of the mouth. Symptoms of severe overdose include respiratory depression, hypotension, coma, convulsions, cardiac arrhythmia, and cardiac tachycardia. In addition, urinary retention (bladder atony), decreased GI motility (paralytic ileus), hyperthermia or hypothermia, hypertension, dilated pupils, and hyperactive reflexes may be present.

For mild overdose, observation and supportive therapy are usually necessary. For severe overdose, medical management consists of aggressive supportive therapy. If the patient is conscious, gastric lavage with appropriate precautions to prevent pulmonary aspiration should be performed, although doxepin is rapidly absorbed. Use of activated charcoal has been recommended, as has been continuous gastric lavage with saline for ≥ 24 h. An adequate airway should be established in comatose patients and assisted ventilation used if necessary. ECG monitoring may be required for several days because relapse after apparent recovery has been reported. Arrhythmia should be treated with appropriate antiarrhythmic agents. Many cardiovascular and CNS symptoms can be reversed by slow IV administration of 1–3 mg of physostigmine salicylate. Because physostigmine is rapidly metabolized, the dose should be repeated as required. Convulsions may respond to standard anticonvulsant therapy; however, barbiturates may potentiate any respiratory depression. Dialysis and forced diuresis generally are not of value because of high tissue and protein binding of doxepin.

PATIENT INFORMATION

Patients should be advised of the typical delay in response to drug action and encouraged to stay on the treatment regimen. Patients should be advised to stay out of the sun and to wear protective clothing and sunglasses.

AVAILABILITY

Capsules—10 mg in 100s, 500s, 1000s, and UD 100s; 25 mg in 30, 50s, 100s, 360s, 500s, 1000s, and UD 100s; 50 mg in 30s, 100s, 360s, 500s, 1000s, and UD 100s; 75 mg in 30s, 100s, 500s, 1000s, and UD 100s; 100 mg in 100s, 500s, 1000s, and UD 100s; and 150 mg in 50s, 100s, 500s, and UD 100s

Oral concentrate—10 mg/mL in 120 mL

IMIPRAMINE HYDROCHLORIDE

(Tofranil)

Imipramine HCl is the original TCA. Its mechanism of action is not definitely known. The clinical effect is hypothesized as being the result of potentiation of adrenergic synapses by blocking uptake of norepinephrine at nerve endings. Imipramine has a similar effect on the serotonin system.

SPECIAL PRECAUTIONS

Caution should be used when this drug is given to patients with cardiovascular conduction defects or those with a history of urinary retention, glaucoma, or seizure disorder.

It is capable of blocking the antihypertensive effect of guanethidine and similarly acting compounds.

An ECG recording should be taken before initiation of larger-than-usual doses and at appropriate intervals thereafter until steady state is achieved.

If patient is suicidal, prescriptions should be written in the smallest amount feasible; close supervision and careful adjustment of dose are required when drug is administered concomitantly with anticholinergic drugs

Caution should be exercised when used with agents that lower blood pressure.

The drug should be discontinued before elective surgery; notify the anesthetist as to when the final dose was taken.

Patients taking the drug should avoid excessive exposure to sunlight because there have been reports of photosensitization.

SPECIAL GROUPS

Children: Safety and efficacy for use as antidepressant in children have not been established. Recommended use is only in adolescents.

Elderly: Elderly patients, especially if they have a history of cardiac disease, are at special risk of developing the cardiac abnormalities associated with use of imipramine. Also, elderly patients are more susceptible to states of confusion when taking this drug.

Renal impairment: Caution should be used in patients with significantly impaired renal function.

Hepatic impairment: Caution should be used in patients with significantly impaired hepatic function.

Pregnancy: Category B drug. No well-controlled studies have been conducted in pregnant women to determine the effect of imipramine on the fetus. There have, however, been clinical reports of congenital malformations associated with use of the drug. Use in pregnant women and women of childbearing age only if the clinical condition clearly justifies the risk to the fetus.

Breast-feeding: Limited data suggest that imipramine is likely to be excreted in human breast milk. Women taking the drug should not nurse because the drug may be excreted in breast milk and may be harmful to the infant.

DOSAGE

Adults: Use parenteral administration for starting therapy only in patients unable or unwilling to use oral medication. Do not administer IV. Initially, up to 100 mg/d IM in divided doses. Oral form should replace parenteral as soon as possible. Dose should be started at 25 to 50 mg and gradually increased until therapeutic effect or 300 mg/d is reached. Can be given in one dose at bedtime.

(Continued on next page)

In Brief

INDICATIONS
Relief of symptoms of depression (endogenous depression is more likely to be alleviated than are other depressive states)

CONTRAINDICATIONS
During the acute recovery period after myocardial infarction

INTERACTIONS
Alcohol, barbiturates and other CNS depressants, hepatic enzyme inhibitors, MAO inhibitors
Drug/laboratory test interactions: Increased metanephrine (Pisano test); decreased urinary 5-HIAA

ADVERSE EFFECTS
Most are rare. Observed in patients taking imipramine but causal link not established. Orthostatic hypotension, hypertension, tachycardia, palpitations, myocardial infarction, arrhythmias, heart block, ECG changes, precipitation of congestive heart failure, stroke, confusional states (especially in elderly), delusions, anxiety, agitation, insomnia and nightmares, exacerbation of psychosis, numbness, tingling, incoordination, ataxia, tremors, extrapyramidal symptoms, tinnitus, seizures, dry mouth, blurred vision, mydriasis, constipation, paralytic ileus, urinary retention, delayed micturition, dilation of urinary tract, petechiae, urticaria, photosensitization, edema, drug fever, marrow depression, nausea, vomiting, anorexia, diarrhea, peculiar taste, black tongue, impotence, testicular swelling, gynecomastia in the male, breast enlargement in the female, jaundice, altered liver function, perspiration, flushing, urinary frequency, drowsiness, dizziness, weakness and fatigue, headache, parotid swelling, alopecia, proneness to falling

PHARMACOKINETICS AND PHARMACODYNAMICS
Onset of action: about 2 wk (sometimes longer)
Peak plasma levels: about 2–8 h, but it may be as long as 12 h
Plasma half-life: 11–25 h (mean, 18 h) for parent drug; about 22 h for major metabolite (desipramine)
Bioavailability: about 40% (both parent drug and major metabolite)
Metabolism: metabolized in the liver; major route is to active product desipramine; biotransformation of either compound occurs largely by oxidation to 2-hydroxy metabolites; unknown to what extent the demethylated metabolites of imipramine have antidepressant activity
Excretion: excreted in urine; less than 2% unchanged drug
Protein binding: more than 90% plasma protein bound
Renal impairment: amount of major active metabolite bound to plasma protein is altered with uremia

PROLONGED USE
Not systemically studied; it appears safe after 30 years of use.

OVERDOSAGE
Symptoms vary according to the amount of drug absorbed, age of patient, and interval between drug ingestion and start of treatment. CNS abnormalities include drowsiness, stupor, coma, ataxia, restlessness, agitation, hyperactive reflexes, muscle rigidity, athetoid and choreiform movements, and convulsions. Cardiac abnormalities include arrhythmia, tachycardia, ECG evidence of impaired conduction, and signs of congestive heart failure. Respiratory depression, cyanosis, hypotension, shock, vomiting, hyperpyrexia, mydriasis, and diaphoresis also may be present.
The recommended treatment for overdose may change periodically. It is recommended that the physician contact a poison control center for current information on treatment.

IMIPRAMINE HYDROCHLORIDE
(CONTINUED)

DOSAGE (CONTINUED)
Elderly: Initially, 30 to 40 mg/d orally; generally it is not necessary to exceed 100 mg/d.
Children: Not recommended for children younger than 12 years. For adolescents aged 12 to 18, initially 30 to 40 mg/d orally; generally, it is not necessary to exceed 100 mg/d.

AVAILABILITY
Tablets—10 mg in 30s, 100s, 1000s, and UD 100s; 25 mg in 30s, 40s, 50, 60s, 100s, 1000s, UD 32s, UD 100s, and Gy-Pak 100s; 50 mg in 30s, 40s, 50s, 60s, 90s, 100s, 1000s, UD 100s, and Gy-Pak 100s
Injection—25 mg/mL in 2-mL amps with ascorbic acid, sodium bisulfite, and anhydrous sodium sulfite

NORTRIPTYLINE HYDROCHLORIDE
(Pamelor Aventyl)

Nortriptyline HCl is a TCA that has moderate anticholinergic and sedative effects but slight orthostatic hypotensive effects.

SPECIAL PRECAUTIONS
Patients with cardiovascular disease should be given nortriptyline only under close supervision because the drug may produce sinus tachycardia and prolong the conduction time. Myocardial infarction, arrhythmia, and strokes have occurred. In addition, the antihypertensive action of guanethidine and similar agents may be blocked. Because of its anticholinergic activity, nortriptyline should be used with great caution in patients who have glaucoma or a history of urinary retention.

Patients with a history of seizures should be followed closely when nortriptyline is administered because this drug lowers the convulsive threshold.

Close supervision and careful adjustment of the dose are required when nortriptyline is used with other anticholinergic drugs and sympathomimetic drugs.

Concurrent administration of cimetidine and nortriptyline can produce significant increases in plasma concentration of nortriptyline.

In Brief

INDICATIONS
Relief of symptoms of depression; endogenous depression is more likely to be alleviated than are other depressive states

CONTRAINDICATIONS
During recovery period following myocardial infarction

INTERACTIONS
Anticholinergic drugs, cimetidine, MAO inhibitors, reserpine, sympathomimetic drugs

ADVERSE EFFECTS
Most are rare. Observed in patients taking nortriptyline, but causal link has not been established. Hypotension, hypertension, tachycardia, palpitation, myocardial infarction, arrhythmias, heart block, stroke, confusional states, disorientation, delusions, anxiety, restlessness, agitation, insomnia, panic, nightmares, hypomania, exacerbation of psychosis, numbness, tingling, paresthesias of extremities, incoordination, ataxia, tremors, peripheral neuropathy, extrapyramidal symptoms, seizures, tinnitus, dry mouth, blurred vision, constipation, urinary retention, dilation of urinary tract, skin rash, urticaria, photosensitization, edema, bone marrow depression, nausea and vomiting, anorexia, diarrhea, stomatitis, abdominal cramps, black tongue, gynecomastia in the male, breast enlargement and galactorrhea in the female, increased or decreased libido, testicular swelling, elevation or depression of blood sugar levels, jaundice, altered liver function, weight gain or loss, perspiration, flushing, urinary frequency, nocturia, drowsiness, dizziness, weakness, fatigue, headache, parotid swelling, alopecia

PHARMACOKINETICS AND PHARMACODYNAMICS
Plasma half-life: 18–44 h
Bioavailability: about 50%
Metabolism: metabolized in the liver; undergoes preferential oxidation at the 10 position; the 10-hydroxy metabolites may have some biologic activity; conjugation of hydroxylated metabolites with glucuronic acid extinguishes any remaining biologic activity
Excretion: about 1%–3% of dose excreted in urine
Protein binding: about 92%; increases in presence of hyperlipoproteinemia
Renal impairment: prolonged half-life and lower clearance in presence of uremia

PROLONGED USE
Anecdotal information suggests that it is safe long term.

(Continued on next page)

SPECIAL GROUPS

Children: Safety and efficacy for use in children have not been established. Use only in adolescents.

Elderly: Generally, lower doses are recommended for the elderly. Elderly patients are more susceptible to confusion when given this drug.

Pregnancy: Safe use during pregnancy has not been established; use only if clearly needed. Animal reproduction studies have yielded inconclusive results.

Breast-feeding: Safe use during lactation has not been established. Administer to nursing mothers only if potential benefits justify potential hazards to fetus.

DOSAGE

Adults: Usual dose is 25 mg three or four times daily. Begin at a low level and increase as required. Doses of 150 to 200 mg/d may be required. May be given in a single dose at bedtime.

Elderly: Administer 30 to 50 mg daily in divided doses.

Children: Not recommended for children. For adolescents, administer 30 to 50 mg daily in divided doses.

OVERDOSAGE

Toxic overdose may result in confusion, restlessness, agitation, vomiting, hyperpyrexia, muscle rigidity, hyperactive reflexes, tachycardia, ECG evidence of impaired conduction, shock, congestive heart failure, stupor, coma, and CNS stimulation with convulsions followed by respiratory depression. Deaths have occurred.

No antidote is known. General supportive measures are indicated, with gastric lavage. Respiratory assistance is apparently the most effective measure when indicated. Use of CNS depressants may worsen the prognosis. Administration of barbiturates for control of convulsions alleviates an increase in cardiac workload but should be undertaken with caution to avoid potentiation of respiratory depression. Use of digitalis or physostigmine can be considered in case of serious cardiovascular abnormalities or cardiac failure. Value of dialysis has not been established.

PATIENT INFORMATION

Patients should be advised to wear protective clothing when exposed to sunlight.

AVAILABILITY

Capsules—10 and 25 mg in 100s, 500s, and UD 100s; 50 mg in 100s and UD 100s; 75 mg in 100s

Solution—10 mg/5 mL in pint with and without 4% alcohol and sorbitol

PROTRIPTYLINE HYDROCHLORIDE

(Vivactil)

Protriptyline HCl is a TCA with significant anticholinergic effects but low sedative and orthostatic hypotensive effects.

SPECIAL PRECAUTIONS

Protriptyline should be used with caution in patients with a history of seizures and, because of its autonomic activity, patients with a tendency toward urinary retention or increased intraocular tension.

Tachycardia and postural hypotension may occur more frequently with protriptyline than with other antidepressant drugs. The drug should be used with caution in patients with cardiovascular disorders; such patients should be observed closely because the drug may produce tachycardia, hypotension, arrhythmias, and prolonged conduction time. Myocardial infarction and stroke have occurred.

Hyperpyrexia has been reported when it is administered with anticholinergic agents or neuroleptic drugs, particularly during hot weather.

Protriptyline should be discontinued several days before elective surgery, if possible.

In Brief

INDICATIONS

Treatment of symptoms of mental depression in patients who are under close medical supervision

CONTRAINDICATIONS

During acute recovery following myocardial infarction

INTERACTIONS

Anticholinergic agents, barbiturates, cimetidine, MAO inhibitors

ADVERSE EFFECTS

Most are infrequent. Have been observed in patients taking tricyclics, but causal link has not been established.

Myocardial infarction, stroke, heart block, arrhythmias, hypotension (particularly orthostatic hypotension), hypertension, tachycardia, palpitation, confusional states with hallucinations, delusions, anxiety, agitation, hypomania, exacerbation of psychosis, insomnia, panic, nightmares, seizures, ataxia, tremor, numbness, paresthesias of extremities, extrapyramidal symptoms, drowsiness, dizziness, weakness and fatigue, headache, syndrome of inappropriate antidiuretic hormone secretion, tinnitus, alteration in EEG patterns, urinary retention, delayed micturition, dilation or urinary tract, constipation, blurred vision, mydriasis, dry mouth, drug fever, petechiae, skin rash, urticaria, photosensitization, edema, agranulocytosis, bone marrow depression, leukopenia, thrombocytopenia, purpura, eosinophilia, nausea and vomiting, anorexia, epigastric distress, diarrhea, stomatitis, abdominal cramps, black tongue, impotence, increased or decreased libido, jaundice, parotid swelling, nocturia, urinary frequency, perspiration

(Continued on next page)

PROTRIPTYLINE HYDROCHLORIDE (CONTINUED)

SPECIAL GROUPS
Children: Safety and efficacy for use in children have not been established. Use in adolescents only.
Elderly: Because the elderly are more likely to have cardiac impairment, generally lower doses of protriptyline are administered. The elderly seem more susceptible to states of confusion when given this drug.
Pregnancy: Safe use during pregnancy has not been established.
Breast-feeding: Safe use during lactation has not been established; use in nursing mothers requires that possible benefits be weighed against possible hazards to the infant.

DOSAGE
Adults: Administer 15 to 40 mg/d in three or four doses. Can increase to 60 mg/d. Any increases should be made in the morning dose. Doses higher than 60 mg/d are not recommended.
Elderly: Initially, 5 mg three times per day. Increase gradually, if necessary. Monitor the cardiovascular system closely if dose exceeds 20 mg/d.
Children: Not recommended for children. In adolescents, initially, 5 mg three times per day. Increase gradually if necessary.

PHARMACOKINETICS AND PHARMACODYNAMICS
Onset of action: not clearly established; approximately 26 wk
Plasma half-life: 67–89 h
Bioavailability: about 14%
Metabolism: oxidized by hepatic microsomal enzymes followed by conjugation with glucuronic acid
Excretion: partially secreted into the hepatobiliary circulation and stomach and then resorbed; minimal excretion in urine
Protein binding: 92%–98% plasma protein bound

PROLONGED USE
Like the other tricyclics, which have been available for more than 30 years, anecdotal observation suggests that they are safe long term.

OVERDOSAGE
High doses may cause temporary confusion, disturbed concentration, or transient visual hallucinations. Overdose may cause drowsiness, hypothermia, tachycardia, and other arrhythmic abnormalities. Other symptoms include ECG evidence of impaired conduction, congestive heart failure, convulsions, severe hypotension, stupor, and coma.
Agitation, hyperactive reflexes, muscle rigidity, vomiting, hyperpyrexia, and any symptoms listed under Adverse Effects.
Experience in the management of overdose with protriptyline is limited. Dialysis is of no value because of low plasma concentrations of the drug. Close monitoring of cardiac function for not fewer than 5 d is advisable. Because overdose is often deliberate, patients may attempt suicide by other means during the recovery phase. Deaths by deliberate or accidental overdose have occurred.

PATIENT INFORMATION
Patients should be advised to wear protective clothing when exposed to sunlight.

AVAILABILITY
Tablets—5 mg in 100s; 10 mg in 100s and UD 100s

TRIMIPRAMINE MALEATE

(Surmontil)

Trimipramine maleate is a TCA that causes moderate anticholinergic and orthostatic hypotensive effects and significant sedative effects.

SPECIAL PRECAUTIONS
Extreme caution should be used when this drug is given to patients with any evidence of cardiovascular disease because conduction defects may be exacerbated.

Caution is advised in patients with increased intraocular pressure, history of urinary retention, or history or narrow-angle glaucoma because of the drug's anticholinergic properties.

Particular care should be exercised when administering trimipramine with sympathomimetic amines, local decongestants, local anesthetics that contain epinephrine, atropine, or drugs with an anticholinergic effect.

Elevated and lowered blood sugar have been reported with use of trimipramine maleate.

In Brief

INDICATIONS
Relief of symptoms of depression (endogenous depression more likely to be alleviated than are other depressive states)

CONTRAINDICATIONS
During acute recovery following myocardial infarction

INTERACTIONS
Anticholinergic agents, atropine, catecholamines, cimetidine, local anesthetics, local decongestants, MAO inhibitors, sympathomimetic amines

(Continued on next page)

SPECIAL PRECAUTIONS *(CONTINUED)*

Leukocyte and differential counts should be performed in any patient who develops fever and sore throat during therapy. Trimipramine should be discontinued if there is evidence of pathologic neutrophil depression.

SPECIAL GROUPS

Children: Safety and efficacy for use in children have not been established. Use in adolescents only.
Elderly: Generally, lower doses are prescribed for the elderly.
Hepatic impairment: Use with caution in patients with impaired liver function.
Pregnancy: Category C drug. No adequate and well-controlled studies in pregnant women. Use during pregnancy only if potential benefit justifies potential risk to fetus.
Breast-feeding: Safe use during lactation has not been established; use only if clearly necessary.

DOSAGE

Adults: Start with 25 to 30 mg/d. Gradually increase until therapeutic effect or a dose of 300 mg is reached. *Maintenance*—Medication may be required at the lowest dose that maintains remission. Administer as single bedtime dose.
Elderly: Initially, 50 mg/d with gradual increments up to 100 mg/d. See Adults for maintenance instructions.
Children: Not recommended. For adolescents, initially 50 mg/d with gradual increments up to 100 mg/d. See Adults dosage for maintenance instructions.

ADVERSE EFFECTS

Most are rare; have been observed in patients taking TCAs but causal link may not have been established
Numbness, tingling, paresthesias of extremities, ataxia, tremors, seizures, alterations in EEG patterns, tinnitus, disorientation, delusions, restlessness, agitation, nightmares, hypomania, hypotension, hypertension, tachycardia, myocardial infarction, heart block, stroke, nausea and vomiting, anorexia, diarrhea, peculiar taste, abdominal cramps, dry mouth, blurred vision, mydriasis, constipation, urinary retention, delayed micturition, dilation of urinary tract, bone marrow depression, jaundice, altered liver function, weight gain or loss, perspiration, flushing, urinary frequency, drowsiness, dizziness, weakness, fatigue, headache, parotid swelling, alopecia

PHARMACOKINETICS AND PHARMACODYNAMICS

Onset of action: 2–6 d
Plasma half-life: 7–30 h
Bioavailability: rapidly absorbed from the GI tract
Metabolism: oxidized by hepatic microsomal enzymes followed by conjugation wit glucuronic acid
Excretion: partially excreted into hepatobiliary circulation and stomach and then reabsorbed; small percentage excreted in urine
Protein binding: extensively bound to plasma proteins
Hepatic impairment: hepatic congestion, fatty infiltration, increased serum liver enzymes

PROLONGED USE

Use for > 4 consecutive months has not been systematically studied.

OVERDOSAGE

Response of patients to toxic overdose may vary in severity and is conditioned by such factors as age, amount ingested, amount absorbed, and interval between ingestion and start of treatment. if a child accidentally ingests any amount, it should be regarded as serious and potentially fatal. Hospitalization of the child with continuous monitoring for up to 4 days is recommended. Hemodialysis, peritoneal dialysis, exchange transfusions, and forced diuresis have been reported as ineffective. Physicians can contact poison control centers for specific treatment procedures.

AVAILABILITY

Capsules—25 and 50 mg in 100s and Redipak 100s; 100 mg in 100s

ISOCARBOXAZID

(Marplan)

Isocarboxazid is a hydrazide derivative MAO inhibitor. MAO inhibitors are chemically heterogeneous drugs that can block oxidative deamination of naturally occurring monoamines.

SPECIAL PRECAUTIONS

Use with caution in combination with antihypertensive drugs, including thiazide diuretics, because hypotension may result.

Use with caution in schizophrenic patients because it can cause excessive stimulation.

The drug appears to have varying effects in epileptic patients.

All patients should be watched for symptoms of postural hypotension; if such hypotension occurs, the dose should be reduced.

The drug should not be used in combination with fluoxetine or other SSRIs. Fluoxetine and its major metabolite have very long half-lives, and at least 5 weeks should elapse between stopping fluoxetine and starting isocarboxazid.

SPECIAL GROUPS

Children: Safety and efficacy for use in patients younger than 16 years have not been established because there are no controlled studies in this group.

Elderly: Because the most serious reactions to this drug relate to effects on blood pressure, it is not advisable to use this drug in elderly patients.

Renal impairment: Use cautiously in patients with impaired renal function.

Hepatic impairment: Clinical evidence indicates a low incidence of altered liver function or jaundice in patients. Because it is difficult to differentiate most cases of drug-induced hepatocellular jaundice from viral hepatitis (histopathologically and biochemically indistinguishable), watch for hepatic complications. Use of the drug should be discontinued with the first sign of hepatic dysfunction.

Pregnancy: Safe use during pregnancy has not been established. The potential benefit of the drug should be weighed against its possible hazard to mother and child.

Breast-feeding: Safe use during lactation has not been established.

DOSAGE

Adult: Individualize doses. Usual starting dose is 10 mg/d. Dose can be gradually increased in single or divided doses. Because daily doses greater than 30 mg may cause increase in incidence or severity of side effects, patients taking doses greater than this should be monitored carefully. As soon as clinical improvement is observed, reduce the dose to a maintenance level of 10 to 20 mg/d. If no favorable response is seen within 4 weeks, continued administration is unlikely to help.

Elderly: Not advisable to use this drug.

Children: Not recommended for patients younger than 16 years. For patients aged 16 to 18 years, use adult dosage.

In Brief

INDICATIONS

The FDA has classified this drug as "probably" effective for treatment of depressed patients who are refractory to TCAs or electroconvulsive therapy and depressed patients in whom TCAs are contraindicated.

CONTRAINDICATIONS

Severe impairment of liver or renal function and other antidepressants

INTERACTIONS

Alcohol, barbiturates, buspirone, caffeine, clomipramine HCl, dextromethorphan, dibenzazepines, food with high concentrations of tryptophan or tyramine, narcotics, other MAO inhibitors, sympathomimetic drugs, thiazide diuretics and other antihypertensive drugs

ADVERSE EFFECTS

Orthostatic hypotension disturbances in cardiac rate and rhythm, dizziness, vertigo, constipation, headache, overactivity, hyperreflexia, tremors and muscle twitching, mania, hypomania, jitters, confusion and memory impairment, insomnia, peripheral edema, weakness, fatigue, dry mouth, blurred vision, hyperhidrosis anorexia and body weight changes, gastrointestinal disturbances, skin rashes, akathisia, ataxia, black tongue, coma, dysuria, euphoria, hematologic changes, incontinence, neuritis, photosensitivity, sexual disturbances, spider telangiectases, urinary retention, hallucinations, toxic amblyopia, impaired water excretion

PHARMACOKINETICS AND PHARMACODYNAMICS

Onset of action: about 3–4 wk

Metabolism: believed to be cleaved with resultant liberation of active products (eg, hydrazines); inactivated primarily by acetylation.

Excretion: metabolized by the liver

Effect of food: should not be taken with any foods containing tryptophan (broad beans) or tyramine (cheese, beer, wine, alcohol-free and reduced-alcohol beer and wine products, pickled herring, chicken liver, yeast extract); also excessive amount of caffeine should be avoided.

Renal impairment: accumulation can occur with multiple doses.

Hepatic impairment: drug-induced hepatocelluar jaundice can occur.

Lethal dose is unknown. Major overdose may be evidenced by tachycardia, hypotension, coma, convulsions, respiratory depression, sluggish reflexes, pyrexia, and diaphoresis; these may persist for 8–14 d. General supportive measures should be followed, along with immediate gastric lavage or emetics. An adequate airway should be maintained with supplemental oxygen if necessary. The mechanism by which amine-oxidase inhibitors produce hypotension is not fully understood, but there is evidence that the vascular bed response is blocked. Thus, plasma may be of value in the management of hypotension. Liver function tests are recommended during the 4–6 wk after recovery and at the time of overdose.

PATIENT INFORMATION

All patients should be warned against self-medication with proprietary cold, hay fever, weight-reducing preparations or any sympathomimetic drug. Patients should be warned against eating foods that contain high concentrations of tyramine or tryptophan. Beverages containing caffeine should be used in moderation. Patients should be instructed to report promptly the occurrence of headache or other unusual symptoms

AVAILABILITY

Tablets—10 mg in 100s

PHENELZINE SULFATE

(Nardil)

Phenelzine sulfate is a hydrazine analog of phenethylamine, a substrate for MAO. MAO inhibitors are heterogenous drugs that can block oxidative deamination of naturally occurring monoamines.

SPECIAL PRECAUTIONS

The most serious reaction to phenelzine involves changes in blood pressure, especially hypertensive crises, which have sometimes been fatal. In addition to tachycardia or bradycardia, intracranial bleeding has been reported in association with the increase in blood pressure. Therapy should be discontinued immediately if palpitation or sudden onset of severe headache occurs. Such patients should be evaluated in a hospital emergency room as soon as possible.

In depressed patients, the possibility of suicide should always be considered and adequate precautions taken. Patients undergoing treatment should be monitored carefully until depression is controlled.

All patients should be followed closely for symptoms of postural hypotension. Hypotension side effects have occurred in hypertensive, normal, and hypotensive patients.

Because the effect of phenelzine on the convulsive threshold may vary, adequate precautions should be taken when treating epileptic patients.

Hypomania has been reported.

Phenelzine can cause excessive stimulation in schizophrenic patients; in manic-depressive patients, it may result in a swing from a depressive to a manic state.

Because it is a hydrazine derivative, phenelzine has induced pulmonary and vascular tumors in mice.

In Brief

INDICATIONS

Depressed patients clinically characterized as atypical, nonendogenous, or neurotic with mixed anxiety and depression and phobic or hypochondriacal features; rarely the first antidepressant drug used but more suitable for use in treatment-resistant patients

CONTRAINDICATIONS

Contraindicated in patients with history of liver disease or abnormal liver function tests, patients taking other antidepressants (including other MAO inhibitors), buspirone HCl, guanethidine, SSRIs, or meperidine

INTERACTIONS

Alcohol, amoxapine, amitriptyline HCl, bupropion HCl, carbamazepine, clomipramine HCl, cyclobenzaprine, desipramine HCl, dextromethorphan, doxepin, food with high concentrations of tryptophan or tyramine, guanethidine, imipramine HCl, maprotiline HCl, nortriptyline HCl, other MAO inhibitors, perphenazine HCl, protriptyline HCl, sympathomimetic drugs and related compounds, trimipramine maleate, mirtazepine, and meperidine

ADVERSE EFFECTS

Common: dizziness, headache, drowsiness, sleep disturbances, fatigue, weakness, tremors, twitching, myoclonic movements, hyperreflexia, constipation, dry mouth, GI disturbances, elevated serum transaminase, weight gain, postural hypotension, edema, sexual disturbances

Less common: jitters, palilalia, euphoria, nystagmus, paresthesias, urinary retention, hypernatremia, skin rash, sweating, blurred vision, glaucoma

Less frequent: ataxia, shocklike coma, toxic delirium, manic reaction, convulsions, acute anxiety reaction, precipitation of schizophrenia, transient respiratory and cardiovascular depression, fatal progressive necrotizing hepatocellular damage, reversible jaundice, leukopenia, hypermetabolic syndrome, edema of the glottis, fever associated with increased muscle tone

PHARMACOKINETICS AND PHARMACODYNAMICS

Onset of action: 5–10 d; up to 5–6 wk
Bioavailability: absorbed readily
Metabolism: believed to be cleaved, with resultant liberation of active products (eg, hydrazines); inactivated primarily by acetylation
Excretion: metabolized by the liver.

PROLONGED USE

Drug should be continued for as long as required.

(Continued on next page)

PHENELZINE SULFATE
(CONTINUED)

SPECIAL GROUPS
Children: Safety and efficacy for use in patients younger than 16 years have not been established.
Elderly: Use with caution.
Hepatic impairment: Drug should not be prescribed for patients with a history of liver disease or with abnormal liver function tests.
Pregnancy: Category C drug. No adequate and well-controlled studies in pregnant women. Use during pregnancy only if the potential benefit justifies the potential risk to the fetus. The drug has an adverse effect in mice when given in doses well exceeding the maximum recommended human dose. In addition, growth of young dogs and rats has been retarded by doses exceeding the maximum human dose.
Breast-feeding: It is unknown whether this drug is excreted in human breast milk. Because of the potential for serious adverse reactions in nursing infants a decision should be made whether to discontinue the drug or discontinue nursing, taking into account the importance of the drug to the mother.

DOSAGE
Adult: Initial dose of 15 mg daily. Increase dose to at least 60 mg/d. It may be necessary to increase dose up to 90 mg/d. After maximum benefit is achieved, reduce dose slowly over several weeks. Maintenance dose should be the lowest that controls symptoms.
Elderly: Same as adult dosage.
Children: Not recommended for patients younger than 16 years. For patients aged 16 to 18 years, same as adult dosage.

OVERDOSAGE
Accidental or intentional overdose may be more common in patients who are depressed. Depending on amount of overdose, symptoms might involve the CNS and cardiovascular stimulation or depression. Symptoms may be absent during the initial 12 h following ingestion and may develop slowly thereafter, reaching a maximum in 24–48 h. Death has been reported; immediate hospitalization with continuous patient observation and monitoring throughout the period is essential. Symptoms include (alone or in combination) drowsiness, dizziness, faintness, irritability, hyperactivity, agitation, severe headache, rigidity, hallucinations, trismus, opisthotonus, convulsions and coma, rapid and irregular pulse, hypertension, hypotension and vascular collapse, precordial pain, respiratory depression and failure, hyperpyrexia, diaphoresis, and cool clammy skin. Intensive symptomatic and supportive treatment may be required. Induction of emesis or gastric lavage with instillation of charcoal slurry may be helpful in early poisoning, provided the airway has been protected against aspiration. Symptoms of CNS stimulation should be treated with diazepam given slowly IV. Phenothiazine derivatives and CNS stimulants should be avoided. Hypotension and vascular collapse should be treated with IV fluids and blood pressure titration with IV infusion of dilute pressor agent. Adrenergic agents may produce a markedly increased pressor response. Respiration should be supported by appropriate measures, including management of the airway, use of supplemental oxygen, and mechanical ventilatory assistance, as required. Body temperature should be monitored closely. Intensive management of hyperpyrexia may be required. Maintenance of fluid and electrolyte balance is essential. There are no data regarding the lethal doses in humans. The pathophysiologic effects of massive overdose may persist for several days. With symptomatic and supportive measures, recovery from mild overdose may be expected within 3 to 4 days. Hemodialysis, peritoneal dialysis, and charcoal hemoperfusion may be of value, but sufficient data are not available to recommend their routine use. Toxic blood levels of phenelzine have not been established, and assay methods are not practical for clinical or toxicologic use.

PATIENT INFORMATION
All patients should be given a list of the specific foods and medications to avoid. Patients under the care of another physician or dentist should inform each one that they are taking phenelzine. Patients should be instructed to report promptly the occurrence of headache or other unusual symptoms.

AVAILABILITY
Tablets—15 mg in 100s

TRANYLCYPROMINE SULFATE
(Parnate)

Tranylcypromine sulfate is a nonhydrazine MAO inhibitor that is the result of cyclization of the side chain of amphetamine.

Tranylcypromine increases the concentration of epinephrine, norepinephrine, and serotonin in storage sites throughout the nervous system; this increased concentration of MAOs in the brain stem is believed to be the basis for the drug's antidepressant activity.

In Brief

INDICATIONS
FDA-approved: Treatment of major depressive episode without melancholia in adult patients who can be closely supervised and have failed to respond to drugs more commonly used for depression; effectiveness in patients with endogenous depression has not been established

CONTRAINDICATIONS
Patients with a history of liver disease or abnormal liver function tests, patients taking antiparkinsonism drugs, meperidine, CNS depressants

INTERACTIONS
Anesthetics, antihistamines, antihypertensives, buspirone, cheese or other foods with high tyramine content, CNS depressants (including narcotics and alcohol), dextromethorphan, dibenzazepine derivatives, disulfiram, diuretics, excessive quantities of caffeine, meperidine, metrizamide, other MAO inhibitors, sedatives, SSRIs, sympathomimetics (including amphetamines)

(Continued on next page)

SPECIAL PRECAUTIONS

Hypertensive crises, which have sometimes been fatal, can occur in association with the drug. All patients taking this drug should have their blood pressure monitored closely to detect evidence of any pressor response.

Hypotension has been observed during drug therapy. Symptoms of postural hypotension are most common in patients with preexistent hypertension; blood pressure usually returns rapidly to pretreatment levels when the drug is discontinued. When tranylcypromine is combined with phenothiazine derivatives or other compounds known to cause hypotension, the possibility of addictive hypotensive effects should be considered.

There have been reports of drug dependency in patients using doses in excess of the therapeutic range. Use with caution in patients with a history of previous substance abuse.

Tranylcypromine should not be used with metrizamide and should be discontinued at least 48 hours before myelography (gradual withdrawal) and not resumed for at least 24 hours after the procedure.

In depressed patients, the possibility of suicide should always be considered and adequate precautions taken.

The drug may have the capacity to suppress anginal pain that would otherwise be a warning of myocardial ischemia.

Use with caution in diabetic patients because it may contribute to hypoglycemic episodes.

Administer with caution to patients receiving disulfiram because severe toxicity, including convulsions and death, may occur.

Before prescribing this drug, physicians should be completely familiar with the full material on doses, side effects, and contraindiations. Physicians should be familiar with the symptoms of various mental depressions and alternate methods of treatment.

SPECIAL GROUPS

Children: Safety and efficacy have not been established.

Elderly: Older patients may suffer more morbidity than younger patients during and after an episode of hypertension or malignant hyperthermia. Older patients also have less compensatory reserve to cope with any serious adverse reactions. Therefore, tranylcypromine should be used with caution in the elderly population.

Renal impairment: The usual precautions should be observed in patients with impaired renal function.

Hepatic impairment: Contraindicated in patients with a history of liver disease or with abnormal liver function tests.

Pregnancy: Use during pregnancy or in women of childbearing age only if potential benefits of the drug are weighed against possible hazards to mother and child. Animal reproductive studies show that tranylcypromine passes through the placental barrier into the fetus of rats.

Breast-feeding: Excreted in human milk. Use during lactation requires that the potential benefits of the drug be weighed against its possible hazards to mother and child.

DOSAGE

Adult: Individualize dose. Usual effective dose is 30 mg/d in divided doses. If there is no improvement after 2 weeks, increase dose in 10 mg/d increments of 1 to 3 weeks. Dose range may be extended to 60 mg/d. Withdrawal should be gradual.

Elderly: Use with extreme caution, and use the low end of dose range.

Children: Not recommended.

ADVERSE EFFECTS

Increased anxiety, agitation, manic symptoms, restlessness or insomnia, weakness, drowsiness, episodes of dizziness, dry mouth, nausea, diarrhea, abdominal pain, constipation, tachycardia, significant anorexia, edema, palpitations, blurred vision, chills, impotence, headaches, hepatitis, skin rash, impaired water excretion, tinnitus, muscle spasm, tremors, myoclonic jerks, numbness, paresthesia, urinary retention, retarded ejaculation, anemia, leukopenia, agranulocytosis, thrombocytopenia, localized scleroderma, cystic acne flareup, ataxia, confusion, disorientation, memory loss, urinary frequency, urinary incontinence, urticaria, fissuring in corner of mouth, akinesia

PHARMACOKINETICS AND PHARMACODYNAMICS

Onset of action: 48 h–3 wk
Bioavailability: readily absorbed
Renal impairment: accumulation with chronic administration

PROLONGED USE

Anecdotal observation suggests it is safe.

OVERDOSAGE

Symptoms of overdose are intensification of the adverse effects listed, depending on degree of overdose and individual susceptibility. Some patients exhibit insomnia, restlessness, and anxiety, progressing in severe cases to agitation, mental confusion, and incoherence. Hypotension, dizziness, weakness, and drowsiness may occur, progressing in severe cases to extreme dizziness and shock. A few patients may have hypertension with severe headache. In rare instances, the hypertension is accompanied by twitching or myoclonic fibrillation of skeletal muscles with hyperpyrexia, sometimes progressing to generalized rigidity and coma.

Gastric lavage is helpful if performed early. Treatment should normally consist of general supportive measures, close observation of vital signs, and steps to counteract specific symptoms as they occur. Barbiturates have been reported to help relieve myoclonic reactions. If pressor agents are used for hypotension, the rate of infusion should be regulated by careful observation of the patient, because an exaggerated pressor response may occur. The toxic effect of tranylcypromine may be delayed or prolonged following the last dose of the drug. The patient should be observed closely for at least 1 week. It is unknown whether tranylcypromine is dialyzable.

PATIENT INFORMATION

Patients should be instructed to report promptly the occurrence of headache or other unusual symptoms, such as palpitations or tachycardia, sense of constriction in the throat or chest, sweating, dizziness, neck stiffness, nausea, or vomiting. Patients should receive a list of foods to avoid and be told not to drink alcoholic beverages. The patient also should be warned about the possibility of hypotension, faintness, and drowsiness sufficient to impair performance during potentially hazardous tasks. Caution patients not to take concomitant medications, whether prescription or over-the-counter drugs, and not to consume excessive amounts of caffeine in any form. Patients should inform other physicians and their dentist that they are taking tranylcypromine.

AVAILABILITY

Tablets—10 mg in 100s and 1000s

MAPROTILINE HYDROCHLORIDE

(Ludiomil)

Maprotiline HCl is a tetracyclic compound with many similarities to tricyclic drugs. It causes moderate sedative, anticholinergic, and orthostatic hypotensive effects. The mechanism of action is not known. Maprotiline apparently acts primarily by potentiation of central adrenergic synapses by blocking reuptake of norepinephrine at nerve endings.

SPECIAL PRECAUTIONS

Seizures have been associated with the use of maprotiline. Most of the seizures have occurred in patients with a known history of seizures. The risk of seizures may be increased when the drug is taken concomitantly with phenothiazines, the dose of benzodiazepine is rapidly tapered in patients receiving maprotiline, or the recommended dose is exceeded.

The possibility of suicide in seriously depressed patients is inherent in the illness and may persist until significant remission occurs. Such patients should be supervised carefully during the early phase of treatment and may require hospitalization. Prescriptions should be written for the smallest amount feasible.

Concurrent administration with electroshock therapy may increase the hazards; such treatment should be limited to patients for whom it is essential because there is limited clinical experience.

Maprotiline can enhance the response to alcohol and the effects of barbiturates and other CNS depressants. In patients who may use alcohol excessively, the potentiation may increase the danger inherent in any suicide attempt or overdose.

Before elective surgery, the drug should be discontinued for as long as clinically feasible because little is known about the interaction between the drug and general anesthetics.

Caution should be exercised when administering the drug to hyperthyroid patients or those taking thyroid medication.

Extreme caution should be used when this drug is given to patients with a history of myocardial infarction and patients with a history or presence of cardiovascular disease because of the possibility of conduction defects, arrhythmias, myocardial infarction, strokes, and tachycardia.

Hypomanic or manic episodes have occurred in some patients taking this drug, particularly in patients with cyclic disorders.

SPECIAL GROUPS

Children: Safety and efficacy in children younger than 18 years have not been established.
Elderly: In general, lower doses are used in the elderly patient.
Pregnancy: Category B drug. No adequate and well-controlled studies in pregnant women. Use during pregnancy only if clearly needed.
Breast-feeding: Maprotiline is excreted in breast milk. At steady state, the concentrations in breast milk correspond closely to the concentrations in whole blood. Caution should be exercised when administered to a nursing mother.

In Brief

INDICATIONS
Treatment of depressive illness

CONTRAINDICATIONS
Known hypersensitivity to the individual drug or any tricyclic compound. Concomitant use of MAO inhibitors and tricyclic compounds also is contraindicated. Hyperpyretic crises or severe convulsive seizures may occur in patients receiving such combinations. The potentiation of adverse effects can be serious or even fatal. When it is desired to substitute a tricyclic compound in patients receiving an MAO inhibitor, as long an interval should elapse as the clinical situation will allow, with a minimum of 14 days. Initial doses should be low, and increases should be gradual and cautiously prescribed.

INTERACTIONS
Anticholinergic or sympathomimetic drugs, benzodiazepines, guanethidine or similar agents, hepatic enzyme inducers, hepatic enzyme inhibitors, phenothiazines, thyroid medication

ADVERSE EFFECTS
Most are rare. Have been observed in patients taking maprotiline or tricyclics, but causal link has not always been established. Rare occurrences of hypotension, hypertension, tachycardia, palpitation, arrhythmia, heart block, and syncope. Other effects include nervousness, anxiety, insomnia, agitation, hallucinations, disorientation, nightmares, exacerbation of psychosis, hypomania, mania, drowsiness, dizziness, tremor, dry mouth, constipation, blurred vision, rare instances of skin rash, petechiae, nausea, epigastric distress, diarrhea, bitter taste, abdominal cramps, dysphagia, rare instances of increased or decreased libido, rare instances of impotence, weakness and fatigue, headache, rare instances of altered liver function and jaundice, weight loss or gain, perspiration, flushing, urinary frequency, increased salivation, nasal congestion, and alopecia.

PHARMACOKINETICS AND PHARMACODYNAMICS
Onset of action: a minimum of 2 wk
Peak plasma levels: 12 h
Plasma half-life: 21–25 h
Bioavailability: readily absorbed from the GI tract
Metabolism: metabolized in the liver by hepatic microsomal enzymes
Protein binding: significantly bound to plasma proteins

PROLONGED USE
Monitor patients carefully; adjust doses downward.

OVERDOSAGE
Symptoms include drowsiness, tachycardia, ataxia, vomiting, cyanosis, hypotension, shock, restlessness, agitation, hyperpyrexia, muscle rigidity, athetoid movements, mydriasis, cardiac arrhythmias, and impaired cardiac condition. In severe cases, loss of consciousness and generalized convulsions may occur.
The recommended treatment for overdose may change periodically. Therefore, it is recommended that the physician contact a poison control center for current information on treatment. Because it has been reported that physostigmine increases the risk of seizures, its use is not recommended in cases of overdose with maprotiline. Digitalis may increase conduction abnormalities and further irritate an already sensitized myocardium. Dialysis is of little value because of the low plasma concentration of this drug.

(Continued on next page)

DOSAGE

Adults: *Initial dose for mild to moderate depression*—75 mg/d is suggested for outpatients. In some patients, initial dose of 25 mg daily can be used. Maintain initial dose for 2 weeks. Dose can then be increased gradually in 25-mg increments as required and tolerated. Most patients respond to 150 mg/d, but doses as high as 225 mg/d may be required. Most hospitalized patients respond to a daily dose of 150 mg, although doses as high as 225 mg may be required. Most hospitalized patients respond to a daily dose of 150 mg, although doses as high as 225 mg may be required. Do not exceed 225 mg/d. *Maintenance*—Dose during prolonged maintenance therapy should be kept at the lowest effective level. Dose can be reduced to 75 to 150 mg/d with adjustment, depending on therapeutic response.
Elderly: Initial dose of 25 mg daily for 2 weeks. Maintenance doses of 50 to 75 mg/d are satisfactory for patients who do not tolerate higher amounts.
Children: Not recommended.

PATIENT INFORMATION

Patients should be warned of the association between seizures and the use of maprotiline. Patients should exercise caution about performing potentially hazardous tasks or operating automobiles or machinery because the drug can impair mental and physical abilities. Caution patients against taking this medication concomitantly with alcohol or barbiturates and other CNS depressants.

AVAILABILITY

Tablets—25, 50, and 75 mg in 20s, 100s, 500s, 1000s, UD 100s, and Accu-Pak 100s

CITALOPRAM

Citalopram is the most selective inhibitor of serotonin reuptake yet studied and has little or no affinity for adrenergic, dopaminergic, histaminergic, and muscarinic cholinergic receptors. Currently, citalopram is under review at the United States FDA for the treatment of major depression; the compound is also being investigated for the treatment of panic disorder, obsessive-compulsive disorder, poststroke depression, and the behavioral disturbance of dementia. Its chemical structure is unrelated to those of other antidepressants, including tricyclic and tetracyclic antidepressants, as well as other SSRIs.

SPECIAL GROUPS

Elderly: The adverse-effect profile observed in clinical trials in the elderly was similar to that of younger patients. Citalopram demonstrates linear pharmacokinetics, and the pharmacokinetic profile of citalopram in elderly subjects is similar to that seen in younger patients, although plasma concentrations are somewhat higher in the elderly. Citalopram has little or no effect on cytochrome P450 enzymes, and thus has a low potential for drug interactions
Renal impairment: No statistically significant differences in clearance of citalopram have been observed between subjects with normal or mild to moderate impaired renal function.
Hepatic impairment: Subjects with severely reduced hepatic function clear citalopram more slowly than do subjects with normal liver function. Therefore, lower doses of citalopram should be administered to patients with liver disease.
Pregnancy: Safety of citalopram in pregnancy has not been studied.
Breast-feeding: The concentration of citalopram excreted in breast milk is not known; therefore, caution should be exercised when administering to nursing mothers.

In Brief

INDICATIONS
Treatment of depression

CONTRAINDICATIONS
Concomitant administration with MAO inhibitors

INTERACTIONS
Citalopram is not highly protein bound and has been shown not to interfere with the metabolism of highly protein-bound drugs such as warfarin and digoxin; citalopram has little or no effect on cytochrome P450 isoenzyme and thus had a low potential for drug interactions

ADVERSE EFFECTS
Data from controlled clinical trials show nausea, dry mouth, somnolence, and increased sweating to be the most frequently reported adverse effects

PHARMACOKINETICS AND PHARMACODYNAMICS
Onset of action: 1–4 wk
Plasma half-life: 35 h
Bioavailability: complete (at least 80%) after oral administration
Metabolism: extensively metabolized in the liver, with successive N-demethylations to demethylcitalopram and didemethylcitalopram
Excretion: 13% recovered unchanged in urine; almost 70% was not detected as parent drug or metabolites, suggesting significant faccal excretion or alternative metabolic breakdown
Effect of food: none
Protein binding: approximately 80% plasma protein bound

PROLONGED USE
Effectiveness of citalopram in the treatment of depression and prevention of relapse has been established in two 24-week studies.

(Continued on next page)

CITALOPRAM
(CONTINUED)

DOSAGE

Adults: *Initial dose*—20 mg taken once daily is the recommended initial dose. The dose can be increased in 20-mg increments to a maximum recommended dosage of 60 mg/d.

Elderly: Same as adult dosage, with maximum recommended dosage of 40 mg/d.

Children: Adequate clinical trials have not been conducted to assess citalopram use in children.

OVERDOSAGE

The safety of citalopram in overdose is consistent with that of other SSRIs. Nonfatal overdoses of up to 5200 mg have been described. Common symptoms included nausea, vomiting, convulsions, tremor, dizziness, hyperventilation, tachycardia, drowsiness, somnolence, and coma, which generally resolve with supportive care. A single fatality has been reported following an ingestion of 3290 mg of citalopram alone (the equivalent of 200 times the common daily dose of 20 mg). Citalopram in overdose in combination with alcohol or other drugs may cause serious symptoms and can be fatal; therefore, any overdose situation should be treated carefully. An adequate airway should be maintained, and adequate ventilation and oxygenation should be ensured. Cardiac and vital signs should be monitored, along with necessary general supportive measures. Gastric evacuation should be performed. The physician should contact a poison control center for the most recent information on the treatment of overdose of this drug.

AVAILABILITY

Currently available in more than 50 countries; not yet available in the United States
Tablets—10, 20, and 40 mg
IV and oral liquid form

FLUOXETINE HYDROCHLORIDE

(Prozac)

Fluoxetine HCl is an antidepressant that is not chemically related to tricyclic, tetracyclic, or other antidepressants. The effect is believed to be the result of inhibition of uptake of serotonin into CNS neurons.

SPECIAL PRECAUTIONS

During premarketing testing, about 4% of patients developed a rash or urticaria. Clinical findings reported in association with the rash include fever, leukocytosis, arthralgias, edema, carpal tunnel syndrome, respiratory distress, lymphadenopathy, proteinuria, and mild transaminase elevation. Whether the systemic events and rash have a common underlying cause or are attributable to different causes or pathogenic processes is unknown.

Anxiety, nervousness, and insomnia have been reported.

During premarketing testing, hypomania or mania occurred.

Drug should be introduced with caution in patients with a history of seizures.

Because of the long elimination half-lives of the parent drug and its major active metabolite, changes in dose will not be fully reflected in plasma for several weeks, affecting both strategies for titration to final dose and withdrawal from treatment.

In patients with diabetes, fluoxetine can alter glycemic control. Hypoglycemia has occurred during therapy, and hyperglycemia has developed following discontinuation of the drug.

Several cases of hyponatremia have been reported, particularly in patients taking diuretics or who were otherwise volume depleted.

There have been rare reports of altered platelet function or abnormal results from laboratory studies in patients taking fluoxetine. Although there have been reports of abnormal bleeding, it is unclear whether the drug had a causative role.

(Continued on next page)

In Brief

INDICATIONS

Treatment of depression in outpatients (antidepressant action of fluoxetine in hospitalized patients has not been adequately studied), obsessive-compulsive disorder, bulimia nervosa

CONTRAINDICATIONS

Known hypersensitivity to fluoxetine and concomitant administration with MAO inhibitors. Should wait 5 weeks after discontinuing before starting an MAOI.

INTERACTIONS

Antidepressants, diazepam, drugs tightly bound to plasma proteins, MAO inhibitors, tryptophan, CNS-activated drugs, warfarin drugs metabolized by cytochrome $P_{450}IID_6$, drugs metabolized by cytochrome $P_{450}IIIA_4$

ADVERSE EFFECTS

Associated with discontinuation of treatment: insomnia and sweating

Most common in controlled trials: nausea, anorexia, dry mouth, insomnia, anxiety, nervousness, somnolence, tremor, asthenia.

Frequent: chills, increased appetite, weight loss, abnormal dreams, agitation, bronchitis, rhinitis, yawning

Infrequent: chills, fever, cyst, face edema, hangover effect, jaw pain, malaise, neck pain, neck rigidity, pelvic pain, angina pectoris, arrhythmia, hemorrhage, hypertension, hypotension, migraine, postural hypotension, syncope, tachycardia, aphthous stomatitis, dysphagia, eructation, esophagitis, gastritis, gingivitis, glossitis, melena, stomatitis, thirst, hypothyroidism, anemia, lymphadenopathy, generalized edema, hypoglycemia, peripheral edema, weight gain, arthritis, bone pain, bursitis, tenosynovitis, twitching, abnormal gait, acute brain syndrome, akathisia, amnesia, apathy, ataxia, buccoglossal syndrome, CNS stimulation, convulsion, delusions, depersonalization, emotional lability, euphoria, hallucinations, hostility, hyperkinesia, hypesthesia, incoordination, libido increased, manic reaction, neuralgia,

(Continued on next page)

SPECIAL GROUPS

Elderly: The effects of age on the metabolism of fluoxetine have not been fully explored. The disposition of single doses in healthy subjects older than 65 years did not differ significantly from that in younger normal patients. Given the long half-life and nonlinear disposition of the drug, however, a single-dose study is not adequate to rule out the possibility of altered pharmacokinetics in the elderly, particularly if they have systemic illness or are receiving multiple drugs for concomitant diseases.

Renal impairment: The use of a lower or less frequent dose is not routinely necessary.

Hepatic impairment: Fluoxetine must be used with caution in patients with liver disease. If fluoxetine is administered to such patients, a lower or less frequent dose should be used.

Pregnancy: Category C. Fluoxetine should be used during pregnancy only if the potential benefit justifies the potential risk to the fetus.

Breast-feeding: Because fluoxetine is excreted in human breast-milk, nursing while taking fluoxetine is not recommended. In one breast milk sample, the concentration of fluoxetine plus its major metabolite, norfluoxetine, was 70.4 ng/mL. The concentration in the mother's plasma was 295 ng/mL. No adverse effects on the infant were reported.

ADVERSE EFFECTS *(CONTINUED)*

neuropathy, paranoid reaction, psychosis, vertigo, asthma, epistaxis, hiccups, hyperventilation, pneumonia, acne, alopecia, contact dermatitis, dry skin, herpes simplex, maculopapular rash, urticaria, amblyopia, conjunctivitis, ear pain, eye pain, mydriasis, photophobia, tinnitus, abnormal ejaculation, amenorrhea, breast pain, cystitis, dysuria, fibrocystic breast, impotence, leukorrhea, menopause, menorrhagia, ovarian disorder, urinary incontinence, urinary urgency, urination impaired, vaginitis

Rare: increased bleeding time, blood dyscrasia, leukopenia, lymphocytosis, petechia, purpura, increased sedimentation rate, thrombocythemia, goiter, hyperthyroidism, bone necrosis, chondrodystrophy, muscle hemorrhage, myositis, osteoporosis, pathologic fracture, rheumatoid arthritis, abnormal EEG, chronic brain syndrome, antisocial reaction, circumoral paresthesia, CNS depression, coma, dysarthria, dystonia, extrapyramidal syndrome, hypertonia, hysteria, myoclonus, nystagmus, paralysis, decreased reflexes, stupor, torticollis, apnea, hemoptysis, hypoxia, larynx edema, lung edema, lung fibrosis, pleural effusion, eczema, erythema multiforme, fungal dermatitis, herpes zoster, hirsutism, psoriasis, purpuric rash, pustular rash, seborrhea, skin discoloration, skin hypertrophy, subcutaneous nodule, vesiculobullous rash, blepharitis, cataract, corneal lesion, deafness, diplopia, eye hemorrhage, glaucoma, iritis, ptosis, strabismus, taste loss, abortion, albuminuria, breast enlargement, dyspareunia, epididymitis, female lactation, hematuria, hypomenorrhea, kidney calculus, metrorrhagia, orchitis, polyuria, pyelonephritis, pyuria, salpingitis, urethral pain, urethritis, urinary tract disorder, urolithiasis, uterine hemorrhage, uterine spasm, vaginal hemorrhage

PHARMACOKINETICS AND PHARMACODYNAMICS

Onset of action: $\geq$ 4 wk (depression); $\geq$ 5 wk (OCD)

Peak plasma levels: 6–8 h

Plasma half-life: fluoxetine, 1–3 d after acute administration and 4–6 d after chronic administration; major metabolite norfluoxetine, 4–16 d after acute and chronic administration

Bioavailability: > 60%

Metabolism: extensively metabolized in the liver to norfluoxetine, a metabolite with equal potency to fluoxetine; norfluoxetine further metabolized by liver to inactive metabolites

Excretion: primary route of elimination, hepatic metabolism to inactive metabolites excreted by kidneys; < 2.5% unchanged drug excreted in urine

Effect of food: food does not affect systemic bioavailability but may delay absorption; can be administered with or without food

Protein binding: about 94.5% bound to serum proteins, including albumin and α1-glycoprotein; interaction between fluoxetine and other highly protein-bound drugs has not been fully evaluated but may be important.

Renal impairment: in depressed patients on dialysis (n = 12), 20 mg of fluoxetine per day taken for 2 months produces comparable steady-state fluoxetine and norfluoxetine plasma concentrations to depressed patients with normal renal function

Hepatic impairment: liver impairment can affect elimination; half-life prolonged in study of cirrhotic patients, with mean of 7.5 d compared with range of 2–3 d.

PROLONGED USE

Systematic evaluation of fluoxetine has shown that its antidepressant efficacy is maintained for up to 38 wk following 12 wk of open treatment (total, 50 wk) at a dose of 20 mg/d.

(Continued on next page)

FLUOXETINE HYDROCHLORIDE (CONTINUED)

DOSAGE

Adults: *Initial treatment*—20 mg/d in the morning is the recommended initial dose. A dose increase can be considered after several weeks if no clinical improvement is observed. Doses higher than 20 mg/d should be administered once a day (morning) or twice a day (morning and noon) and should not exceed 80 mg/d. *Maintenance, continuation, and extended treatment*—Optimum duration of therapy is inconclusive. It is unknown whether the dose of antidepressant needed to induce remission is identical to the dose needed to maintain or sustain euthymia.
Elderly: *See Adults.* Elderly patients should receive lower or less frequent doses.
Children: Not recommended.
Hepatic impairment: A lower or less frequent dose should be used.

OVERDOSAGE

Two deaths among about 38 reports of acute overdose with fluoxetine, either alone or in combination with other drugs or alcohol, have been recorded. Nausea and vomiting are prominent in overdoses. Other symptoms include agitation, restlessness, hypomania, and other signs of CNS excitation. Except for the two deaths noted above, all other overdose cases recovered without residue.
Management of an overdose includes establishing and maintaining an airway and ensuring adequate oxygenation and ventilation. Activated charcoal, with or without sorbitol, may be as or more effective than emesis or lavage and should be considered. Cardiac and vital signs monitoring is recommended, along with general symptomatic and supportive measures. There are no specific antidotes. Because of the large volume of distribution of the drug, forced diuresis, dialysis, hemoperfusion, and exchange transfusion are unlikely to be of benefit. Physicians should consider contacting a poison control center for the most recent information on this drug.

AVAILABILITY

Pulvules—20 mg in 100s and 10 mg
Liquid—20 mg/5 mL in mint flavor in 120 mL with 0.23% alcohol and sucrose

FLUVOXAMINE HYDROCHLORIDE

(Luvox)

Fluvoxamine HCl is a potent and selective inhibitor of presynaptic neuronal reuptake of serotonin. It is chemically unrelated to other SSRIs.

SPECIAL PRECAUTIONS

In preclinical studies, hypomania and mania were reported in 1% of depressed patients. Seizures occurred in 0.2% of patients. Fluvoxamine should be used with caution in patients with a history of mania or seizures. Treatment should be discontinued in any patient who develops seizures. Caution is advised in administering to patients with conditions or diseases that could affect hemodynamic responses or metabolism. Fluvoxamine should be slowly titrated in patients with liver dysfunction during the initiation of therapy.

Fluvoxamine has not been systematically evaluated or used to any appreciable extent in patients with a recent history of myocardial infarction or unstable heart disease. Evaluation of the ECGs for patients with depression or obsessive-compulsive disorder who participated in premarketing studies revealed no differences between fluvoxamine and placebo in the emergence of clinically important ECG changes. Fluvoxamine clearance was decreased by approximately 30% in patients with liver dysfunction; initiation of treatment should be slowly titrated in these patients.

In Brief

INDICATIONS
Treatment of major depression and obsessive-compulsive behavior

CONTRAINDICATIONS
Concomitant use in patients taking MAO inhibitors, terfenadine, astemizole, or cisapride

INTERACTIONS
β-Adrenergic blockers, atenolol, warfarin, propranolol

ADVERSE EFFECTS
Controlled trials: nausea, vomiting, somnolence, dry mouth, headache, constipation, agitation, anorexia, insomnia, dizziness, syncope, tremor, hypokinesia, asthenia, abnormal liver function tests, mania
Frequent: increased cough, sinusitis, edema, weight gain, weight loss, amnesia, apathy, hyperkinesia, hypokinesia, manic reaction, myoclonus, psychotic reaction, elevated liver transaminases, accidental injury, malaise
Infrequent: asthma, bronchitis, abnormal accommodation, conjunctivitis, deafness, diplopia, dry eyes, ear pain, eye pain, mydriasis, otitis media, parosmia, photophobia, taste loss, visual-field defect epistaxis, hoarseness, hyperventilation, agoraphobia, akathisia, ataxia, CNS depression, convulsion, delirium, delusion, depersonalization, drug dependence, dyskinesia, dystonia, emotional lability, euphoria, extrapyramidal syndrome, unsteady gait, hallucinations, hemiplegia, hostility, hypersomnia, hypochondriasis, hypotonia, hysteria, incoordination, increased salivation, increased libido, neuralgia, paralysis, paranoid reaction, phobia, psychosis, sleep disorder, stupor, twitching, vertigo arthralgia, arthritis, bursitis, generalized muscle spasm, myasthenia, tendinous contracture, tenosynovitis, acne, alopecia, dry skin, eczema, exfoliative dermatitis, furunculosis, seborrhea, skin discoloration, urticaria, dehydration, hypercholesterolemia, hypothyroidism, anemia, ecchymosis, leukocytosis, lymphadenopathy, thrombocytopenia, colitis, eructation, esophagitis, gastritis, gastroenteritis, gastrointestinal hemorrhage, gastrointestinal ulcer, gingivitis, glossitis, hemorrhoids, melena, rectal hemorrhage, stomatitis, angina pectoris,

(Continued on next page)

(Continued on next page)

SPECIAL GROUPS

Children: Safety and effectiveness of fluvoxamine in individuals younger than 18 years of age have not been established.

Elderly: No overall differences in safety were observed between patients 65 years of age and older and younger patients. Other reported clinical experience has not identified differences in response between the elderly and younger patients. However, the clearance of fluvoxamine is decreased by about 50% in the elderly compared with younger patients; therefore, fluvoxamine should be slowly titrated during initiation of therapy.

Hepatic impairment: Initiation of treatment should be slowly titrated.

Pregnancy: There are no adequate and well-controlled studies in pregnant women. Fluvoxamine should be used during pregnancy only if the potential benefit justifies potential risk to the fetus.

Breast-feeding: Fluvoxamine is secreted in human breast milk. The decision of whether to discontinue nursing or to discontinue the drug should take into account the potential for serious adverse effects in the infant as well as the potential benefits to the mother.

DOSAGE

The recommended starting dose is 50 mg, administered as a single daily dose at bedtime. The dose should be increased in 50-mg increments every 4 to 7 days, as tolerated, until maximum therapeutic benefit is achieved, not to exceed 300 mg/d. It is advisable that a total daily dose of more than 100 mg should be given in two divided doses. *Maintenance*—Dosage adjustments should be made to maintain the patient on the lowest effective dosage, and patients should be periodically reassessed to determine the need for continued treatment.

Elderly: Initiation of treatment should be slowly titrated.

Hepatic impairment: Initiation of treatment should be slowly titrated.

ADVERSE EFFECTS *(CONTINUED)*

bradycardia, cardiomyopathy, cardiovascular disease, cold extremities, conduction delay, heart failure, myocardial infarction, pallor,pulse irregular, ST segment changes, hypertension, hypotension, syncope, tachycardia, allergic reaction, neck pain, anuria, breast pain, cystitis, delayed menstruation, dysuria, female lactation, hematuria, menopause, menorrhagia, metrorrhagia, nocturia, polyuria, premenstrual syndrome, urinary incontinence, urinary tract infection, urinary urgency, urination impaired, vaginal hemorrhage, vaginitis, neck rigidity, overdose, photosensitivity reaction, suicide attempt

Rare: apnea, congestion of upper airway, hemoptysis, hiccups, laryngismus, obstructive pulmonary disease, pneumonia arthrosis, myopathy, pathologic fracture, goiter, leukopenia, purpura, diabetes mellitus, hyperglycemia, hyperlipidemia, hypoglycemia, hypokalemia, lactate dehydrogenase, increased biliary pain, cholecystitis, cholelithiasis, fecal incontinence, hematemesis, intestinal obstruction, jaundice, atrioventricular block, cerebrovascular accident, coronary artery disease, embolus, pericarditis, phlebitis, pulmonary infarction, supraventricular extrasystoles, cyst, pelvic pain, corneal ulcer, retinal detachment, kidney calculus, hematospermia, oliguria, sudden death

PHARMACOKINETICS AND PHARMACODYNAMICS

Onset of action: about 4 wk
Peak plasma levels: 3–8 h
Plasma half-life: 15 h
Bioavailability: 53%
Metabolism: metabolized in the liver; four major metabolic pathways identified
Excretion: 94% recovered in urine in form of at least 11 inactive metabolites; no unchanged drug recovered
Effect of food: time to peak and peak plasma levels unaffected by food
Protein binding: average of 80% plasma protein bound
Elderly: mean maximum plasma concentrations in patients 66–73 y old were 40% higher than in patients 19–35 y. The multiple dose elimination half-life of fluvoxamine was 17.4 and 25.9 h in the elderly compared with 13.6 and 15.6 h in the young subjects at steady state for 50 and 100 mg doses, respectively; the clearance of fluvoxamine is decreased by about 50% in the elderly compared with younger patients
Hepatic impairment: there is a 30% decrease in fluvoxamine clearance in patients with hepatic dysfunction compared with healthy subjects

PROLONGED USE

Effectiveness for use > 10 wk has not been systematically evaluated in controlled trials. Patients should be maintained on the lowest possible dose and should be periodically reassessed to determine the need for continued treatment.

OVERDOSAGE

Adverse events associated with overdose include drowsiness, vomiting, diarrhea, and dizziness. Other signs include coma, tachycardia, bradycardia, hypotension, ECT abnormalities, liver function abnormalities, and convulsions. In addition, aspiration, pneumonitis, respiratory difficulties or hypokalemia may occur secondary to loss of consciousness or vomiting.

Administration of activated charcoal may be as effective as emesis or lavage in treating overdose. Since absorption with overdose may be delayed, measures to minimize absorption may be necessary for up to 24 hours postingestion. An unobstructed airway should be established with maintenance of respiration as required. Dialysis is not believed to be beneficial.

AVAILABILITY

Tablets—50 and 100 mg in 100s and 1000s.

PAROXETINE HYDROCHLORIDE

(Paxil)

Paroxetine HCl is an antidepressant that inhibits neuronal uptake of serotonin in the CNS, resulting in potentiation of serotoninergic activity. It appears to have weak effects on neuronal uptake of norepinephrine and dopamine.

SPECIAL PRECAUTIONS

During premarketing testing, hypomania or mania occurred in about 1% of patients treated with paroxetine. In addition, seizures occurred in 0.1% of patients. The drug should be used with caution in patients with a history of mania or seizures. The drug should be discontinued in any patient who develops seizures.

Several cases of hyponatremia have been reported. Patients who are taking diuretics or are volume depleted should be monitored closely.

Paroxetine has not been evaluated or used to any appreciable extent in patients with a recent history of myocardial infarction or unstable heart disease. Physicians should monitor these patients carefully.

SPECIAL GROUPS

Elderly: In clinical trials in patients aged 65 years and older, no overall differences in the adverse event profile between elderly and younger patients were noted. Effectiveness was similar in younger and older patients. Because pharmacokinetic studies revealed a decreased clearance in the elderly, a lower starting dose is recommended.

Renal impairment: Initial dose should be reduced in patients with severe renal impairment, and upward titration should be at increased intervals.

Hepatic impairment: Initial dose should be reduced in patients with severe hepatic impairment, and upward titration, if necessary, should be at increased intervals.

Breast-feeding: Paroxetine is secreted in human breast milk; caution should be exercised when administered to nursing mothers.

(Continued on next page)

In Brief

INDICATIONS
Treatment of major depressive episodes in outpatients (antidepressant action in hospitalized depressed patients has not been adequately studied), panic disorder, and obsessive-compulsive disorder

CONTRAINDICATIONS
Concomitant use in patients taking MAO inhibitors

INTERACTIONS
Alcohol, cimetidine, cytochrome $P_{450}IID_6$, diazepam, digoxin, drugs highly bound to plasma proteins, lithium, MAO inhibitors, phenobarbital, phenytoin, procyclidine, propranolol, warfarin

ADVERSE EFFECTS
Associated with discontinuation of treatment: somnolence, insomnia, agitation, tremor, anxiety, nausea, diarrhea, dry mouth, vomiting, asthenia, abnormal ejaculation, sweating
Most common in controlled trials: asthenia, sweating, nausea, decreased appetite, somnolence, dizziness, insomnia, tremor, nervousness, ejaculatory disturbance and other male genital disorders
Frequent in controlled trials: chills, malaise, hypertension, syncope, tachycardia, edema, weight gain, weight loss, amnesia, CNS stimulation, impaired concentration, depression, emotional lability, vertigo, increased cough, rhinitis, pruritus
Infrequent: allergic reaction, carcinoma, face edema, moniliasis, neck pain, bradycardia, conduction abnormalities, abnormal electrocardiogram, migraine, peripheral vascular disorder, bruxism, dysphagia, eructation, gastritis, glossitis, increased salivation, mouth ulceration, rectal hemorrhage, anemia, leukopenia, lymphadenopathy, purpura, hyperglycemia, peripheraledema, thirst, arthralgia, arthritis, abnormal thinking, akinesia, ataxia, convulsion, depersonalization, hallucinations, hyperkinesia, hypertonia, incoordination, lack of emotion, manic reaction, paranoid reaction, asthma, bronchitis, dyspnea, epistaxis, hyperventilation, pneumonia, respiratory flu, sinusitis, acne, alopecia, dry skin, ecchymosis, eczema, furunculosis, urticaria, abnormality of accommodation, ear pain, eye pain, mydriasis, otitis media, taste loss, tinnitus, abortion, amenorrhea, breast pain, cystitis, dysuria, nocturia, polyuria, urethritis, incontinence, urinary retention, vaginitis
Rare: abscess, adrenergic syndrome, cellulitis, neck rigidity, pelvic pain, peritonitis, ulcer, angina pectoris, arrhythmia, atrial fibrillation, bundle branch block, cerebral ischemia, cerebrovascular accident, congestive heart failure, low cardiac output, myocardial infarction, myocardial ischemia, pallor, phlebitis, pulmonary embolus, supraventricular extrasystoles, thrombosis, varicose veins, vascular headache, ventricular extrasystoles, bloody diarrhea, bulimia, colitis, duodenitis, esophagitis, fecal impactions, fecal incontinence, gastritis, gastroenteritis, gingivitis, hematemesis, hepatitis, ileus, jaundice, melena, peptic ulcer, salivary gland enlargement, stomach ulcer, stomatitis, tongue edema, tooth caries, diabetes mellitus, hyperthyroidism, hypothyroidism, thyroiditis, abnormal erythrocytes, eosinophilia, leukocytosis, lymphedema, abnormal lymphocytes, lymphocytosis, microcytic anemia, monocytosis, normocytic anemia, alkaline phosphatase increased, bilirubinemia, dehydration, gout, hypercholesteremia, hypocalcemia, hypoglycemia, hypokalemia, hyponatremia, arthrosis, bursitis, myositis, osteoporosis, tetany, abnormal electroencephalogram, abnormal gait, antisocial reaction, choreoathetosis, delirium, delusions, diplopia, dysarthria, dyskinesia, dystonia, euphoria, fasciculation, grand mal convulsion, hostility, hyperalgesia, hypokinesia, hysteria, increased libido, manic-depressive reaction, meningitis, myelitis, neuralgia, neuropathy, nystagmus, paralysis, psychosis, psychotic depression, increased reflexes, stupor, withdrawal syndrome, carcinoma of lung, hiccups, lung fibrosis,

(Continued on next page)

DOSAGE

Adults: *Usual initial dose*—Administer as single daily dose, usually in the morning. Recommended initial dose is 20 mg/d. In clinical trials, patients took 20 to 50 mg/d. Some patients not responding to 20-mg dose may benefit from dose increases in 10 mg/d increments to 50 mg/d. Dose changes should occur at intervals of at least 1 week. *Patients with severe renal or hepatic impairment*—10 mg/d; increase as indicated, but do not exceed 40 mg/d. *Maintenance therapy*—Evidence is available to indicate how long treatment should last. Systematic evaluation indicates an average of about 30 mg for maintenance purposes.
Elderly: Follow adult dose for patients with severe renal or hepatic impairment.
Children: Not recommended.

ADVERSE EFFECTS *(CONTINUED)*

angioedema, contact dermatitis, erythema nodosum, maculopapular rash, photosensitivity, skin discoloration, skin melanoma, amblyopia, cataracts, conjunctivitis, corneal ulcer, exophthalmos, eye hemorrhage, glaucoma, hyperacusis, breast atrophy, breast carcinoma, breast neoplasm, female lactation, hematuria, kidney calculus, kidney pain, mastitis, nephritis, oliguria, prostatic carcinoma, vaginal moniliasis

PHARMACOKINETICS AND PHARMACODYNAMICS

Onset of action: about 10 d
Plasma half-life: 1 h
Bioavailability: completely absorbed from GI tract; distributed throughout body, including CNS, with only 1% remaining in plasma; plasma levels increase in elderly patients
Metabolism: extensively metabolized in the liver to inactive metabolites, primarily polar and conjugated products of oxidation and methylation
Excretion: two thirds excreted in urine (2% as parent compound and 62% as metabolites); one third excreted in feces (mostly metabolites and < 1% as parent compound)
Protein binding: 93%–95% plasma protein bound
Renal impairment: increased plasma concentrations in renal impairment; mean plasma concentrations in patients with creatinine clearance below 30 mL/min about four times greater than in normal volunteers
Hepatic impairment: patients with hepatic functional impairment had about twofold increase in plasma concentrations

PROLONGED USE

Efficacy in maintaining antidepressant response for ≤ 1 y was demonstrated in controlled trial; nevertheless, physicians who elect to use drug for extended periods should periodically reevaluate long-term usefulness.

OVERDOSAGE

No deaths have been reported following acute overdose. Symptoms include nausea, vomiting, drowsiness, sinus tachycardia, and dilated pupils. There have been no reports of ECG abnormalities, coma, or convulsions.
Treatment should consist of establishing and maintaining an airway and ensuring adequate oxygenation and ventilation. There are no specific antidotes. Gastric evacuation should be performed. Supportive care with frequent monitoring of vital signs and careful observation is indicated. Forced diuresis, dialysis, hemoperfusion, and exchange transfusion are unlikely to be of benefit. The physician should contact the local poison control center for additional information on the treatment of any overdose of this drug.

AVAILABILITY

Tablets—20 mg in 30s, 100s, and UD 100s; 30 mg in 30s

SERTRALINE HYDROCHLORIDE

(Zoloft)

Sertraline HCl is an antidepressant believed to act by inhibiting CNS neuronal uptake of serotonin. The drug is not believed to have any significant affinity for adrenergic cholinergic, dopaminergic, histaminergic, serotoninergic, GABA, or benzodiazepine receptors.

SPECIAL PRECAUTIONS

During premarketing testing, hypomania or mania occurred in about 0.4% of patients treated with sertraline. Activation of mania or hypomania also has been reported in a small proportion of patients with major affective disorder.

Significant weight loss results.

Sertraline has not been evaluated in patients with seizure disorder. The drug therefore should be introduced with care in epileptic patients.

There have been rare reports of altered platelet function or abnormal results from laboratory studies in patients taking sertraline. Although there have been reports of abnormal bleeding or purpura in several patients taking this drug, it is unclear whether it had a causative role.

SPECIAL GROUPS

Elderly: The pattern of adverse reactions in the elderly has been similar to that of younger patients in clinical trials. Sertraline plasma clearance in elderly patients can, however, be about 40% lower than in younger individuals. Decreased clearance of the major metabolite may occur in older men but does not occur in older women.

Renal impairment: Any effect on patients with impaired renal function has not been determined.

Hepatic impairment: Use of sertraline in patients with liver disease must be approached with caution. If the drug is administered, a lower or less frequent dose should be used.

Breast-feeding: It is unknown whether, and in what amount, sertraline or its metabolites are excreted in human breast milk. Caution should be exercised when administered to nursing mothers.

In Brief

INDICATIONS
Treatment of major depressive episode in outpatients

CONTRAINDICATIONS
MAO inhibitors

INTERACTIONS
Alcohol, atenolol, cimetidine, CNS active drugs, drugs highly bound to plasma proteins, hypoglycemic drugs

ADVERSE EFFECTS
Frequent: dry mouth, increased sweating, palpitations, chest pain, headache, dizziness, tremor, paresthesia, hypoesthesia, twitching, hypertonia, rash, nausea, diarrhea, constipation, dyspepsia, vomiting, flatulence, anorexia, abdominal pain, increased appetite, fatigue, fever, back pain, thirst, flushing, myalgia, insomnia, sexual dysfunction, somnolence, agitation, nervousness, anxiety, yawning, sexual dysfunction (female), impaired concentration, menstrual disorder, rhinitis, pharyngitis, abnormal vision, tinnitus, taste perversion, micturition frequency, micturition disorder

Less frequent: mydriasis, increased saliva, cold clammy skin, postural dizziness, hypertension, hypotension, edema, periorbital edema, peripheral ischemia, syncope, tachycardia, ataxia, abnormal coordination, abnormal gait, hyperesthesia, hyperkinesia, migraine, nystagmus, vertigo, acne, alopecia, pruritus, dry skin, dysphagia, eructation, malaise, rigors, weight decrease, weight increase, lymphadenopathy, purpura, arthralgia, arthrosis, dystonia, muscle cramps, muscle weakness, abnormal dreams, aggressive reaction, amnesia, apathy, delusion, depersonalization, depression, emotional lability, euphoria, hallucination, neurosis, paranoid reaction, suicide ideation, suicide attempt, teeth-grinding, abnormal thinking, dysmenorrhea, intermenstrual bleeding, bronchospasm, coughing, dyspnea, epistaxis, abnormal accommodation, conjunctivitis, diplopia, earache, eye pain, xerophthalmia, dysuria, nocturia, polyuria, urinary incontinence

Rare: pallor, precordial chest pain, substernal chest pain, aggravated hypertension, myocardial infarction, varicose veins, local anesthesia, coma, convulsions, dyskinesia, dysphonia, hyporeflexia, hypotonia, ptosis, dermatitis, erythema, multiforme, abnormal hair texture, hypertrichosis, photosensitivity reaction, follicular rash, skin discoloration, abnormal skin odor, urticaria, diverticulitis, fecal incontinence, gastritis, gastroenteritis, glossitis, gum hyperplasia, hemorrhoids, hiccups, melena, hemorrhagic peptic ulcer, proctitis, stomatitis, tenesmus, tongue edema, tongue ulceration, enlarged abdomen, halitosis, otitis media, aphthous stomatitis, anemia, anterior chamber eye hemorrhage, dehydration, hypercholesterolemia, hypoglycemia, hernia, hysteria, somnambulism, withdrawal syndrome, amenorrhea, balanoposthitis, breast enlargement, female breast pain, leukorrhea, menorrhagia, atrophic vaginitis, bradypnea, hyperventilation, sinusitis, stridor, abnormal lacrimation, photophobia, visual field defect, oliguria, renal pain, urinary retention

(Continued on next page)

DOSAGE

Adults: Use lower or less frequent doses in patients with hepatic impairment. Use care in patients with renal impairment until adequate studies have been completed. *Initial treatment*—50 mg once daily. In clinical trials, patients responded to doses ranging from 50 to 200 mg/d. Dose changes should not occur at intervals less than 1 week and should be longer for patients with hepatic impairment. Do not exceed 200 mg/d. *Maintenance*—Dose needed is undetermined because there are insufficient data to indicate whether dose needed to maintain or sustain euthymia and that needed to induce remission are identical.

Elderly: Same as adult dosage.

Children: Not recommended.

PHARMACOKINETICS AND PHARMACODYNAMICS

Onset of action: about 14 d but may take as long as 4–6 wk

Peak plasma levels: about 8.4 h

Plasma half-life: about 26 h for parent drug; 62–104 h for metabolite *N*-desmethylsertraline

Bioavailability: completely absorbed

Metabolism: extensive first-past metabolism with principal initial pathway being *N*-demethylation. Parent drug and *N*-desmethylsertraline undergo oxidative deamination and subsequent reduction, hydroxylation, and glucuronide conjugation.

Excretion: about 40%–45% recovered in urine, with no unchanged drug detectable; about 40%–45% recovered in feces, including 12%–14% unchanged drug

Effect of food: AUC slightly increases with food but C_{max} 25% greater and time to reach peak plasma concentration decreases

Protein binding: highly bound (98%) to serum proteins

Renal impairment: pharmacokinetics in patients with significant renal dysfunction not determined

Hepatic impairment: liver impairment can affect elimination; half-life prolonged in study of patients with mild stable cirrhosis with mean of 52 h

PROLONGED USE

Effectiveness for use > 16 wk has not been evaluated systematically in controlled trials; physicians who elect to use this drug for extended periods should periodically reevaluate long-term usefulness.

OVERDOSAGE

About 80 reports of nonfatal acute overdoses have been reported. Symptoms include somnolence, nausea, vomiting, tachycardia, ECG changes, anxiety, and dilated pupils. Although there were no reports of death when sertraline has been taken alone, there have been deaths reported when taken in combination with other drugs or alcohol. Therefore, any overdose should be treated aggressively.

An airway should be established and maintained and adequate oxygenation and ventilation ensured. Activated charcoal may be as or more effective than emesis or lavage. Cardiac and vital signs monitoring is recommended, along with general symptomatic and supportive measures. There are no antidotes. Forced diuresis, dialysis, hemoperfusion, and exchange transfusion are probably not beneficial. The physician should contact a poison control center before treating an overdose with this drug.

AVAILABILITY

Tablets—50 and 100 mg in 50s

BUPROPION HYDROCHLORIDE

(Wellbutrin)

Bupropion HCl is an antidepressant of the aminoketone class and is chemically unrelated to tricyclic, tetracyclic, or other known antidepressant agents. Its structure closely resembles that of diethylpropion; it is related to the phenylethylamines. The drug does not inhibit MAO and only weakly blocks neuronal uptake of epinephrine, serotonin, and dopamine. Although its mechanism of action is not known, it is presumed to be mediated by noradrenergic or dopaminergic mechanisms.

SPECIAL PRECAUTIONS

Bupropion is associated with seizures; the incidence may exceed that of other marketed antidepressants by as much as fourfold. The risk of seizure appears to be strongly associated with dose and predisposing factors. Sudden and large increments in dose may contribute to increased risk. Although many seizures occur early in the course of treatment, some seizures may occur after several weeks at a fixed dose. History of head trauma or prior seizure, CNS tumor, concomitant mediations that lower seizure threshold, and other significant predisposing factors were present in about half of the patients experiencing seizures.

A substantial proportion of patients experience some degree of increased restlessness, agitation, anxiety, and insomnia, especially shortly after initiation of treatment.

Patients have been reported to show a variety of neuropsychiatric symptoms, including delusions, hallucinations, psychotic episodes, confusion, and paranoia.

The drug can precipitate manic episodes in patients with bipolar manic depression during the depressed phase of illness and may activate latent psychosis in other susceptible patients.

A weight loss of more than 5 lb occurred in 28% of patients; this incidence is about double that seen in comparable patients treated with tricyclics. If weight loss is a major presenting sign of a patient's depressive illness, the anorectic or weight-reducing potential of bupropion should be considered.

The possibility of suicide attempt is inherent in depression and may persist until significant remission occurs. Prescriptions should be written for the smallest number of tablets consistent with good patient management.

No clinical experience establishes the safety of bupropion in patients with a recent history of myocardial infarction or unstable heart disease. Care should be exercised if the drug is used in these patients.

In Brief

INDICATIONS
Treatment for depressed inpatients and outpatients

CONTRAINDICATIONS
Patients with seizure disorder. Patients with current or prior diagnosis of bulimia or anorexia nervosa. Concurrent administration of MAO inhibitor without at least 14 days between discontinuing an MAO inhibitor and initiating treatment with bupropion. Known hypersensitivity to bupropion and patients taking any other medication that contains bupropion.

INTERACTIONS
No systematic data have been collected on the consequences of concomitant administration of bupropion and other drugs. Animal data suggest that the drug may induce drug-metabolizing enzymes, which may be of potential clinical importance because the blood levels of coadministered drugs may be altered. Because the drug is metabolized extensively, coadministration of other drugs may affect its clinical activity. Concurrent administration of bupropion and agents that lower seizure threshold should be undertaken only with extreme caution.

ADVERSE EFFECTS
Frequent: edema, nonspecific rashes, nocturia, ataxia, incoordination, seizure, myoclonus, dyskinesia, dystonia, mania or hypomania, increased libido, hallucination, decrease in sexual function, depression, stomatitis, flu-like symptoms
Infrequent: chest pain, ECG abnormalities, shortness of breath or dyspnea, alopecia, dry skin, gynecomastia, dysphagia, thirst disturbance, liver damage or jaundice, vaginal irritation, testicular swelling, urinary tract infection, painful erection, retarded ejaculation, mydriasis, vertigo, dysarthria, memory impairment, depersonalization, psychosis, dysphoria, mood instability, paranoia, formal thought disorder, frigidity, toothache, bruxism, gum irritation, oral edema, bronchitis, visual disturbance, nonspecific pain
Rare: flushing, pallor, phlebitis, myocardial infarction, change in hair color, hirsutism, acne, glycosuria, hormone level change, rectal complaints, colitis, GI bleeding, intestinal perforation, stomach ulcer, dysuria, enuresis, urinary incontinence, menopause, ovarian disorder, pelvic infection, cystitis, dyspareunia, painful ejaculation, lymphadenopathy, anemia, pancytopenia, musculoskeletal chest pain, EEG abnormality, abnormal neurologic exam, impaired attention, sciatica, aphasia, suicidal ideation, glossitis, epistaxis, respiratory rate or rhythm disorder, pneumonia, pulmonary embolism, diplopia, body odor, surgically related pain, infection, medication reaction
Causal relationship unknown: orthostatic hypotension, third-degree heart block, esophagitis, hepatitis, syndrome of inappropriate antidiuretic hormone secretion, ecchymosis, leukocytosis, leukopenia, arthralgia, myalgia, muscle rigidity, fever, rhabdomyolysis, coma, delirium, dream abnormalities, paresthesia, unmasking of tardive dyskinesia, Steven-Johnson syndrome, angioedema, exfoliative dermatitis, urticaria, tinnitus

PHARMACOKINETICS AND PHARMACODYNAMICS
Onset of action: ≤ 4 wk
Peak plasma levels: 2 h followed by biphasic decline
Plasma half-life: 8–24 h with average half-life of second (postdistribution) phase of 14 h; steady-state half-life, 21 h
Bioavailability: absolute bioavailability has not been determined because an IV formulation for human use is not available. It appears likely, however, that only a small proportion of an orally administered dose reaches systemic circulation intact. The absolute bioavailability in animals (rats and dogs) is 5%–20%.

(Continued on next page)

(Continued on next page)

SPECIAL GROUPS

Children: Safety and efficacy for use in children younger than 18 years have not been established.

Elderly: Drug has not been systematically evaluated. In general, older patients are known to metabolize drugs more slowly and to be more sensitive to the anticholinergic, sedative, and cardiovascular side effects of antidepressants. Clinical trials showed no difference between these patients and younger ones.

Renal impairment: Initial doses in patients with renal impairment should be reduced because the drug and its metabolites may accumulate in these patients beyond concentrations expected in patients without renal impairment. The patient should be closely monitored for possible toxic effects and elevated blood and tissue levels of drug and metabolites.

Hepatic impairment: Although scattered abnormalities in liver function tests were detected in patients participating in clinical trials, there is no clinical evidence that the drug acts as a hepato-toxin in humans. Initial doses in patients with hepatic impairment should be reduced because the drug and its metabolites may accumulate in these patients beyond concentrations expected in patients without hepatic impairment. The patient should be closely monitored for possible toxic effects of elevated blood and tissue levels of drug and metabolites.

Pregnancy: Category B drug. No adequate and well-controlled studies in pregnant women. Use during pregnancy only if clearly needed. The effect on labor and delivery in humans is unknown.

Breast-feeding: Because of the potential for serious adverse reactions in nursing infants, a decision should be made whether to discontinue nursing or discontinue the drug, taking into account the importance of the drug to the mother.

DOSAGE

Adult: Use with caution and at reduced doses in patients with cardiovascular, hepatic, or renal impairment. It is particularly important to administer bupropion in a manner most likely to minimize risk of seizure. Do not exceed dose increases of 100 mg/d in a 3-day period. Gradual escalation also is important to minimize agitation, motor restlessness, and insomnia often seen during the initial days of treatment. If necessary, these effects can be managed by temporary reduction of dose or short-term administration of an intermediate to long-acting sedative-hypnotic. No single dose should exceed 150 mg. Administer three times daily, preferably with at least 6 hours between successive doses. Normal adult dose is 300 mg/d given three times daily. Dosing should begin at 200 mg/d, given as 100 mg twice a day. Based on clinical response, dose can be increased to 300 mg/d no sooner than 3 days after beginning therapy. An increase in dose up to 450 mg/d given in divided doses of not more than 150 mg each can be considered for patients in whom no clinical improvement is noted after several weeks of treatment at 300 mg/d. Dosing above 300 mg/d can be accomplished using the 75-mg or 100-mg tablets. The 100-mg tablets must be administered four times daily with at least 4 hours between successive doses not to exceed 150 mg in a single dose. Discontinue in patients who do not demonstrate an adequate response after an appropriate period of 450 mg/d. For maintenance, use the lowest dose that maintains remission.

Elderly: Use adult dose with caution and constant monitoring.

Children: Not recommended.

PHARMACOKINETICS AND PHARMACODYNAMICS
(CONTINUED)

Metabolism: extensively metabolized in the liver. Several metabolites are pharmacologically active, but their potency and toxicity relative to bupropion have not been fully characterized; however, because of their longer elimination half-lives, plasma concentrations of at least two known metabolites are much higher than plasma concentration of bupropion. Plasma and urinary metabolites so far identified include biotransformation products formed through reduction of the carbonyl group or hydroxylation of the tert-butyl group of bupropion. Four basic metabolites have been identified: erythro- and threo-amino alcohols, erythro-amino diol, and a morpholinol metabolite.

Excretion: eliminated in kidneys with 87% of dose recovered in urine and 10% recovered in feces; 0.5% excreted unchanged

Protein binding: *in vitro* tests show that bupropion is 80% or more bound to human albumin at plasma concentrations up to 800 micromolar (200 µg/mL)

Renal impairment: elimination of major metabolites may be affected by reduced renal function

Hepatic impairment: preliminary results of comparative single-dose pharmacokinetic study in normal versus cirrhotic patients indicated that half-lives of the metabolites were prolonged by cirrhosis and the metabolites accumulated to levels two to three times normal; elimination of major metabolites may be affected by reduced hepatic function because they are moderately polar compounds and are likely to undergo conjugation in the liver prior to urinary excretion

PROLONGED USE

Effectiveness in use for > 6 wk has not been systematically evaluated in controlled trials; physicians who elect to use bupropion for extended periods should periodically reevaluate the long-term usefulness of the drug for individual patients.

OVERDOSAGE

There has been limited clinical experience. Thirteen overdoses occurred during clinical trials. Twelve patients recovered without significant sequelae. Another patient experienced a grand mal seizure and recovered without further sequelae. Seizure was reported in about one third of all cases that have been reported since clinical trials. Other serious reactions reported include hallucinations, loss of consciousness, and tachycardia. Fever, muscle rigidity, rhabdomyolysis, hypotension, stupor, coma, and respiratory failure have been reported when bupropion was part of multiple overdoses. Deaths associated with overdoses of the drug alone have been reported rarely. Multiple uncontrolled seizures, bradycardia, cardiac failure, and cardiac arrest prior to death were reported.

Hospitalization is advised following suspected overdose. If the patient is conscious, vomiting should be induced by syrup of ipecac. Activated charcoal also can be administered every 6 h during the first 12 h after ingestion. Baseline laboratory values should be obtained. ECG and EEG monitoring also are recommended for the next 48 h. Adequate fluid intake should be provided. If the patient is stuporous, comatose, or convulsing, airway intubation is recommended before undertaking gastric lavage. There is no experience with the use of diuresis, dialysis, or hemoperfusion in the management of bupropion overdose. Because diffusion from tissue to plasma may be slow, dialysis may be of minimal benefit several hours after overdose. Further information about the treatment of overdoses can be obtained from a poison control center.

(Continued on next page)

57

BUPROPION HYDROCHLORIDE
(CONTINUED)

PATIENT INFORMATION
Physicians are advised to discuss the following issues with patients: (1) take bupropion in equally divided doses three or four times a day to minimize the risk of seizure; (2) the drug may impair ability to perform tasks requiring judgment or motor cognitive skills; (3) the use and cessation of use of alcohol may alter the seizure threshold and the consumption of alcohol should be minimized and, if possible, avoided completely; (4) inform the physician if you are taking or plan to take any prescription of over-the-counter drugs; and (5) notify the physician if you become pregnant or intend to become pregnant or intend to become pregnant during therapy.

AVAILABILITY
Tablets—75 and 100 mg in 100s

MIRTAZAPINE
(Remeron)

Mirtazapine has a tetracyclic chemical structure unrelated to SSRIs, tricyclics, and MAO inhibitors. It belongs to the iperazine-azepine group of compounds.

The mechanism of action is unknown. It is believed that mirtazapine enhances central noradrenergic and serotonergic activity by acting antagonistically at central presynaptic $\alpha 2$ adrenergic inhibitory autoreceptors and heteroreceptors. Mirtazapine is a potent antagonist of $5-HT_2$ and $5-HT_3$ receptors, with no significant affinity for the $5-HT_{1A}$ and $5-HT_{1B}$ receptors. It is a potent antagonist of histamine (H_1) receptors, a property that may explain its prominent sedative effects; a moderate peripheral $\alpha 1$ adrenergic antagonist, a property that may explain occasional orthostatic hypotension reported; and a moderate antagonist at muscarinic receptors, a property that may explain the relatively low incidence of anticholinergic side effects associated with its use.

SPECIAL PRECAUTIONS

In premarketing clinical trials, two (one with Sjögren's syndrome) out of 2796 patients treated developed agranulocytosis with associated signs and symptoms (eg, fever, infection), and a third patient developed severe neutropenia without any associated symptoms. All three patients recovered after treatment with remeron was stopped. If a patient develops a sore throat, fever, stomatitis, or other signs of infection, along with a low leukocyte count, treatment with remeron should be discontinued, and the patient should be closely monitored.

Mirtazapine should not be used in combination with an MAO inhibitor, or within 14 days of initiating or discontinuing therapy with an MAO inhibitor. Somnolence was reported in 54% of patients treated with mirtazapine, compared with 18% of those taking placebo and 60% of those taking amitriptyline. Dizziness was reported in 7% of patients treated with mirtazapine, compared with 3% of those taking placebo and 14% of those taking amitriptyline. Appetite increase was reported in 17% of patients treated with mirtazapine, compared with 2% of those taking placebo and 6% of those taking amitriptyline. In these same trials, weight gain of $\geq 7\%$ of body weight was reported in 7.5% of patients treated with mirtazapine, compared with 0% of those taking placebo and 5.9% of those taking amitriptyline.

Nonfasting cholesterol increases to $\geq 20\%$ above the upper limits of normal were observed in 15% of patients treated with mirtazapine, compared with 7% of those taking placebo and 8% of those taking amitriptyline. In these same studies, nonfasting triglyceride increases to ≥ 500 mg/dL were observed in 6% of patients treated with mirtazapine, compared with 3% of those taking placebo and 3% of those taking amitriptyline.

(Continued on next page)

In Brief

INDICATIONS
Treatment of depression. Its efficacy in hospitalized depressed patients has not been adequately studied

CONTRAINDICATIONS
Contraindicated in patients with a known hypersensitivity to mirtazapine

INTERACTIONS
Drugs affecting hepatic metabolism, drugs that are metabolized by or inhibit cytochrome P_{450} enzymes, alcohol, diazepam

ADVERSE EFFECTS
Associated with discontinuation treatment: somnolence and nausea

Most common in controlled trials: somnolence, increased appetite, weight gain, dizziness

Frequent: malaise, abdominal pain, acute abdominal syndrome, hypertension, vasodilatation, vomiting, anorexia, thirst, myasthenia, arthralgia, hypesthesia, apathy, depression, hypokinesia, vertigo, twitching, agitation, anxiety, amnesia, hyperkinesia, paresthesia, increased cough, sinusitis, pruritus, rash, urinary tract infection

Infrequent: chills, fever, face edema, ulcer, photosensitivity reaction, neck rigidity, neck pain, enlarged abdomen, angina pectoris, myocardial infarction, bradycardia, ventricular extrasystoles, syncope, migraine, hypotension, eructation, glossitis, cholecystitis, nausea and vomiting, gum hemorrhage, stomatitis, colitis, abnormal liver function tests, dehydration, weight loss, arthritis, tenosynovitis, ataxia, delirium, delusions, depersonalization, dyskinesia, extrapyramidal syndrome, increased libido, coordination abnormal, dysarthria, hallucinations, manic reaction, neurosis, dystonia, hostility, increased reflexes, emotional lability, euphoria, paranoid reaction, epistaxis, bronchitis, asthma, pneumonia, acne exfoliative dermatitis, dry skin, herpes simplex, alopecia, eye pain, abnormality of accommodation, conjunctivitis, deafness, keratoconjunctivitis, lacrimation disorder, glaucoma, hyperacusis, ear pain, kidney calculus, cystitis, dysuria, urinary incontinence, urinary retention, vaginitis, hematuria, breast pain, amenorrhea, dysmenorrhea, leukorrhea, impotence

Rare: cellulitis, chest pain substernal, atrial arrhythmia, bigeminy, vascular headache, pulmonary embolus, cerebral ischemia, cardiomegaly, phlebitis, left heart failure, tongue discoloration, ulcerative stomatitis, salivary gland enlargement, increased salivation, intestinal obstruction, pancreatitis, aphthous stomatitis, cirrhosis of liver, gastritis, gastroenteritis, oral moniliasis, tongue edema, goiter, hypothyroidism, lymphadenopathy, leukopenia, petechia, anemia, thrombocytopenia, lymphocytosis, pancytopenia, gout, increased serum glutamic-oxaloacetic transaminase (SGOT), abnormal healing, increased acid phosphatase, increased SGPT, diabetes mellitus, pathologic fracture, osteoporosis fracture, bone pain, myositis, tendon rupture, arthrosis, bursitis, aphasia, nystagmus, akathisia,

(Continued on next page)

58

SPECIAL PRECAUTIONS (CONTINUED)

Clinically significant ALT (serum glutamate pyruvate transaminase [SGPT]) elevations (≥ three times the upper limit of the normal range) were observed in 2.0% of patients treated with mirtazapine compared with 0.3% of those taking placebo and 2.0% of those taking amitriptyline. Most of these patients with ALT increases did not develop signs or symptoms associated with compromised liver function. Although some patients were discontinued for the ALT increases, in other cases the enzyme levels returned to normal despite continued treatment. Mirtazapine should be used with caution in patients with impaired hepatic function.

Mania or hypomania occurred in approximately 0.2% of mirtazapine-treated patients in United States studies.

Mirtazapine has not been systematically evaluated in patients with a recent history of myocardial infarction or other significant heart disease. It was not associated with clinically significant ECG abnormalities in placebo controlled trials. Mirtazapine was associated with significant orthostatic hypotension in early clinical pharmacology trials with normal volunteers. Orthostatic hypotension was infrequently observed in clinical trials with depressed patients. Mirtazapine should be used with caution in patients with known cardiovascular or cerebrovascular disease that could be exacerbated by hypotension (history of myocardial infarction, angina, or ischemic stroke) and conditions that predispose patients to hypotension (dehydration, hypovolemia, and treatment with antihypertensive medication).

SPECIAL GROUPS

Elderly: No unusual adverse age-related phenomena were identified in individuals 65 years of age or older. However, since pharmacokinetic studies revealed a decreased clearance in the elderly, caution is indicated in administering to elderly patients.

Renal impairment: Mirtazapine should be used with caution in patients with renal impairment.

Hepatic impairment: Mirtazapine should be used with caution in patients with hepatic impairment.

Pregnancy: There are no adequate and well-controlled studies in pregnant women. This drug should be used during pregnancy only if clearly needed.

Breast-feeding: It is not known whether mirtazapine is excreted in human breast milk. Because many drugs are excreted in human breast milk, caution should be exercised. Tablets are administered to nursing women.

DOSAGE

Adults: Start with 15 mg/d, administered in a single dose, preferably in the evening prior to sleep. Mirtazapine has an elimination half-life of approximately 20–40 hours; therefore, changes in dose should not be made for 1 to 2 weeks in order to allow sufficient time for therapeutic response to a given dose. Therapeutic dose ranges from 15–45 mg/d. *Maintenance*—There is no body of evidence available from controlled trials to indicate how long the depressed patient should be treated with mirtazapine. It is not known whether the dose of antidepressant needed to induce remission is identical to the dose needed to maintain euthymia.

ADVERSE EFFECTS (CONTINUED)

stupor, dementia, diplopia, drug dependence, paralysis, grand mal convulsion, hypotonia, myoclonus, psychotic depression, withdrawal syndrome, asphyxia, laryngitis, pneumothorax, hiccup, urticaria, herpes zoster, skin hypertrophy, seborrhea, skin ulcer, blepharitis, partial transitory deafness, otitis media, taste loss, parosmia, polyuria, urethritis, metrorrhagia, menorrhagia, abnormal ejaculation, breast engorgement, breast enlargement, urinary urgency

PHARMACOKINETICS AND PHARMACODYNAMICS

Peak plasma levels: approximately 2 h
Plasma half-life: 20–40 h; females of all ages exhibit significantly longer elimination half-lives than do males (mean half-life of 37 h for females vs 26 h for males)
Bioavailability: approximately 50%
Metabolism: mirtazapine is extensively metabolized after oral administration; major pathways of biotransformation are demethylation and hydroxylation followed by glucuronide conjugation; *in vitro* data from human liver microsomes indicate that whereas cytochromes 2D6 and 1A2 are involved in the formation of the 8-hydroxy metabolite of mirtazapine, cytochrome 3A is considered to be responsible for the formation of the N-desmethyl and N-oxide metabolite
Excretion: eliminated predominantly via urine (75%) and also in feces (15%)
Protein binding: approximately 85% bound to plasma proteins
Renal impairment: patients with moderate and severe renal impairment had reductions in mean clearance of mirtazapine of about 30% and 50%, respectively, compared with normal subjects; caution is indicated in administering mirtazapine to patients with compromised renal function
Hepatic impairment: the clearance of mirtazapine was decreased by approximately 30% in hepatically impaired patients compared with normal subjects; caution is indicated in administering mirtazapine to patients with compromised hepatic function
Elderly: clearance of mirtazapine was reduced in the elderly compared with the younger subjects; the differences were most striking in males, with a 40% lower clearance in elderly males compared with younger males; the clearance in elderly females was only 10% lower compared with younger females; caution is indicated in administering mirtazapine to elderly patients

PROLONGED USE

Use for > 6 wk has not been systematically evaluated in controlled trials; physicians who elect to use for extended periods should periodically evaluate the long-term usefulness.

OVERDOSAGE

In premarketing clinical studies, there were eight reports of mirtazapine overdose alone or in combination with other pharmacologic agents. The only drug overdose death was in combination with amitriptyline and chlorprothixene in a non–United States clinical study. Signs and symptoms reported in association with overdose included disorientation, drowsiness, impaired memory, and tachycardia. There were no reports of ECG abnormalities, coma, or convulsions following overdose with mirtazapine taken alone. There are no specific antidotes for overdose. If the patient is unconscious, establish and maintain an airway to ensure adequate oxygenation and ventilation. Gastric evacuation either by the induction of emesis, lavage, or both should be considered. Activated charcoal should also be considered for overdose. Cardiac and vital signs monitoring is recommended.

PATIENT INFORMATION

Patients should be warned about the risk of developing agranulocytosis and advised to contact their physician if they experience any indication of infection, such as fever, chills, sore throat, mucous membrane ulceration, or other possible signs of infection. Although patients may notice improvement with mirtazapine therapy in 1 to 4 weeks, they should be advised to continue therapy as directed. Patients should be advised to avoid alcohol while taking mirtazapine.

AVAILABILITY

Tablets—15 and 30 mg in 20s and 100s

NEFAZODONE HYDROCHLORIDE
(Serzone)

Nefazodone HCl has a chemical structure unrelated to selective serotonin reuptake inhibitors, tricyclics, tetracyclics, and MAO inhibitors. It is a synthetically derived phenylpiperazine. The mechanism of action of nefazodone is unknown. Preclinical studies have shown that nefazodone inhibits neuronal reuptake of both serotonin and norepinephrine.

SPECIAL PRECAUTIONS

Nefazodone should not be used in combination with an MAO inhibitor or within 14 days of discontinuing therapy with an MAO inhibitor. At least 1 week should elapse after stopping therapy with nefazodone and starting therapy with an MAO inhibitor.

There is some risk of postural hypotension in association with nefazodone.

During premarketing testing, hypomania or mania occurred in 0.3% of nefazodone-treated unipolar patients, compared with 0.3% of tricyclic- and 0.4% of placebo-treated patients.

Although priapism did not occur during pre-marketing experience with nefazodone, priapism has been reported with a structurally related drug, trazodone. If patients present with prolonged or inappropriate erections, they should discontinue therapy immediately.

Nefazodone has not been evaluated or used to any appreciable extent in patients with a recent history of myocardial infarction or unstable heart disease; such patients should be treated with caution. Evaluation of ECGs in patients who received nefazodone in 6- to 8-week, double-blind, placebo-controlled trials did not indicate that nefazodone is associated with the development of clinically important ECG abnormalities. However, sinus bradycardia was observed in 1.5% of nefazodone-treated patients compared with 0.4% of placebo-treated patients.

In patients with cirrhosis of the liver, the AUC values of nefazodone and hydroxynefazodone (HO-NEF) were increased by approximately 25%.

In Brief

INDICATIONS
Treatment of depression

CONTRAINDICATIONS
Coadministration of terfenadine, astemizole, or cisapride; contraindicated in patients with known hypersensitivity to nefazodone or other phenylpiperazine antidepressants.

INTERACTIONS
MAO inhibitors, drugs highly bound to plasma protein, CNS-active drugs, cardiovascular-active drugs that inhibit or are metabolized by cytochrome P_{450} isozymes

ADVERSE EFFECTS
Commonly observed in controlled clinical trials: somnolence, dry mouth, nausea, dizziness, constipation, asthenia, lightheadedness, blurred vision, confusion, abnormal vision
Frequent: gastroenteritis, dyspnea, bronchitis, eye pain, impotence
Infrequent: allergic reaction, malaise, photosensitivity reaction, face edema, hangover effect, enlarged abdomen, hernia, pelvic pain, halitosis, tachycardia, hypertension, syncope, ventricular extrasystoles, angina pectoris, dry skin, acne, alopecia, urticaria, maculopapular rash, vesiculobullous rash, eczema, eructation, periodontal abscess, abnormal liver function test results, gingivitis, colitis, gastritis, mouth ulceration, stomatitis, esophagitis, peptic ulcer, rectal hemorrhage, ecchymosis, anemia, leukopenia, lymphadenopathy, weight loss, gout, dehydration, increased lactic dehydrogenase, increased serum glutamic-oxaloacetic transaminase, increased serum glutamate pyruvate transaminase, arthritis, tenosynovitis, muscle stiffness, bursitis, vertigo, twitching, depersonalization, hallucinations, suicide attempt, apathy, euphoria, hostility, suicidal thoughts, abnormal gait, abnormal thinking, decreased attention, derealization, neuralgia, paranoid reaction, dysarthria, increased libido, suicide, myoclonus, asthma, pneumonia, laryngitis, voice alteration, epistaxis, hiccup, dry eye, ear pain, abnormality of accommodation, diplopia, conjunctivitis, mydriasis, keratoconjunctivitis, hyperacusis, photophobia, cystitis, urinary urgency, metrorrhagia, amenorrhea, polyuria, vaginal hemorrhage, breast enlargement, menorrhagia, urinary incontinence, abnormal ejaculation, hematuria, nocturia, kidney calculus
Rare: cellulitis, atrioventricular block, congestive heart failure, hemorrhage, pallor, varicose vein, glossitis, hepatitis, dysphagia, gastrointestinal hemorrhage, oral moniliasis, ulcerative colitis, hypercholesteremia hypoglycemia, tendinous contracture, hyperkinesia, increased salivation, cerebrovascular accident, hyperesthesia, hypotonia, ptosis, neuroleptic malignant syndrome, hyperventilation yawn, deafness, glaucoma, night blindness, taste loss, enlarged uterine fibroids, uterine hemorrhage, anorgasmia, oliguria

(Continued on next page)

SPECIAL GROUPS

Children: Safety and effectiveness in individuals younger than 18 years of age have not been established.

Elderly: Treatment should be initiated at half the usual dose in elderly patients, especially women, but the therapeutic dose range is similar in younger and older patients. No unusual adverse age-related phenomena were identified in elderly patients treated with nefazodone.

Hepatic impairment: Use cautiously.

Breast-feeding: It is not known whether Nefazodone or its metabolites are excreted in human breast milk. Because many drugs are excreted in human breast milk, caution should be exercised when nefazodone is administered to nursing women.

Pregnancy: There are no adequate and well-controlled studies in pregnant women. Nefazodone should be used during pregnancy only if the potential benefit to the mother justifies the potential risk to the fetus.

DOSAGE

Adults: The recommended starting dosage is 200 mg/d, administered in two divided doses (twice a day). Dose increases should be based on clinical response, and should occur in increments of 100–200 mg/d (on a twice-daily schedule), at intervals of at least 1 week. In controlled clinical trials, the effective dose range was generally 300–600 mg/d. *Maintenance*—Whether the dose of antidepressant needed to induce remission is identical to the dose needed to maintain euthymia is unknown. The safety of nefazodone in long-term use is supported by data from both double-blind and open-label trials involving more than 250 patients treated for at least one year.

Elderly: Treatment should be initiated at half the usual dose, but titration upward should take place over the same range as in younger patients.

PHARMACOKINETICS AND PHARMACODYNAMICS

Peak plasma levels: 1 h

Plasma half-life: 2–4 h

Bioavailability: rapidly and completely absorbed, but subject to extensive metabolism so that its absolute bioavailability is only about 20%, and variable

Metabolism: extensively metabolized after oral administration by dealkylation and aliphatic and aromatic hydroxylation

Excretion: less than 1% is excreted unchanged in urine

Effect of food: delays absorption and decreases bioavailability by 20%

Protein binding: at concentrations of 25–2500 ng/mL, extensively (> 99%) binds to human plasma proteins *in vitro*.

Elderly: after single doses of 300 mg, Cmax and AUC for nefazodone and HO-NEF were up to twice as high in older patients than in younger patients; however, with multiple doses, differences were much smaller (10%–20%)

Renal impairment: nefazodone plasma concentrations are not affected by different degrees of renal impairment

Hepatic impairment: with multiple doses, the AUC for nefazodone and HO-NEF at steady state were approximately 25% greater for patients with liver cirrhosis than for normal volunteers

PROLONGED USE

Use for > 6–8 wk has not been systematically evaluated in controlled trials. The physician who elects to use nefazodone for extended periods should periodically reevaluate the long-term usefulness.

OVERDOSE

There is very limited experience with nefazodone overdose. In premarketing clinical studies, there were seven reports of nefazodone overdose alone or in combination with other pharmacologic agents. None of the patients died. The amount of nefazodone ingested ranged from 1000 to 11,200 mg. Commonly reported symptoms included nausea, vomiting, and somnolence. Overdosage may cause an increase in incidence or severity of any of the reported adverse reactions. There is no specific antidote; treatment should be symptomatic and supportive in the case of hypotension or excessive sedation. Any patient suspected of having taken an overdose should have the stomach emptied by gastric lavage.

AVAILABILITY

Tablets—100, 150, 200, and 250 mg

TRAZODONE HYDROCHLORIDE

(Desyrel)

Trazodone HCl is an antidepressant chemically unrelated to tricyclic, tetracyclic, or other known antidepressant agents. It is a triazolopyridine derivative. Trazodone does not inhibit MOA and is devoid of amphetamine-like effects. The drug may inhibit serotonin uptake by brain cells, therefore increasing serotonin concentrations in the synapse. It also may cause changes in binding of serotonin to receptors. The drug causes moderate sedative and orthostatic hypotensive effects and slight anticholinergic effects.

SPECIAL PRECAUTIONS

Associated with the occurrence of priapism. In about one third of reported cases, surgical intervention was required, and in a portion of these cases, permanent impairment of erectile function or impotence resulted. Male patients with prolonged or inappropriate erections should immediately discontinue the drug and consult the physician.

Not recommended for use during the initial recovery phase of myocardial infarction. Also, caution should be used when administering the drug to patients with cardiac disease; such patients should be monitored. Recent clinical studies in patients with preexisting cardiac disease indicate that trazodone may be arrhythmogenic in some patients in that population.

The possibility of suicide in seriously depressed patients is inherent in the illness and may persist until significant remission occurs. Prescriptions should be written for the smallest number of tablets consistent with good patient management.

Hypotension, including orthostatic hypotension and syncope, has been reported in patients receiving trazodone. Concomitant administration of antihypertensive therapy may require reduction in the dose of the antihypertensive drug.

Little is known about the interaction between trazodone and general anesthetics; before elective surgery, trazodone should be discontinued for as long as clinically feasible.

The expected benefits of trazodone therapy should be weighed against the potential risk factors.

Occasional low white blood cell and neutrophil counts have been noted. These were not considered clinically significant and did not necessitate discontinuation of the drug; however, the drug should be discontinued in any patient whose white blood cell count or absolute neutrophil count falls below normal levels. White blood cell and differential counts are recommended for patients who develop fever and sore throat (or other signs of infection) during therapy.

Concurrent administration of trazodone and electroshock therapy should be avoided because of the absence of experience in this area.

In Brief

INDICATIONS
Treatment of depression in inpatient and outpatient settings and for depressed patients with and without prominent anxiety

CONTRAINDICATIONS
Known hypersensitivity to trazodone

INTERACTIONS
Digoxin, phenytoin. It is unknown whether interactions will occur between MAO inhibitors and trazodone. Because of the absence of clinical experience, if MAO inhibitors are discontinued shortly before or are to be given concomitantly with trazodone, therapy should be initiated cautiously with gradual increases in dose until optimum response is achieved.

ADVERSE EFFECTS
Clinical trial reports: skin condition or edema, blurred vision, constipation, dry mouth, hypertension, hypotension, shortness of breath, syncope, tachycardia and palpitations, anger or hostility, confusion, decreased concentration, disorientation, dizziness or lightheadedness, drowsiness, excitement, fatigue, headache, insomnia, impaired memory, nervousness, abdominal or gastric disorder, bad taste in mouth, diarrhea, nausea or vomiting, musculoskeletal aches and pains, incoordination, paresthesia, tremors, decreased libido, decreased appetite, red eyes, itching eyes, tired eyes, heavy head, malaise, nasal or sinus congestion, nightmares or vivid dreams, sweating and clamminess, tinnitus, weight gain, weight loss, akathisia, allergic reaction, anemia, chest pain, delayed urine flow, early menses, flatulence, hallucinations or delusions, hematuria, hypersalivation, hypomania, impaired speech, impotence, increased appetite, increased libido, increased urinary frequency, missed periods, muscle twitches, numbness, retrograde ejaculation
Postintroduction reports: agitation, alopecia, apnea, ataxia, breast enlargement or engorgement, diplopia, edema, extrapyramidal symptoms, grand mal seizures, hallucinations, hemolytic anemia, hyperbilirubinemia, leukonychia, jaundice, lactation, liver enzyme alterations, methemoglobinemia, nausea or vomiting, paresthesia, priapism, pruritus, psychosis, rash, stupor, inappropriate antidiuretic hormone syndrome, tardive dyskinesia, unexplained death, urinary incontinence, urinary retention, urticaria, vasodilation, vertigo, weakness, conduction block, orthostatic hypotension and syncope, palpitations, bradycardia, atrial fibrillation, myocardial infarction, cardiac arrest, arrhythmia, ventricular ectopic activity

PHARMACOKINETICS AND PHARMACODYNAMICS
Onset of action: range of 1–4 wk
Peak plasma levels: 1 h on empty stomach; 2 h when taken with food
Plasma half-life: initial half-life of 3–6 h followed by slower phase of 5–9 h
Bioavailability: well absorbed without selective localization in any tissue
Metabolism: extensively metabolized in the liver
Excretion: elimination is biphasic; less than 1% excreted unchanged in urine and feces
Effect of food: when taken shortly after ingestion with food there may be an increase in the amount of drug absorbed, a decrease in maximum concentration, and a lengthening in time to maximum concentration; elimination is unaffected by presence or absence of food

(Continued on next page)

SPECIAL GROUPS

Children: Safety and efficacy for use in children younger than 18 years have not been established.

Pregnancy: Category C drug. Trazodone has been shown to cause increased fetal resorption and other adverse effects on the fetus in two rat studies. There also was an increase in congenital anomalies in one of three rabbit studies. There are no adequate and well-controlled studies in pregnant women. Use during pregnancy only if the potential benefit justifies the potential risk to the fetus.

Breast-feeding: Trazodone or its metabolites have been found in the milk of lactating rats, suggesting that the drug may be secreted in human breast milk. Caution should be exercised when administered to nursing mothers.

DOSAGE

Adults: Initiate dose at a low level and increase gradually. Drowsiness may require administration of a major portion of the daily dose at bedtime or a reduced dose. Take shortly after a meal or light snack. Initial dose is 150 mg/d, which can be increased by 50 mg/d every 3 to 4 days. Maximum dose for outpatients should not exceed 400 mg/d in divided doses. Inpatients or more severely depressed individuals may be given up to but not in excess of 600 mg/d in divided doses. For maintenance, keep dose at lowest effective level. Once an adequate response has been achieved, the dose can be gradually reduced with subsequent adjustment depending on response.

Elderly: Same as Adults.

Children: Not recommended.

PROLONGED USE

Although there has been no systematic evaluation of the efficacy of trazodone beyond 6 wk, it is generally recommended that a course of antidepressant drug treatment be continued for several months

OVERDOSAGE

Death from overdose has occurred in patients ingesting trazodone and other drugs concurrently (alcohol, alcohol plus chloralhydrate plus diazepam, amobarbital, chlordiazepoxide, or meprobamate). The most severe reactions that have occurred with overdose of trazodone alone have been priapism, respiratory arrest, seizures, and ECG changes. Reactions reported most frequently have been drowsiness and vomiting. Overdose may cause an increase in incidence or severity of any of the reported adverse reactions.

There is no specific antidote. Treatment should be symptomatic and supportive in the case of hypotension or excessive sedation. Any patient suspected of having taken an overdose should have the stomach emptied by gastric lavage. Forced diuresis may be useful in facilitating elimination of the drug.

PATIENT INFORMATION

Because priapism has been reported, patients who develop prolonged or inappropriate penile erection should immediately discontinue the drug and consult with the physician. The drug can impair the mental or physical ability required for performing potentially hazardous tasks. It can enhance the response to alcohol, barbiturates, and other CNS depressants. Patients should be advised to take each dose after a meal or light snack.

AVAILABILITY

Tablets—50 and 100 mg in 30s, 100s, 250s, 500s, 1000s, and UD 100s; 150 mg in 30s, 100s, 250s, 500s, and 1000s; 300 mg in 100s

VENLAFAXINE HYDROCHLORIDE

(Effexor)

Venlafaxine is an antidepressant chemically unrelated to tricyclics, tetracyclics, and other antidepressants. Venlafaxine is a potent inhibitor of neuronal serotonin and norepinephrine reuptake and a weak inhibitor of dopamine reuptake.

SPECIAL PRECAUTIONS

Venlafaxine treatment may be associated with sustained increases in blood pressure. It is recommended that patients have regular monitoring of blood pressure; patients who experience a sustained increase in blood pressure should have their dose reduced or discontinue treatment. Anxiety, insomnia, and weight loss have been reported. During phase 2 and 3 trials, hypomania or mania occurred. During premarketing testing, seizures were reported in 0.26% of patients. Most occurred in patients receiving doses of 150 mg/d or less. It should be used carefully with patients with a history of seizures and discontinued in any patient who develops seizures.

In Brief

INDICATIONS

Treatment of depression

CONTRAINDICATIONS

Known hypersensitivity to venlafaxine and concomitant administration with MAO inhibitors; should wait at least 7 days after discontinuing before starting an MAO inhibitor

INTERACTIONS

Drugs tightly bound to plasma proteins, lithium, diazepam, cimetidine, alcohol, drugs that metabolized cytochrome $P_{450}IID_6$ and drugs that inhibit its metabolism, MAO inhibitors

(Continued on next page)

VENLAFAXINE HYDEOCHLORIDE (CONTINUED)

SPECIAL GROUPS

Children: Safety and effectiveness < 18 y has not been established.

Elderly: No differences in safety or effectiveness for individuals 65 years and over. However, greater sensitivity in some older individuals cannot be ruled out. No dose adjustment is recommended for elderly patients.

Renal impairment: Total daily dose should be reduced by 25% in patients with mild to moderate renal impairment. It is recommended for patients undergoing hemodialysis that the dose be withheld until dialysis is completed (4 h).

Hepatic impairment: Total daily dose should be reduced by 50% in patients with moderate hepatic impairment.

Pregnancy: No well-controlled studies. Should be used only if clearly needed.

Breast-feeding: It is not known whether venlafaxine or its metabolites are excreted in human breast milk. Because many drugs are, caution should be exercised when used by nursing woman.

DOSAGE

The recommended starting dose is 75 mg/d, administered in two or three divided doses, taken with food. The dose may be increased up to 275 mg/d. When increasing the dose, increments of up to 75 mg/d should be made at intervals of no less than 4 days. In outpatient settings, the therapeutic dose for moderately depressed patients was no more than 225 mg/d, but more severely depressed inpatients responded to a mean dose of 350 mg/d.

(Continued on next page)

ADVERSE EFFECTS

Associated with discontinuation treatment: somnolence, insomnia, dizziness, nervousness, dry mouth, anxiety, nausea, abnormal ejaculation, headache, asthenia, sweating

Most common in controlled trials: asthenia, sweating, nausea, constipation, anorexia, vomiting, somnolence, dry mouth, dizziness, nervousness, anxiety, tremor, blurred vision, abnormal ejaculation or orgasm, impotence

Frequent: accidental injury, malaise, neck pain, migraine, dysphagia, eructation, ecchymosis, emotional lability, trismus, vertigo, bronchitis, dyspnea, abnormal vision, ear pain, anorgasmia, dysuria, hematuria, metrorrhagia, impaired urination, vaginitis

Infrequent: enlarged abdomen, allergic reaction, cyst, face edema, generalized edema, hangover effect, hernia, intentional injury, moniliasis, neck rigidity, overdose, substernal chest pain, pelvic pain, photosensitivity reaction, suicide attempt, angina pectoris, extrasystoles, hypotension, peripheral vascular disorder (mainly cold feet or hands), syncope, thrombophlebitis, colitis, tongue edema, esophagitis, gastritis, gastroenteritis, gingivitis, glossitis, rectal hemorrhage, hemorrhoids, melena, stomatitis, stomach ulcer, mouth ulceration, anemia, leukocytosis, leukopenia, lymphadenopathy, lymphocytosis, thrombocythemia, thrombocytopenia, abnormal leukocyte count, increased alkaline phosphatase, increased creatinine, diabetes mellitus, edema, glycosuria, hypercholesteremia, hyperglycemia, hyperlipemia, hyperuricemia, hypoglycemia, hypokalemia, increased SGOT, thirst, arthritis, arthrosis, bone pain, bone spurs, bursitis, joint disorder, myasthenia, tenosynovitis, apathy, ataxia, circumoral paresthesia, CNS stimulation, euphoria, hallucinations, hostility, hyperesthesia, hyperkinesia, hypertonia, hypotonia, incoordination, increased libido, manic reaction, myoclonus, neuralgia, neuropathy, paranoid reaction, psychosis, psychotic depression, sleep disturbance, abnormal speech, stupor, torticollis, asthma, chest congestion, epistaxis, hyperventilation, laryngismus, laryngitis, pneumonia, voice alteration, acne, alopecia, brittle nails, contact dermatitis, dry skin, herpes simplex, herpes zoster, maculopapular rash, urticaria, cataract, conjunctivitis, corneal lesion, diplopia, dry eyes, exophthalmos, eye pain, otitis media, parosmia, photophobia, subconjunctival hemorrhage, taste loss, visual-field defect, albuminuria, amenorrhea, kidney calculus, cystitis, leukorrhea, menorrhagia, nocturia, bladder pain, breast pain, kidney pain, polyuria, prostatitis, pyelonephritis, pyuria, urinary incontinence, urinary urgency, enlarged uterine fibroids, uterine hemorrhage, vaginal hemorrhage, vaginal moniliasis

Rare: appendicitis, body odor, carcinoma, cellulitis, halitosis, ulcer, withdrawal syndrome, arrhythmia, first-degree atrioventricular block, bradycardia, bundle branch block, mitral valve disorder, mucocutaneous hemorrhage, sinus bradycardia, varicose vein, cheilitis, cholecystitis, cholelithiasis, hematemesis, gum hemorrhage, hepatitis, ileitis, jaundice, oral moniliasis, intestinal obstruction, proctitis, increased salivation, soft stools, tongue discoloration, esophageal ulcer, peptic ulcer syndrome, goiter, hyperthyroidism, hypothyroidism, basophilia, cyanosis, eosinophilia, abnormal erythrocytes, alcohol intolerance, bilirubinemia, increased blood urea nitrogen, gout, hemochromatosis, hyperkalemia, hyperphosphatemia, hypoglycemic reaction, hyponatremia, hypophosphatemia, hypoproteinemia, increased SGPT, uremia, osteoporosis, akathisia, akinesia, alcohol abuse, aphasia, bradykinesia, cerebrovascular accident, loss of consciousness, delusions, dementia, dystonia, hypokinesia, neuritis, nystagmus, increased reflexes, seizures, atelectasis, hemoptysis, hypoxia, pleurisy, pulmonary embolus, sleep apnea, increased sputum, skin atrophy, exfoliative dermatitis, fungal dermatitis, lichenoid dermatitis, hair discoloration, eczema, furunculosis, hirsutism, skin hypertrophy, leukoderma, psoriasis, pustular rash, vesiculobullous rash, blepharitis, chromatopsia, conjunctival edema, deafness, glaucoma, hyperacusis, keratitis, labyrinthitis, miosis, papilledema, decreased pupillary reflex, scleritis, abortion, breast engorgement, breast enlargement, calcium crystalluria, female lactation, hypomenorrhea, menopause, prolonged erection, uterine spasm

PHARMACOKINETICS AND PHARMACODYNAMICS

Plasma half-life: venlafaxine, 3–7 h after acute administration; major metabolite O-desmethylvenlafaxine (ODV), 9–13 h after acute administration

Bioavailability: 100% from a tablet when compared with an oral solution

Metabolism: extensively absorbed in the liver to ODV; based on mass balance studies, at least 92% of a single dose is absorbed

Excretion: approximately 87% of a single dose is recovered in the urine within 48 h as either unchanged venlafaxine (5%), unconjugated ODV (29%), conjugated ODV (26%), or other minor inactive metabolites (27%); renal elimination of venlafaxine and ODV is the primary route of excretion

Effect of food: no significant effect on the absorption of venlafaxine or on the formation of ODV

Protein binding: not highly bound to plasma proteins; protein binding–induced drug interactions with venlafaxine are not expected

Renal impairment: venlafaxine elimination was prolonged by about 50% and clearance was reduced by 24%, and ODV elimination was prolonged by 40% in renally impaired patients compared with normal subjects; in dialysis patients, venlafaxine elimination was prolonged by about 180% and clearance was reduced by 57%, and ODV elimination was prolonged by 142% and clearance was reduced by 56% compared with normal subjects; a large degree of intersubject variability was noted

Hepatic impairment: venlafaxine elimination was prolonged by about 30% and clearance decreased by about 50% in cirrhotic patients; ODV elimination was prolonged by about 60% and clearance decreased by about 30% in cirrhotic patients compared with normal subjects; a large degree of intersubject variability was noted ; patients with more severe cirrhosis had a more substantial decrease in venlafaxine clearance (about 90%) compared with normal subjects

PROLONGED USE

Effectiveness of use for > 4–6 wk has not been systematically evaluated in controlled trials; physicians who elect to use venlafaxine for extended periods should periodically reevaluate long-term usefulness of the drug for patients.

OVERDOSAGE

In premarketing studies, there were 14 reports of acute overdose either alone or in combination with other drugs or alcohol. The majority of the reports involved the total dose no more than several-fold higher than the usual therapeutic dose. All 14 patients recovered. In postmarketing experience, venlafaxine taken alone has not been associated with lethal overdose. However, fatal reactions have been reported in patients taking overdoses of venlafaxine in combination with alcohol or other drugs. To manage overdose, ensure an adequate airway, oxygenation, and ventilation. Monitoring of cardiac rhythm and vital signs is recommended. Use of activated charcoal, induction of emesis, or gastric lavage should be considered. Forced diuresis, dialysis, hemoperfusion, and exchange transfusion are not likely to be of benefit. No specific antidotes are known.

AVAILABILITY

Tablets—25, 37.5, 50, 75, and 100 mg in 100s

Antimanic Agents

Charles L. Bowden

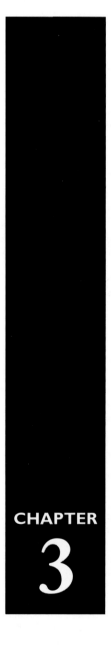

Antimanic drugs are indicated for the treatment of acute manic episodes in patients with bipolar disorder and the prevention of new episodes of mania, and possibly depression, during extended treatment. Manic episodes vary in severity from mild, or hypomanic, episodes to severe episodes with psychotic symptoms and near complete functional impairment. These agents, alone or in combination with adjunctive drugs, are indicated in the spectrum of manic episodes. Each of the three drugs (lithium, valproate, carbamazepine) for which substantial evidence of efficacy exists differs in functional chemical class, known effects on central nervous system (CNS) activity, and adverse effects. Therefore, effective use of these drugs requires knowledge of the unique characteristics of each (Table 3-1).

EFFICACY AND USE

The efficacy of antimanic drugs is best established for alleviating acute manic episodes. When used as monotherapy, 50% to 70% of acutely manic patients have moderate or greater improvement within 3 weeks. When antimanic agents are combined with one another or adjunctive medications are used for impaired sleep or psychotic symptoms, response rates increase in 70% to 80% of patients. Lithium, one of only two FDA-approved drugs for this condition, has been used and studied for more than 25 years. The divalproex form of valproate, which was recently approved by the FDA for the treatment of mania, and carbamazepine have been used less extensively and for a shorter time; therefore, more information regarding benefits and liabilities is available for lithium. Studies of prophylactic efficacy are more difficult to interpret, although there is evidence that each of the drugs provides some protection against recurrences. A discrepancy exists between studies of lithium from 25 to 30 years ago, which generally report substantial protection against relapse, and more recent studies, which indicate low rates of protection for mania and depression [1,2]. Clinical experience suggests that patients with milder episodes of manic behavior, as seen in hypomania or bipolar II disorder and cyclothymia, are responsive to these agents, although no prospective, randomized data are available.

Manic symptomatology encompasses a broad spectrum of psychopathology. Recent data indicate that for divalproex and lithium, symptoms that are specific to mania (*eg*, elation, grandiosity, speeded thought) show greater acute improvement than do symptoms that, although characteristic of mania, are not limited to that disorder (*eg*, motor restlessness, irritability) [3].

MODE OF ACTION

The modes of action responsible for the pharmacodynamic benefits of these drugs are not established. However, several neurochemical effects, unique for each of the three drugs, may be linked to clinical response. Lithium has several effects on intraneuronal signaling systems that are essential to the release of amine neurotransmitters, phosphorylation of proteins, and early gene activation, each of which could contribute to the episodic behavior expression of this disease [4]. Lithium blocks inositol phosphatase, altering levels of inositol, one of the two moieties that forms phosphatidylinositol, as well as levels of inositol triphosphate, which in turn triggers release of intracellular calcium [5]. Lithium causes a reduction in PKC [6].

Valproate augments γ-aminobutyric acid (GABA)–mediated activity in the CNS by inhibiting its degradation and enhancing its synthesis [7]. Pretreatment plasma levels of GABA were inversely related to response to divalproex (but not lithium) in acutely manic patients [8]. Additionally, divalproex significantly reduced plasma GABA, which was not significantly associated with magnitude of response in the patients studied. Valproate, as does lithium, causes a reduction in PKC activity or concentrations that are clinically effective, and the combination of lithium and valproate resulted in greater reduction of PKC than each drug did alone [9].

Carbamazepine has several neurochemical effects that could be associated with antimanic effects, but direct clinical support for such relationships is not available [10]. Carbamazepine inhibits sodium channel activation at the neuronal membrane, thus potentially stabilizing the membrane against wide voltage or agonist-induced changes. Carbamazepine also has reduced turnover of norepinephrine, although it is likely that this is an indirect pharmacodynamic effect [11]. Investigation of the mode of action of these agents has been hampered by the lack of animal models for mania and the inaccessibility of brain tissue in human studies. Most direct clinical studies of possible mechanisms have been in peripheral fluids and cells (eg, platelets), which although important, are limited in the conclusions that can be drawn.

Table 3-1. Factors Associated with Relatively Favorable Outcome with Antimanic Agents

Lithium
  Pure mania
  Few previous episodes
  Mild symptoms
  Previous good response to lithium
Valproate
  Elated (pure) mania
  Depressive (mixed) mania
  Rapid cycling*
  Lithium refractoriness
  Secondary mania*
Carbamazepine
  Lithium refractoriness
  Secondary mania*
  No family history of bipolar disorder*

*Soft evidence.

Valproate and carbamazepine also are effective as anticonvulsants. The mechanisms for the effectiveness of electroconvulsant therapy (ECT) as antimanic therapy may involve its anticonvulsant effects. This suggests that investigation of neuronal mechanisms associated with seizure development may help in understanding the pharmacodynamic effects of valproate, carbamazepine, and other antiepileptic drugs that may prove to be effective for alleviating mania.

PHARMACOKINETICS

Pharmacokinetic properties clinically are important for each of these agents. In the case of lithium, interaction with other monovalent cations (Na^+, K^+) can result in changes in Na^+, K^+, or lithium levels. Many drugs, especially nonsteroidal antiinflammatory drugs, excreted by the kidneys also interact with lithium, increasing lithium levels. Higher lithium levels and rapid rates of increase in levels are associated with more adverse effects. Therefore, loading dose strategies are not feasible for lithium. The slower rate of increase in lithium with sustained-release preparations would presumably be associated with less severe and less frequent side effects, although the question has not been studied. Renal concentrating impairment was less with sustained-release lithium than regular lithium carbonate [12]. Sustained-release preparations of lithium require once- or twice- daily dosing regimens. These may improve compliance without diminishing efficacy [13].

Valproate is highly protein bound. Therefore, it is subject to displacement by other protein-bound drugs or by a high-fat meal with a resultant increase in the free, active component of valproate. As total serum level rises above 100 μg/mL, the free component of valproate increases nonlinearly, which accounts in part for the greater frequency of adverse effects at total serum levels of 125 μg/mL or greater [11]. Although valproate's half-life is less than 24 hours (ie, 10–18 h), many patients are treated effectively with a single daily dosing schedule. In contrast to lithium, which has a large volume of distribution, the volume of distribution of valproate is small (0.1–0.5 L/kg). Valproate has mild hepatic oxidative enzyme-inhibiting properties because it is largely metabolized by glucuronidation.

The pharmacokinetic complexities of carbamazepine stem almost entirely from its strong enzyme-inducing properties, particularly of the P450 3A4 isoenzyme [14,15]. This effect is delayed and gradual, with full effects occurring a few days to a few months following initiation of treatment. Therefore, carbamazepine dosage usually will need to be increased from that initially effective to compensate for the increased carbamazepine clearance consequent to enzymatic induction. Similarly, a wide range of psychotropic and nonpsychotropic drugs that are oxidatively metabolized may be expected to have clinically significant reduction in plasma levels (50% or greater reductions) requiring either a corresponding increase in dosage or a change in treatment modality. In both instances, frequent plasma level monitoring of the drug is essential.

INDICATIONS

Recent studies provide useful direction regarding the clinical characteristics that portend response or nonresponse to each of these drugs. For lithium, acute response is better in patients with mania without concurrent depressive symptomatology [16,17]. Previous response to lithium is directly associated with response in a new manic episode [3]. Studies show that patients with a positive family history for bipolar disorder and several indices of less severe illness (eg, relatively few lifetime episodes, full resolution of symptoms between episodes, healthy profiles on psychologic testing) are likely to respond [18]. Patients with rapid cycling bipolar disorder have relatively poor response in acute and prophylactic treatment [19]. Patients with secondary and comorbid forms of bipolar disorder respond poorly to lithium [20]. The information on lithium suggests that the different forms or presentations of the illness elicit differences in response to lithium; treatment with lithium is suggested for patients with favorable characteristics and should be avoided in patients with characteristics associated with poor response.

For acute treatment of mania, valproate is equally effective in patients with and without concurrent depressive symptoms and in patients with and without rapid cycling variants [3]. Response is equally effective in patients previously responsive and nonresponsive to lithium [3,21]. An open study suggests equivalent prophylactic benefit for rapid cycling and nonrapid cycling patients, although many patients in the study also received other psychotropic drugs, including lithium [22]. Case report data suggest that valproate is relatively effective in some types of secondary mania and in patients with concurrent substance dependence [23–24]. These reports indicate that valproate is approximately equally effective in the various forms of bipolar disorder.

Carbamazepine has been less studied in relation to favorable indications. Most studies of carbamazepine in mania have been of patients previously nonresponsive to lithium, suggesting that lithium failure is either a favorable indicator or at least not an unfavorable prognostic indicator [24,25]. Patients without a family history of bipolar disorder may do relatively well. One prospective study indicated that patients with secondary mania responded better to carbamazepine than to lithium [19].

Because bipolar disorder most commonly has its onset in adolescence or the early 20s, and once present is chronic and recurrent, young and old patients should be studied. No placebo-controlled studies conducted with adolescents have been published for any of the three drugs. Open trials suggest that some adolescents respond to lithium, although response rates are estimated at 40% [26], possibly because adolescent mania often presents with mixed features [27]. Valproate has been effective in open trials [28]. Therefore, although it seems plausible to commence treatment promptly once bipolar disorder is diagnosed in adolescents, evidence of efficacy, tolerability, and optimal dosing strategies is inadequate.

Elderly patients are particularly susceptible to cognitive impairment and other toxicity from lithium, even at serum concentrations in the lower ranges considered therapeutic for younger patients. Similarly, valproate and carbamazepine are often less tolerated in the elderly. Thus, elderly patients warrant more frequent clinical and laboratory monitoring, with particular attention to pharmacokinetic issues and drug interactions of the specific drug, especially considering the greater likelihood of other medical disorders in the elderly.

Each of the drugs may increase risk of fetal abnormalities, particularly for the relatively rare Ebstein atresia with lithium and for neural tube defects with valproate and carbamazepine. Most women should discontinue these drugs during the first trimester of pregnancy, when teratogenic risk is present. Mood state improves during pregnancy in some women, and treatments without teratogenic potential are available (eg, ECT). Neuroleptic use during pregnancy has not been associated with an increased frequency of birth defects, although there has been relatively little experimental study of their possible teratogenicity.

PATIENT INFORMATION

Patients and involved family members need substantial information about bipolar disorder and its treatment. This will assist patients in identifying early signs of relapse and drug toxicity, understanding the role of stressors that may destabilize a controlled illness, and addressing issues of judgment and self-image, which may interfere with treatment compliance. Pamphlets, directed reading, and encouragement to participate in local chapter support groups of the National Depressive and Manic Depressive Association are helpful.

Lithium requires warning regarding the potentially lethal toxicity at plasma levels only 50% or so greater than required clinically. These warnings should emphasize the early signs, generally neuromuscular and cognitive impairment, of impending toxicity. Divalproex should be used with caution in patients with hepatic disease. Pharmacokinetic interactions with carbamazepine require close monitoring of serum levels of carbamazepine and the affected drugs when used concurrently. Carbamazepine has a small but definite risk of agranulocytosis. Carbamazepine should not be used with clozapine due to the risk of agranulocytosis from both drugs. Rashes are common with carbamazepine and can be severe; therefore, patients should be encouraged to contact the physician about all rashes, especially those that are painful or hemorrhagic. Severe adverse effects to any of the agents should generally preclude retreatment with the same medication, particularly in light of the increasing evidence for the effectiveness of valproate and the general evidence for the efficacy of carbamazepine.

ADVERSE EFFECTS

Adverse reactions occur in the majority of lithium-treated patients. Most adverse reactions in lithium are persistent and interfere with patient function or comfort. This contributes to high rates of poor compliance, a particularly difficult problem because of the importance of prophylactic use of mood stabilizers. Both the common and severe adverse reactions occur at serum levels at or close to that needed for therapeutic efficacy; therefore, relatively close monitoring analytically and clinically is necessary. For most patients, lithium is not associated with renal impairment other than reversible impairment of concentrating ability. A small percentage of patients develop progressive impairment, which can be monitored prophylactically by analysis of serum creatinine and creatinine clearance [29,30].

Divalproex and carbamazepine are often better tolerated than is lithium, but each is associated with adverse effects that can be functionally bothersome or potentially serious. At least some adverse effects to valproate are closely related to serum concentrations above 125 µg/mL [31]. Based on evidence from patients with epilepsy, carbamazepine's adverse effects appear to be more frequent at serum levels above 12 to 14 µg/mL. Agranulocytosis and dermatologic reactions from carbamazepine have not been related to serum levels (Table 3-2).

Table 3-2. Serum Level Clinical Response Relationship of Mood Stabilizers in Bipolar Disorder

Lithium	0.8—1.4 mEq/L*
Valproate	45—100, 125 µg/mL
Carbamazepine	Lower threshold for efficacy not established
	Upper threshold, 12—14 µg/L, associated with greater frequency of adverse effects

*Elderly patients may develop toxicity at levels substantially less than 1.4 mEq/L.

REFERENCES

1. Goldberg JF, Harrow M, Grossman LS: Course and outcome in bipolar affective disorder. *Am J Psychiatry* 1995, 152:379–384.

2. Gelenberg AJ, Kane JM, Keller MB, *et al.*: Comparison of standard and low serum levels of lithium for maintenance treatment of bipolar disorder. *N Engl J Med* 1989, 321:1489–1493.

3. Bowden CL, Brugger AM, Swann AC, *et al.*: Efficacy of divalproex vs lithium and placebo in the treatment of mania. *JAMA* 1994, 271:918–924.

4. Goodwin FK, Jamison KR: *Manic-Depressive Illness*. New York: Oxford University Press; 1990:22–49.

5. Jope RS, Song L, Kolasa K, *et al.*: Inositol trisphosphate, cyclic AMP, and cyclic GMP in rat brain regions after lithium and seizures. *Biol Psychiatry* 1992, 31:505–514.

6. Manji H, Potter WA, Lenox RH: Molecular targets for lithium's actions. *Arch Gen Psychiatry* 1995, 52:543.

7. Godin Y, Heiner L, Mark J, *et al.*: Effect of di-*N*-propyl-acetate, an antiepileptic compound, on GABA metabolism. *J Neurochem* 1969, 16:869–873.

8. Petty F, Rush AJ, Davis JM, *et al.*: Plasma GABA predicts acute response to divalproex in mania. *Biol Psychiatry* 1994, 37:593–683.

9. Chen G, Manji HK, Hawver DB, *et al.*: Chronic sodium valproate selectively decreases protein kinase C alpha and epsilon in vitro. *J Neurochem* 1994, 63:61–2364.

10. Post RM, Rubinow DR, Uhde TW, *et al.*: Effects of carbamazepine on noradrenergic mechanisms in affectively ill patients. *Psychopharmacology* 1985, 87:59–63.

11. Zaccara G, Messori A, Moroni F: Clinical pharmacokinetics of valproic acid. *Clin Pharmacokinet* 1988, 15:367–389.

12. Miller AL, Bowden CL, Plewes J: Lithium and impairment of renal concentrating ability. *J Affect Disord* 1985, 9:115–119.

13. Birch NJ, Grof P, Hullin RP, *et al.*: Lithium prophylaxis: proposed guidelines for good clinical practice. *Lithium* 1993, 4:225–230.

14. Eichelbaum M, Thomson T, Tyloring G: Carbamazepine metabolism in man: induction and pharmacogenic aspects. *Clin Pharmacokinet* 1985, 10:80–90.

15. Ketter TA, Jenkins JB, Schroeder DH, *et al.*: Carbamazepine but not valproate induces bupropion metabolism. *J Clin Psychopharmacol* 1995, 15:327–330.

16. Secunda S, Katz MM, Swann A, *et al.*: Mania: Diagnosis, state measurement and prediction of treatment response. *J Affect Disord* 1985, 8:113–121.

17. Prien RJ, Himmelhoch JM, Kupfer DJ: Treatment of mixed mania. *J Affect Disord* 1988, 15:9–15.

18. Grof E, Haag M, Grof P, *et al.*: Lithium response and the sequence of episode polarities: preliminary report on a Hamilton sample. *Prog Neuropsychopharmacol Biol Psychiatry* 1987, 11:199–203.

19. Dunner DL, Fieve RR: Clinical factors in lithium carbonate prophylaxis. Tranylcypromine versus imipramine in anergic bipolar depression. *Am J Psychiatry* 1991, 148:910–916.

20. Himmelhoch JM, Garfinkel ME: Sources of lithium resistance in mixed mania. *Psychopharmacol Bull* 1986, 22:613–620.

21. Pope HG, Jr, McElroy SL, Keck PE, Jr, Hudson JI: Valproate in the treatment of acute mania: a placebo-controlled study. *Arch Gen Psychiatry* 1991, 48:62–68.

22. Calabrese JR, Delucchi GA: Spectrum of efficacy of valproate in 55 patients with rapid-cycling bipolar disorder. *Am J Psychiatry* 1990, 147:431–434.

23. Sival RC, Haffmans PM, van Gent PP, van Nieuwkerk JF: The effect of sodium valproate on disturbed behavior in dementia. *J Am Geriatr Soc* 1994, 42:906–907.

24. Brady KT, Sonne S, Anton R, Ballenger JC: Valproic acid in the treatment of acute bipolar affective episodes complicated by substance abuse. *J Clin Psychiatry* 1995, 56:118–121.

25. Post RM, Uhde TW, Roy-Byrne PP, Joffe RT: Correlates of antimanic response to carbamazepine. *Psychiatry Res* 1987, 21:71–83.

26. Carlson GA, Davenport YB, Jamison K: A comparison of outcome in adolescent and late-onset bipolar manic-depressive illness. *Am J Psychiatry* 1977, 134:919–922.

27. Ryan ND, Puig-Antich J: Affective illness in adolescence. *American Psychiatric Association Annual Review*, vol 5. Edited by Hales RE, *et al.* Washington, DC: American Psychiatric Press; 1986:420–450.

28. Papatheodorou G, Kutcher SP: Divalproex sodium treatment in late adolescent and young adult acute mania. *Psychopharmacol Bull* 1993, 29:213–219.

29. Gitlin M: Lithium-induced renal insufficiency. *J Clin Psychopharmacol* 1993, 13:276–279.

30. Hetmar O, Brun C, Ladefoged J, *et al.*: Long-term effects of lithium on the kidney: functional-morphological correlations. *J Psychiatr Res* 1989, 23:285–297.

31. Bowden CL, Janicak PG, Orsulak P, *et al.*: Relation of serum valproate concentration to response in mania. *Am J Psychiatry* 1996, 153:765–770.

32. Ballenger JC, Post RM: Carbamazepine in manic-depressive illness: a new treatment. *Am J Psychiatry* 1980, 137:782–790.

33. Okuma T, Yamashita I, Takahashi R, *et al.*: Comparison of the antimanic efficacy of carbamazepine and lithium carbonate by double-blind controlled study. *Pharmacopsychiatry* 1990, 23:143–150.

34. Okuma T: Effects of carbamazepine and lithium on affective disorders. *Neuropsychobiology* 1993, 27:138–145.

35. Denicoff KD, Blake KD, Smith-Jackson EE, *et al.*: Depression. 1994, 2:95–104.

36. Post RM, Leverich GS, Rosoff AS, Altshuler LL: Carbamazepine prophylaxis in refractory affective disorders: a focus on long-term follow-up. *J Clin Psychopharmacol* 1990, 10:318–327.

37. Frankenburg FR, Tohen M, Cohen BM, *et al.*: Long-term response to carbamazepine. A retrospective study. *J Clin Psychopharmacol* 1988, 8:130–132.

38. Wilder BJ, Karas BJ, Penry JK, *et al.*: Gastrointestinal tolerance of divalproex sodium. *Neurology* 1983, 33:808–811.

39. Jeavons PM: Valproate: Toxicity. In *Antiepileptic Drugs*. Edited by Woodbury DM, *et al*, New York: Raven, 1982:601–619.

40. Pedersen B, Juuljensen P: Electroencephalographic alterations during intoxication with sodium valproate: a case report. *Epilepsia* 1984, 25:121–124.

41. Gourru JL: Intoxication aigue massive par le valproate de sodium [thesis]. Lyons, France; 1980.

42. Keck PE Jr, McElroy SL, Tugrul KC, Bennett JA: Valproate oral loading in the treatment of mania. *J Clin Psychiatry* 1993, 54:305–308.

43. Lambert PA, Venaud G: Comparative study of valpromide versus lithium in the treatment of affective disorders. *Nervure* 1992, 5:57–65.

CARBAMAZEPINE

(Tegretol)

Note: The following information is based primarily on the drug's disposition as an anticonvulsant agent. All information should be reviewed carefully to determine whether it pertains to doses used for antimanic treatment.

Carbamazepine is not FDA-approved for treating bipolar disorder; however, studies since 1980 indicate that similar percentages of acutely manic patients have moderate improvement with carbamazepine treatment as with lithium or valproate treatment [32,33]. Technical problems with the studies limit generalizability. Most studies have allowed extensive concurrent neuroleptic use, and the equivalence of the dose or serum level of the comparator drug in some studies has been unsatisfactory [33]. Carbamazepine is particularly effective in patients who have failed to respond to lithium and possibly in patients with secondary mania [22]. Carbamazepine is less effective for patients with rapid cycling illness courses [34,35]. It is effective as adjunctive therapy with lithium, valproate, and neuroleptics. Little data are available regarding maintenance therapy effectiveness, although some patients with initial positive responses relapse with continued treatment [36,37]. Carbamazepine is generally well tolerated. Initial obtundation and neuromuscular side effects often can be minimized by slow dosage escalation. Carbamazepine induces its own metabolism and the metabolism of many other oxidatively metabolized drugs; therefore, serum level monitoring during treatment stabilization is particularly important.

SPECIAL PRECAUTIONS

Aplastic anemia and agranulocytosis have been reported. Complete pretreatment hematologic testing should be obtained as a baseline. If a patient in the course of treatment exhibits low or decreased white blood cell or platelet counts, the patient should be monitored closely. Discontinuation of the drug should be considered if any evidence of significant bone marrow depression develops.

Before prescribing, physicians should be thoroughly familiar with the details of the prescribing information, particularly regarding use with other drugs, especially those that accentuate toxicity potential.

Severe dermatologic reactions, including toxic epidermal necrolysis (Lyell syndrome) and Stevens-Johnson syndrome, have been reported. A few fatalities have occurred.

Carbamazepine has mild anticholinergic activity; therefore, patients with increased intraocular pressure should be observed closely during therapy.

The relationship of this drug to tricyclic compounds increases the possibility of activation of latent psychosis.

Use with caution in patients with a mixed seizure disorder that includes atypical absence (petit mal) seizures, because carbamazepine has been associated with increased frequency of generalized convulsions in these patients.

Hyponatremia has been associated with carbamazepine use, either alone or in combination with other drugs.

SPECIAL GROUPS

Children: Safety and efficacy for use in children younger than 6 years have not been established.

Elderly: Confusion or agitation may occur more often.

Renal impairment: Therapy should be prescribed only after critical benefit-to-risk appraisal of patients with a history of renal damage. Baseline and periodic complete urinalysis and blood urea nitrogen (BUN) determination are recommended for patients with renal dysfunction.

(Continued on next page)

In Brief

INDICATIONS

Off-label: Treatment of mania and stabilization of mood in manic-depressive patients, especially those who cannot be controlled adequately with lithium salts.

CONTRAINDICATIONS

Patients with a history of previous bone marrow depression or with hypersensitivity to carbamazepine or tricyclic compounds. Before administration of carbamazepine, monoamine oxidase (MAO) inhibitors should be discontinued for a minimum of 14 d (or longer if the clinical situation permits).

INTERACTIONS

Erythromycin, cimetidine, propoxyphene, isoniazid or calcium channel blockers, lithium, oral contraceptives, MAO inhibitors, alcohol, acetaminophen, valproic acid, succinimides, posterior pituitary hormones, barbiturates, anticoagulants

ADVERSE EFFECTS

Dizziness, drowsiness, unsteadiness, nausea, vomiting, aplastic anemia, agranulocytosis, pancytopenia, bone marrow depression, thrombocytopenia, leukopenia, leukocytosis, eosinophilia, pruritic and erythematous rashes, urticaria, toxic epidermal necrolysis, Stevens-Johnson syndrome, photosensitivity reactions, alterations in skin pigmentation, exfoliative dermatitis, erythema multiforme and nodosum, purpura, aggravation of disseminated lupus erythematosus, alopecia, diaphoresis, congestive heart failure, edema, aggravation of hypertension, hypotension, syncope and collapse, aggravation of coronary artery disease, arrhythmias, primary thrombophlebitis, recurrence of thrombophlebitis, adenopathy, lymphadenopathy, myocardial infarction, abnormalities in liver function tests, cholestatic and hepatocellular jaundice, hepatitis, pulmonary hypersensitivity, urinary frequency, acute urinary retention, oliguria, azotemia, renal failure, impotence, albuminuria, glycosuria, elevated BUN and microscopic deposits in urine, testicular atrophy, disturbances of coordination, confusion, headache, fatigue, blurred vision, visual hallucinations, transient diplopia, oculomotor disturbances, nystagmus, speech disturbances, abnormal involuntary movements, peripheral neuritis and paresthesias, depression with agitation, talkativeness, tinnitus, hyperacusis, gastric distress, abdominal pain, diarrhea, constipation, anorexia, dry mouth and pharynx, cortical lens opacities, aching joints and muscles, leg cramps, fever, chills, and lupus erythematosus–like syndrome

PHARMACOKINETICS AND PHARMACODYNAMICS

Note: The following information is based on doses as anticonvulsant agent; plasma levels, half-life, and other kinetic parameters may vary with antimanic doses.

Onset of action: slow

Peak plasma levels: 4–5 h

Plasma half-life: initially, 25–65 h, then reduces to 12–17 h with repeated doses; half-life of 10,11-epoxide metabolite, 5–8 h

Bioavailability: about 70% for carbamazepine and 90% for 10,11-epoxide metabolite; absorbed slowly and erratically

Metabolism: carbamazepine may induce own metabolism; metabolized in liver to active metabolite, 10,11-epoxide; 10,11-epoxide metabolized further to inactive compounds

Excretion: metabolites excreted 28% through feces and 72% in urine; 3% unchanged; urinary products composed of hydroxylated and conjugated metabolites

Effect of food: none anticipated; drug taken with meals

Protein binding: about 74% plasma protein binding for carbamazepine and about 50% for 10,11-epoxide metabolite

Renal impairment: protein binding altered in patients with uremia; metabolism and excretion prolonged

(Continued on next page)

SPECIAL GROUPS (CONTINUED)

Hepatic impairment: Therapy should be prescribed only after critical benefit-to-risk appraisal of patients with a history of hepatic damage. Baseline and periodic evaluations of liver function must be performed during treatment. The drug should be discontinued immediately in cases of aggravated liver dysfunction or active liver disease.

Pregnancy: Category C drug. No adequate and well-controlled studies in pregnant women. Transplacental passage of drug is rapid (30–60 min); drug accumulates in fetal tissue with higher levels in the liver and kidneys than in the brain. Carbamazepine should be used during pregnancy only if potential benefit justifies potential risk to fetus. The effect of carbamazepine on human labor and delivery is unknown.

Breast-feeding: During lactation, concentration of carbamazepine in human breast milk is about 60% of the maternal concentration. Because of the potential for serious adverse reactions in nursing infants, a decision should be made whether to discontinue nursing or discontinue the drug, taking into account the importance of the drug to the mother.

DOSAGE

Adults: No information found on dosage for antimanic treatment (only for anticonvulsant therapy or for trigeminal neuralgia). Psychiatrists recommend similar dosage (400–1200 mg/d) and plasma concentrations (6–12 mg/mL) for patients with mania.

Children: Not recommended for children younger than 6 years. No information found on dosage as antimanic agent for children older than 6 years.

PHARMACOKINETICS AND PHARMACODYNAMICS (CONTINUED)

Hepatic impairment: protein binding altered in patients with cirrhosis of the liver; metabolism altered

PROLONGED USE

Periodic complete blood cell (CBC) and platelet counts, liver function studies, eye examinations, and urinalysis and BUN determinations are necessary.

OVERDOSAGE

Initial symptoms appear after 1 to 3 hours. Neuromuscular disturbances are most prominent. Cardiovascular disorders are generally milder, and severe cardiac complications occur only when very high doses have been ingested.

The prognosis in cases of severe poisoning depends on prompt elimination of the drug, which is achieved by inducing vomiting, irrigating the stomach, and taking appropriate steps to diminish absorption. If these measures cannot be implemented without risk on the spot, the patient should be transferred to the hospital, ensuring that vital functions are safeguarded. There is no specific antidote. Charcoal is effective for increasing the total body clearance of drug. Dialysis is indicated only in severe poisoning associated with renal failure. Replacement transfusion is indicated in severe poisoning in small children. If evidence of significant bone marrow depression develops, perform CBC, platelet, and reticulocyte counts and a bone marrow aspiration and trephine biopsy immediately. Fully developed aplastic anemia requires intensive monitoring and therapy.

PATIENT INFORMATION

Patients should be aware of the early toxic symptoms of a potential hematologic problem, such as fever, sore throat, ulcers in the mouth, easy bruising, or petechial or purpuric hemorrhage, and should be advised to report to the physician immediately if any such symptoms appear. Because dizziness and drowsiness may occur, patients should be cautioned about the hazards of operating machinery or engaging in potentially hazardous tasks.

AVAILABILITY

Tablets (chewable)—100 mg in 100s and UD 100s
Tablets—200 mg in 30s, 100s, 500s, 1000s, and UD 100s
Suspension—100 mg/5 mL with citrus-vanilla flavor in 450 mL

LITHIUM

(Eskalith CR, Lithonate, Litholoid)

Lithium is an efficacious mood stabilizer that revolutionized the treatment of bipolar disorder. It is relatively inexpensive, although the cost of monitoring the drug is higher than for valproate or carbamazepine. It is effective in elated or pure manic states. It reduces the rate of relapse during maintenance therapy, although the effect is principally on manic episodes [2]. Although recent studies indicate that several more severe or complicated forms of bipolar disorder may not respond as well to lithium, response is not negligible, and lithium as monotherapy or with valproate or carbamazepine should be considered a possible treatment for most patients with bipolar disorder. The adverse effects of lithium that may lead to poor compliance need to be monitored and reduced through dosage reduction, symptomatic therapy, or discontinuation of lithium.

In Brief

INDICATIONS

FDA-approved: Treatment of manic episodes of manic-depressive illness. Maintenance therapy prevents or diminishes the intensity of subsequent episodes in manic-depressive patients with a history of mania.

CONTRAINDICATIONS

Psoriasis

INTERACTIONS

Acetazolamide, carbamazepine, fluoxetine, haloperidol, loop diuretics, methyldopa, nonsteroidal antiinflammatory drugs, osmotic diuretics, theophyllines, thiazide diuretics, urinary alkalinizers, verapamil, iodide salts, neuromuscular blocking agents, phenothiazines, sympathomimetics, tricyclic antidepressants

(Continued on next page)

LITHIUM (CONTINUED)

SPECIAL PRECAUTIONS

The risk of lithium toxicity is very high in patients with significant cardiovascular disease, severe debilitation, and dehydration or sodium depletion and in patients receiving diuretics. Weekly serum lithium determinations are recommended until the serum level and the clinical condition of the patient are stabilized; hospitalization is necessary.

An encephalopathic syndrome characterized by weakness, lethargy, fever, tremulousness, confusion, extrapyramidal symptoms, leukocytosis, and elevated serum enzymes has occurred.

Because of the sedative effects, patients should use caution while performing potentially hazardous tasks.

Hypothyroidism occurs frequently with long-term lithium administration.

Because lithium decreases sodium resorption, sodium depletion could occur.

Laboratory tests, including serum creatinine, CBC, urinalysis, sodium and potassium testing, ECG, and thyroid function tests, should be done periodically.

SPECIAL GROUPS

Children: Safety and efficacy for use in children younger than 12 years have not been established.

Elderly: Decreased rate of excretion in the elderly contributes to a high incidence of toxic effects. Also, elderly patients often require lower lithium doses to achieve therapeutic serum levels. Use lower doses and monitor more frequently.

Renal impairment: Risk of lithium toxicity is very high in patients with significant renal disease. Acquired nephrogenic diabetes insipidus unresponsive to vasopressin has been associated with chronic lithium administration.

Pregnancy: Category D drug. Lithium crosses the placenta; serum concentration is equal in mother and fetus. Lithium may cause fetal harm; data suggest increases in cardiac anomalies and Ebstein anomaly. Lithium toxicity in newborns includes cyanosis, hypotonia, GI bleeding, cardiomegaly, bradycardia, thyroid depression, ECG abnormalities, and diabetes insipidus. Do not use in pregnancy, especially during the first trimester, unless potential benefits outweigh potential hazards.

Breast-feeding: Lithium is excreted in breast milk at about 40% concentration of maternal serum. Do not allow mother to nurse during lithium therapy except when potential benefits to mother outweigh possible hazards to infant.

DOSAGE

Adults: Use with extreme caution in patients with cardiovascular or renal disease. Individualize dosage according to serum levels and clinical response. Draw blood samples immediately before the next dose (8–12 h after previous dose) when lithium concentrations are relatively stable. Do not rely on serum levels alone. *Acute mania:* Optimum patient response is usually established and maintained with 600 mg three times daily or 900 mg twice daily for slow-release form. Such doses normally produce effective serum lithium levels ranging between 0.8 and 1.2 mEq/L. *Long-term use*—Desirable serum levels are 0.6 to 1.2 mEq/L. Doses vary, but 300 mg three to four times daily usually maintains this level. Monitor serum levels in uncomplicated cases on maintenance therapy during remission every 2 to 4 months.

Elderly: Use at lower doses and monitor frequently.

(Continued on next page)

ADVERSE EFFECTS

Arrhythmia, hypotension, peripheral circulatory collapse, bradycardia, sinus node dysfunction, reversible flattening of T waves, tremors, muscle hyperirritability, ataxia, choreoathetoid movements, blackout spells, epileptiform seizures, slurred speech, dizziness, vertigo, incontinence of urine or feces, somnolence, psychomotor retardation, restlessness, confusion, stupor, coma, acute dystonia, downbeat nystagmus, blurred vision, startled response, hypertonicity, hallucinations, poor memory, tongue movements, tics, tinnitus, cogwheel rigidity, anorexia, nausea and vomiting, diarrhea, dry mouth, gastritis, salivary gland swelling, abdominal pain, excessive salivation, flatulence, indigestion, albuminuria, oliguria, polyuria, glycosuria, decreased creatinine clearance, drying and thinning of hair, anesthesia of skin, chronic folliculitis, xerosis cutis, alopecia, exacerbation of psoriasis, acne, angioedema, euthyroid goiter or hypothyroidism, diffuse slowing of EEG, widening of frequency spectrum of EEG, potentiation of EEG, disorganization of background rhythm of EEG, fatigue, lethargy, sleepiness, dehydration, weight loss, transient scotomata, impotence, dysgeusia, tightness in chest, hypercalcemia, hyperparathyroidism, salty-taste thirst, swollen lips, swollen and painful joints, fever, polyarthralgia, dental caries, leukocytosis, headaches, diffuse nontoxic goiter, transient hyperglycemia, cutaneous ulcers, excessive weight gain, edematous swelling of ankles or wrists, thirst of polyuria, metallic taste, painful discoloration of fingers and toes, coldness of extremities

PHARMACOKINETICS AND PHARMACODYNAMICS

Onset of action: oral, 8 h; slow-release oral, 5–14 d
Peak plasma levels: 1–4 h
Plasma half-life: 24 h
Bioavailability: readily absorbed from GI tract; distribution approximates total body water; distribution across blood–brain barrier is slow, but CSF lithium level about 40% of plasma concentration
Metabolism: 80% of lithium resorbed in kidneys; lithium and sodium compete for reabsorption in proximal renal tubule
Excretion: about 95% eliminated by kidneys
Effects of food: absorption not significantly impaired by food
Protein binding: not protein bound
Renal impairment: renal clearance varies with age and renal dysfunction, elimination half-life prolonged

PROLONGED USE

Maintenance therapy for manic episodes and manic-depressive patients.

OVERDOSAGE

Toxic lithium levels are close to therapeutic. Likelihood of toxicity increases with increasing serum lithium levels. Early symptoms include diarrhea, vomiting, nausea, drowsiness, muscular weakness, and lack of coordination. More severe symptoms include giddiness, ataxia, blurred vision, tinnitus, vertigo, increasing confusion, slurred speech, blackouts, fasciculations, myoclonic twitching, choreoathetoid movements, urinary or fecal incontinence, agitation, hyperreflexia, hypertonia, and dysarthria. Severe toxicity symptoms involve multiple organs; seizures, arrhythmias, hypotension, peripheral vascular collapse, stupor, muscle group twitching, spasticity, and coma may occur.

Early symptoms of toxicity can be treated by dose reduction or cessation and resumption at lower dose after 24–48 h. In severe cases, eliminate the ion from the patient. Treatment is essentially the same as that used in barbiturate toxicity.

DOSAGE *(CONTINUED)*

Children: Safety and efficacy for children younger than 12 years have not been established. For adolescents, *see* adult dose.

Impaired renal function: Essentially all lithium is cleared by the kidneys. Impairment of urinary concentrating ability is because of interference with sleep due to frequent voiding. A small percentage of patients develop parenchymal renal impairment, evidenced by progressive impairment of creatinine clearance. Other mood-stabilizing drugs should be used in such patients.

PATIENT INFORMATION

Outpatients and their families should be warned that the patient must discontinue therapy and contact the physician if clinical signs of toxicity occur: diarrhea, vomiting, tremor, mild ataxia, drowsiness, or muscular weakness. Patients can take lithium immediately after meals or with food or milk to avoid stomach upset. Patients should be advised to drink 8–12 glasses of water or other liquid every day and to contact the physician if fever or diarrhea develops.

AVAILABILITY

Capsules—150 mg in 100s, 1000s, and UD 100s; 300 mg in 100s, 500s, 1000s, and UD 100s; 600 mg in 100s, 1000s, and UD 100s
Tablets—300mg in 100s, 1000s, and UD 100s (slow release); 300 mg in 100s, 1000s, and UD 100s (sustained release); 450 mg in 100s
Syrup—8 mEq/5 mL in 480 and 500 mL, 480 mL with raspberry flavor, and UD 5 and 10 mL.

DIVALPROEX SODIUM

(Depakote)

Divalproex sodium is FDA-approved for the treatment of mania. This 1995 approval was based on recent well-designed placebo-controlled studies that provide evidence for the efficacy of divalproex sodium in treatment of acute manic episodes [3,22]. Although divalproex sodium is equally effective as lithium, for patients with mixed mania and previous nonresponse to lithium, divalproex sodium may provide better results than lithium [3]. Divalproex sodium is generally well tolerated. Fewer gastrointestinal side effects occur with the divalproex formulation than with valproic acid [38]. Divalproex sodium may impair liver function, but this is rare in patients without prior hepatic disease or younger than 2 years. Although hyperammonemia occurs occasionally, it is rarely clinically significant. For patients older than 10 years with bipolar disorder, systematic repeated monitoring of hepatic laboratory tests or CBC is not indicated. For patients with liver disease or who develop hepatic or hematologic symptomatology during therapy with valproate, laboratory testing should be initiated and repeated periodically. Divalproex sodium appears to be relatively safe even with a large overdose. There are reports of the ingestion of 30,000 mg and 75,000 mg of valproate with recovery without sequelae [39]. One patient died following ingestion of valproate, which resulted in a serum level of 1970 mg [40,41]. Divalproex sodium may be administered in a loading dose (20 mg/kg/d) in acutely manic patients, and relief of manic symptoms occurs earlier than with lithium [42]. Maintenance phase effectiveness has been less extensively studied, although open randomized trials and a recent placebo-controlled comparison with lithium indicate somewhat better outcomes and a broader spectrum of efficacy with valproate than with lithium [22,43]. As with the other mood stabilizers, optimal control of bipolar symptomatology is often achieved by concurrent use with other mood stabilizers and adjunctive medications (eg, benzodiazepines for sleep, neuroleptics for psychotic symptomatology).

In Brief

INDICATIONS

FDA-approved: Treatment of mania associated with bipolar disorder
Off-label: Agitation and aggression, borderline personality disorder, panic attack, and post-traumatic stress disorders

CONTRAINDICATIONS

Patients with hepatic disease or significant hepatic dysfunction, known hypersensitivity to valproic acid derivatives

INTERACTIONS

CNS depressants, aspirin, carbamazepine, dicumarol, phenytonin, phenobarbital, primidone, phenytoin, conazepam, warfarin, anticoagulants, oral contraceptives

ADVERSE EFFECTS

Nausea, vomiting, indigestion, diarrhea, abdominal cramps, constipation, anorexia, increased appetite, tremor, hallucinations, ataxia, headache, nystagmus, diplopia, asterixis, dysarthria, dizziness, uncoordination, coma, encephalopathy, transient hair loss, skin rash, photosensitivity, generalized pruritus, erythema multiforme, Stevens-Johnson syndrome, epidermal necrolysis, emotional upset, depression, psychosis, aggression, hyperactivity, behavioral deterioration, musculoskeletal weakness, thrombocytopenia, petechiae, bruising, hematomas, frank hemorrhage, macrocytosis, hypofibrinogenemia, leukopenia, eosinophilia, anemia, bone marrow suppression, acute intermittent porphyria, hepatotoxicity, irregular menses, secondary amenorrhea, breast enlargement, galactorrhea, parotid gland, swelling, abnormal thyroid function tests, acute pancreatitis, hyperammonemia, hyponatremia, decreased carnitine concentrations, hyperglycemia, enuresis, hearing loss, edema of the extremities, fever, lupus erythematosus

(Continued on next page)

DIVALPROEX SODIUM (CONTINUED)

SPECIAL PRECAUTIONS

The frequency of adverse effects (particularly elevated liver enzymes) may be dose related. The benefit of improved manic control that may accompany any high doses should be weighed against the possibility of a greater incidence of adverse effects.

Because of reports of thrombocytopenia, inhibition of the secondary phase of platelet aggregation, and abnormal coagulation parameters, platelet counts and coagulation tests are recommended before initiating therapy and at periodic intervals. Patients receiving valproate derivatives should be monitored for platelet count and coagulation parameters. Evidence of hemorrhage, bruising, or disorder of hemostasis or coagulation is indication for reduction of dose or withdrawal of therapy.

Hyperammonemia with or without lethargy or coma has been reported and may be present in the absence of abnormal liver function tests. Asymptomatic elevations of ammonia are more common and when present, require more frequent monitoring. If clinically significant symptoms occur, the drug dose should be modified or discontinued. Because valproate derivatives may interact with antiepileptic drugs, periodic plasma concentration determinations of all drugs used are recommended during the early course of therapy.

SPECIAL GROUPS

Children: Use with caution in children younger than 2 years, because they are at greater risk for developing fatal hepatotoxicity.
Elderly: Geriatric patients should receive a lower daily dose because they may have increased free unbound levels of the drug in the serum.
Renal impairment: None observed.
Hepatic impairment: Hepatic failure resulting in fatalities has occurred in patients receiving these drugs. Caution should be observed when administering these drugs to patients with history of hepatic disease. Patients on multiple anticonvulsants, children, patients with congenital metabolic disorders, patients with severe seizure disorders accompanied by mental retardation, and patients with organic brain disease may be at particular risk. Liver function tests should be performed prior to therapy and at frequent intervals thereafter. Physicians should not, however, rely totally on serum biochemistry, because these tests may not be abnormal in all instances; instead, physicians also should consider the results of careful interim medical history and physical examination.
Pregnancy: Category D drug. According to published and unpublished reports, valproic acid derivatives can produce teratogenic effects in the offspring of women receiving the drug during pregnancy. Hepatic failure resulting in the death of newborns has been reported after use of valproic acid derivatives during pregnancy.
Breast-feeding: Valproate derivatives are excreted in breast milk. Concentrations in breast milk have been reported to be 1% to 10% of serum concentrations. It is unknown what effect this might have on nursing infants. Caution should be exercised when administering these drugs to nursing women.

DOSAGE

Adults: Usually stated at 250 mg three times daily with dosage adjustment as needed to provide a trough serum level of 45 to 125 mg/mL. Acutely manic patients have tolerated an intial loading dose of 20 mg/kg body weight daily. Maintenance dosage is similar to acute mania dosages, ranging from 1000 to 2500 mg/d for most patients.
Elderly: Owing to the possibility of higher percentages of the free or unbound form of valproate, dosing should be initiated more cautiously in these patients.
Children: Dosages and serum levels in adolescents have been similar to those reported in adults, although data are limited.

PHARMACOKINETICS AND PHARMACODYNAMICS

Note: The following information is based on doses as an anticonvulsant and a mood stabilizer; plasma levels, half-life, and other kinetic parameters may vary according to dose levels as antimanic agents.
Onset of action: rapid, with improvement in 2–7 d with adequate dosing.
Peak plasma levels: valproate, 1–4 h
Plasma half-life: 9–16 h (reduced in patients also taking anticonvulsant medication)
Bioavailability: 100%
Metabolism: metabolized in the liver; majority of the drug is converted to conjugate ester of glucuronic acid; mitochondrial metabolism accounts for the remainder; major metabolites are glucuronide conjugate, 2-propyl-3-keto-pentanoic acid, and 2-prophylhydroxypentanoic acids; other unsaturated metabolites reported
Excretion: almost no (1.8%) valproate excreted unchanged in urine and feces; primarily excreted in urine
Effect of food: food slows absorption process but not extent of absorption
Protein binding: about 93% plasma protein bound
Hepatic impairment: protein binding, drug clearance, distribution, and half-life altered with accumulation of drug and metabolites with prolonged therapy

PROLONGED USE

Periodic liver function studies, CBC and platelet counts, and physical examinations are necessary.

OVERDOSAGE

Overdose may result in somnolence, heart block, and deep coma. Fatalities have been reported.

Because valproate derivatives are absorbed rapidly, the benefit of gastric lavage or emesis varies with the time since ingestion. General supportive measures should be applied, particularly maintaining adequate urinary output. Naloxone has been reported to reverse the CNS-depressant effects of overdose of these drugs. Because naloxone could theoretically also reverse the antiepileptic effects of these drugs, it should be used with caution.

PATIENT INFORMATION

Because valproate derivatives may produce CNS depression, especially when combined with CNS depressants, patients should be advised not to engage in hazardous activities, such as driving an automobile or operating dangerous machinery, until it is known that they do not become drowsy from the drug. Patients should advise the physician immediately if they suspect they are pregnant or if any adverse side effects develop. Patients should not increase or decrease doses, including doses of other concomitant anticonvulsant drugs prescribed by the physician.

AVAILABILITY

Divalproex sodium
Sprinkle capsule—125 mg in 100s and Abbo-Pac (Abbott Laboratories, Abbott Park, IL) UD 100s
Tablets (delayed-release)—125 mg in 100s and Abbo-Pac UD 100s; 250 mg in 100s, 500s, and Abbo-Pac UD 100s; 500 mg in 100s, 500s, and Abbo-Pac UD 100s

Sedative-Hypnotics

Eric J. Heyer

David C. Adams

Sedative-hypnotic drugs produce states of antianxiety (anxiolytic), drowsiness, or sleep. In the past, an antianxiety effect sometimes was achieved by inducing sleepiness; however, some anxiolytic agents produce minimal sedation. Hypnotics, conversely, are designed specifically to produce sleep. Other drugs in this class achieve different pharmacologic states; some are used principally for this purpose and produce sedative-hypnotic effects secondarily.

ELECTROPHYSIOLOGIC, NEUROANATOMIC, AND NEUROCHEMICAL FACTORS ASSOCIATED WITH SLEEP

The electroencephalogram (EEG) associated with sleep states is generated from neurotransmitters located in specific areas of the brain. Many of the sedative-hypnotic drugs used therapeutically act on these specific transmitters and probably on others not yet identified.

The neurotransmitters associated with wakefulness include acetylcholine, glutamate, and norepinephrine [1]. Wakefulness is enhanced by histamine release from posterior hypothalamic neurons and other neurons containing neuropeptides (substance P, corticotropin-releasing factor, thyrotropin-releasing factor, and vasoactive intestinal peptide). Sleep arises not only from a decreased release of these neurotransmitters but also from an increase release of other transmitters, such as adenosine, γ-aminobutyric acid (GABA), serotonin, and a variety of peptides after activation of specific areas of the brain [2,3].

This simplified summary provides a menu of possible neurotransmitters involved in maintaining wakefulness or sleep. Each neurotransmitter has multiple receptor types. For example, it was believed that glutamate did not play a role in wakefulness because it was so short acting. However, with the discovery of metabotropic receptors, activation of glutamate receptors can produce long-lasting actions [4].

Sedative-hypnotic drugs may affect the state of consciousness, either by altering one of these neurotransmitter systems or by working through entirely different mechanisms. This effect may occur during nonrapid eye movement (NREM) or rapid eye movement (REM) sleep, during administration of the drug, and for some drugs, even after cessation.

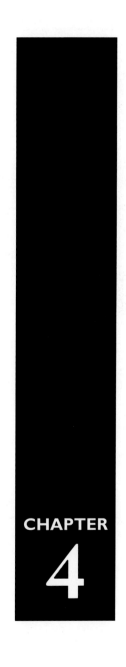

CHAPTER

4

CHEMICAL MODIFICATIONS

Although barbiturates were the first drugs to be used as sedative-hypnotics, they have been superseded by an array of nonbarbiturates. Currently, the benzodiazepines are the most commonly used sedative-hypnotic agents. Balancing the sedative (anxiolytic) and the hypnotic properties determines whether a specific benzodiazepine is used primarily as a sedative-hypnotic or an anxiolytic agent. Several new classes of drugs, such as imidazopyridines and azapirones, have fewer hypnotic effects but good anxiolytic properties. The sedative-hypnotic drugs can be divided into four groups (Table 4-1) [5].

Barbiturates

The barbiturates are derived from barbituric acid (2,4,6-trioxohexahydropyrimidine), which has no central nervous system (CNS) activity. Substitution of specific groups at certain locations on the parent compound confer distinct properties on the compound. For example, lipid solubility is one important factor in determining duration of action, latency of onset, and speed of metabolism. If the oxygen at C-2 is replaced by a sulfur atom, the compound becomes more lipid soluble and is referred to as a *thiobarbiturate* rather than an oxybarbiturate.

Thiobarbiturate compounds have a shorter duration of action, a faster onset of activity, and an increased rate of metabolism, which causes greater hypnotic activity. Addition of polar groups, such as ether, keto, hydroxyl, amino, and carboxyl groups, decreases lipid solubility and hypnotic activity [5].

Therapeutically useful barbiturates reversibly depress the CNS in a dose-dependent manner ranging from sedation to general anesthesia. However, some barbiturate compounds have convulsant properties. These have large aliphatic groups (more than 7 carbons) added at C-5 of the barbiturate backbone [5].

Benzodiazepines

The most commonly used sedative-hypnotic agents, in part because of their safety, are the benzodiazepines. They are all 1,4-benzodiazepines. Substitution of a halogen (diazepam, chlordiazepoxide, flurazepam, desmethyldiazepam, oxazepam, and lorazepam) or nitro (nitrazepam) at position 7 confers sedative-hypnotic activity. Most benzodiazepines contain a carboxamide group in the seven-membered ring. Triazolam and alprazolam have 1,2-annelation of a triazole ring.

Miscellaneous Drugs

Other sedative-hypnotic agents have been developed to minimize side effects; they all have similar pharmacologic properties to the barbiturates and benzodiazepines, including their side effects. These "nonbarbiturates" include piperidinediones (*eg*, glutethimide), propanediol carbamates, (*eg*, meprobamate), alcohols (*eg*, chloral hydrate, paraldehyde), and imidazopyridines (*eg*, zolpidem tartrate). Buspirone is the first of a new class of anxiolytics, called azapirones, which have very little hypnotic effect. Some β-blocking drugs are effective in anxiety states, presumably because they block the autonomic components.

Over-the-Counter Drugs

Many of the over-the-counter drugs are primarily antihistaminic agents. Their side effects arise primarily from their autonomic actions. However, they are safe because they do not produce general anesthesia or addiction.

EFFICACY AND USE

Anxiety

Anxiety is one of the most common of all symptoms in patients with generalized anxiety and panic from panic disorder. Treatment of anxiety is one of the most common indications for use of sedative-hypnotic agents. Because anxiety frequently is associated with psychiatric or medical disorders, other factors must be evaluated before prescribing these agents. The benzodiazepines are most commonly used for this symptom. There is no evidence that any particular benzodiazepine is better than another. The choice is frequently made based on pharmacokinetic considerations; agents with short half-lives are preferred for short-duration treatment, and agents with long half-lives are preferred for long-duration treatment. Although it is controversial and has not been incorporated into common practice, alprazolam may have antidepressant and anxiolytic efficacy [5].

Insomnia

Sleep disorders are common. Approximately 30% of all adults in the United States have difficulty sleeping. All of the barbiturates and benzodiazepines produce hypnotic effects. They prolong the NREM stage 2 phase of sleep and decrease REM sleep. The benzodiazepines may have less effect on REM sleep. These agents

Table 4-1. Sedative-Hypnotic Drugs

Barbiturates	Benzodiazepines	Miscellaneous Drugs	Nonprescription Sleep Aids
Long acting	*Long acting*	Aldehyde	*Antihistamines*
Phenobarbital (phenobarbital sodium)	Chlorazepate	Paraldehyde	Doxylamine
Intermediate acting	Diazepam	Azapirones	Diphenhydramine
Aprobarbital (aprobarbital sodium)	Flurazepam	Buspirone	
Butabarbital (butabarbital sodium)	Quazepam	*Chloral derivatives*	
Mephobarbital	*Intermediate acting*	Chloral hydrate	
Pentobarbital (pentobarbital sodium)	Chlordiazepoxide	*Imidazopyridines*	
Talbutal (talbutal sodium)	Estazolam	Zolpidem tartrate	
Short acting	Lorazepam	*Piperidine derivatives*	
Amobarbital (amobarbital sodium)	Temazepam	Glutethimide	
Secobarbital (secobarbital sodium)	*Short acting*	*Propanediol carbamate*	
Ultrashort acting	Midazolam	Meprobamate	
Thiopental sodium	Oxazepam	*Tertiary acetylenic alcohols*	
Methohexital sodium	Triazolam	Ethchlorvynol	

become less effective after about 1 week of use, and thus should not be used for long-term treatment of insomnia. Abnormalities of the sleep cycle are induced by these drugs, and after cessation of therapy, rebound is manifest as increased REM state with increased dreaming.

Epilepsy

Depending on their physiologic half-life, specific barbiturates or benzodiazepines can be used to stop status epilepticus or for chronic treatment of epilepsy. These drugs act as anticonvulsants through the inhibitory neurotransmitter $GABA_A$ channel, but they act on different components of the channel.

Anesthesia (Sedation and Amnesia)

Certain agents are used for induction or maintenance of general anesthesia. In addition, they may be used for conscious sedation during surgery not requiring general anesthesia. The barbiturates, although not analgesic, produce and may maintain a sufficient plane of anesthesia. On the other hand, the benzodiazepines cannot provide complete anesthesia. However, sedative-hypnotic agents are frequently used at induction of anesthesia to produce amnesia and a state of deep anesthesia sufficient for endotracheal intubation. The agents most commonly used are the benzodiazepines for amnesia and the barbiturates for a deep state of anesthesia.

Muscle Relaxation

Muscle relaxation varies from decreasing muscle tone or rigidity to complete paralysis. The barbiturates and benzodiazepines are used for this purpose because they augment the responsiveness of the intrinsic neurotransmitters, such as $GABA_A$. Barbiturates also attenuate the responsiveness of the excitatory neurotransmitter glutamate. Therefore, they should decrease muscle tone and rigidity by acting on motor-associated neurons in the spinal cord [6]. Benzodiazepines are used extensively for muscle relaxation with doses that do not depress cerebral activity.

Treatment of Withdrawal

After long-term use, the abrupt withdrawal of agents that depress the CNS, such as alcohol and sedative-hypnotics, may have severe and even life-threatening consequences. The benzodiazepines, such as chlordiazepoxide and diazepam, sometimes are used to decrease the intensity of the withdrawal and allow a gradual tapering of the addicting agent.

MODE OF ACTION AND PHARMACODYNAMICS

Sedative-hypnotic drugs, as typified by the barbiturates, depress CNS activity in a dose-dependent manner so that states of sedation and hypnosis are seen with low doses and general anesthesia at much higher doses.

The original description of the benzodiazepine receptor complex ($GABA_A$) indicated a close correlation between the affinities of benzodiazepines and their relative potencies as anxiolytics, anticonvulsants, and muscle relaxants. However, the mechanism by which the benzodiazepines provide sedation or hypnosis is poorly understood. When the benzodiazepine flurazepam was given in conjunction with the $GABA_A$ agonist muscimol, measures related to sleep were not altered, even when paroxysmal EEG activity related to seizures was produced [3]. Studies with the $GABA_A$ antagonists picrotoxin and bicuculline confirmed these results [3].

The $GABA_A$ receptor has two subtypes, I and II. The benzodiazepine quazepam and the imidazopyridine zolpidem bind relatively selectively to the type I receptors [3]. Type I receptors are associated with sleep maintenance and type II receptors with sleep induction. A

benzodiazepine may act on calcium-dependent functions, but this is controversial [7].

The barbiturates act on membranes in multiple ways. For example, at low concentrations, they increase the membrane sensitivity to GABA through the GABA-chloride iontophore, and at higher concentrations, they open chloride channels directly [8,9]. In addition, they directly inhibit the action of the excitatory amino acid, glutamate [6].

The membrane effects of many other drugs in this class are less understood. Buspirone interacts with several neurotransmitter systems. However, its clinically relevant effects are probably mediated through interactions with the serotonin 5-HT$_{1A}$ receptors, where it acts as a partial agonist [10]. Several H_1 histamine antagonists, such as diphenhydramine, promethazine, and hydroxyzine, produce sedation as a side effect of antihistaminic activity. The β-adrenergic antagonists treat anxiety characterized by somatic symptoms, but it is doubtful that they do more than control the peripheral symptoms.

PHARMACOKINETICS

Absorption and Distribution

The benzodiazepines and barbiturates are usually administered orally. Benzodiazepines are readily absorbed in the small intestine because they are weak bases and because of the alkaline environment of this region. In contrast, the barbiturates are weak acids and are absorbed in the acidic environment of the stomach. Both classes of drugs are administered parenterally. Once they are absorbed, their rapidity of action on the

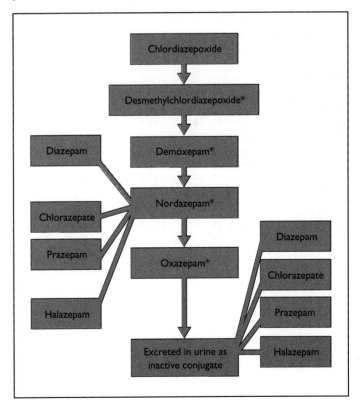

FIGURE 4-1.

Metabolic relationship among benzodiazepines. Modification or removal of a substituent of the diazepine ring, most commonly dealkylation, produces nordazepam, which is an active derivative and an intermediate for diazepam, chlorazepate, prazepam, halazepam, and chlordiazepoxide metabolism. Hydroxylation of nordazepam leads to oxazepam, which is an active derivative. Oxazepam, flurazepam, triazolam, alprazolam, and midazolam are hydroxylated and conjugated with glucuronic acid to be excreted. *Asterisks* indicate active metabolic products. (*From* Rall [5] and Dailey [10].)

CNS and their duration of action depend largely on lipid solubility. This redistribution away from the CNS accounts for the rapid termination of the pharmacologic responses of, many of these drugs. For example, the thiobarbiturates are lipid soluble; therefore, they are absorbed rapidly and distributed through the body, producing a short duration of effect.

Biotransformation and Metabolism

Many benzodiazepines undergo extensive biotransformation by dealkylation and conjugation reactions. Furthermore, dealkylation results in the formation of many pharmacologically active compounds (Fig. 4-1) [10]. Few serious toxicities are associated with administering benzodiazepines or barbiturates, even in patients with impaired liver function, but the dose should be reduced [5].

The bartiturates are organic acids; urine pH influences their rate of excretion. The more alkaline, the higher the concentration of ionized and nonresorbable drug in the urine.

Buspirone is absorbed well from the gastrointestinal system and is extensively metabolized, mainly by hepatic microsomal oxidation [11]. At least one metabolic product is biologically active [10].

	Benzodiazepines	Barbiturates	Azapirones	Imidazopyridines	OTC
Anxiety	++	++	++	+	+/--
Insomnia	++	++	--	++	+
Epilepsy/seizures	++	+++	--	--	--
Sedation/amnesia	+++	++	--	--	--
Anesthesia	--	++	--	--	--
Muscle relaxation	++	--	--	--	--

+,++, and +++ *Indicate appropriate uses for these drugs; more pluses mean the drug is more appropriate. OTC—nonprescription drugs obtained over the counter.*

PATIENT INFORMATION

Elderly patients may be sensitive to sedative-hypnotic drugs because of age-related changes in pharmacodynamics and pharmacokinetics, such as the volume of distribution (V_d) and the relative fraction of total body weight that is lipid. As a result, elderly people suffer an increased incidence of confusion, falls and resulting injuries (*eg*, subdural hematomas or hip fractures). Pharmacologic considerations have been studied in most detail with the benzodiazepines [11]. Hepatic biotransformation is the principal route of clearance for sedative-hypnotic drugs; therefore, the effect of age on drug metabolism capacity is important. Higher plasma concentrations are seen in the elderly with low-clearance drugs, such as some benzodiazepines (triazolam and midazolam) and the azapirones (buspirone). In addition, the same plasma concentration may have a more profound pharmacologic effect because of age-related changes in the brain. Triazolam is especially likely to alter the mental state of elderly patients [12].

Many of these issues also are a concern for children who have different pharmacokinetic and pharmacodynamic considerations. This is because the volume of distribution of the drugs and lipid component of body weight differ from those of adults.

SPECIAL GROUPS

Race: Generally effective regardless of race

Children: Routine use of this class of drugs is not recommended in children; however, in some circumstances, they can be used effectively, especially for amnesia after induction of anesthesia. Some of these drugs (estazolam, flurazepam, lorazepam, temazepam, triazolam, quazepam) are not recommended for use in children. Some of these drugs (chlordiazepoxide, diazepam) are used for children. Others (halazepam, midazolam, oxazepam, prazepam) have no established dosage or record of safety.

Elderly: The elderly may be particularly sensitive to the effects of these drugs. Dosages should be initiated cautiously.

Renal impairment: Many of the metabolites of the benzodiazepines and bartiturates are excreted in the urine. These drugs should be initiated cautiously in patients with renal insufficiency.

Hepatic impairment: Many of the benzodiazepines, barbiturates, and azapirones are metabolized extensively by the liver. These drugs should be given cautiously and in lower-than-usual dosages to patients with hepatic insufficiency.

Pregnancy: Some sedative-hypnotic drugs (*eg*, diazepam, meprobamate, chlordiazepoxide) have been associated with teratogenic effects, especially cleft lip and palate [13–16].

Breast-feeding: There is a risk of accumulation in breast milk for some sedative-hypnotic drugs. Use with caution.

SPECIAL PRECAUTIONS

Careful supervision by medical personnel is essential to prevent tolerance, addiction, and abuse. Sometimes treatment for addiction and withdrawal may be needed. The clinical effectiveness of these agents decreases with time. In general, the benzodiazepines should be prescribed for about 1 month to treat insomnia. They may be required longer for some conditions, such as chronic anxiety. Withdrawal of these drugs, especially when given for insomnia, frequently results in increased difficulty of sleep onset.

CONTRAINDICATIONS

Because of the actions of these drugs on hepatic metabolism, renal excretion, and binding to plasma proteins, the sedative-hypnotic drugs interact extensively with other classes of drugs. These interactions should be monitored by serum levels and secondary measures as appropriate, such as prothrombin time when administering the anticoagulant coumadin.

INTERACTIONS

Many of the older sedative-hypnotic drugs, such as barbiturates, are effective inducers of hepatic drug metabolizing enzymes. In contrast, benzodiazepines only weakly induce hepatic microsomal enzymes.

The barbiturates increase the metabolism of oral contraceptives, phenytoin, digitoxin, quinidine, β-adrenergic blockers, and oral anticoagulants. Therefore, the dosage of these other drugs may have to be adjusted to attain therapeutic levels. Also, the barbiturates bind avidly to plasma proteins and displace other drugs from binding sites. This competition may raise the blood level of these other drugs and result in accelerated clearance by metabolism or excretion.

ADVERSE EFFECTS

These drugs can cause dizziness, light-headedness, or headaches. They have the potential for abuse, dependence, and withdrawal symptoms.

OVERDOSE AND ACCIDENTAL POISONING

All of the benzodiazepines and barbiturate drugs depress the CNS, and the depression is additive. Patients taking one of these drugs should be warned about the additive effect of drinking ethanol-containing beverages, which may result in profound CNS depression. However, barbiturates can be used for anesthesia. Overdose produces death from respiratory depression with barbiturates but not benzodiazepines. There are no antidotes for the barbiturates. In contrast, flumazenil is an effective antibenzodiazepine receptor antagonist [17,18]. Buspirone is unique among the sedative-hypnotic drugs because it does not potentiate the CNS depression seen with the drugs mentioned previously or with alcohol [19].

REFERENCES

1. Steriade M: Basic mechanisms of sleep generation [review]. *Neurology* 1992, 42(suppl 6):9.

2. Culebras A: Neuroanatomic and neurologic correlates of sleep disturbances [review]. *Neurology* 1992, 42(suppl 6):19.

3. Mendelson WB: Neuropharmacology of sleep induction by benzodiazepines [review]. *Crit Rev Neurobiol* 1992, 6:221.

4. McCormick D, van Krosigk M: Corticothalamic activation modulates thalamic firing through glutamate metabotropic receptors. *Proc Natl Acad Sci USA* 1992, 89:2774.

5. Rall TW: Hypnotics and sedatives: ethanol. In *Goodman and Gilman's The Pharmacological Basis of Therapeutics*, edn 8. Edited by Gilman AG, Rall TW, Nies AS, Taylor P. New York: Pergamon; 1990:345.

6. Macdonald RL, Barker JL: Enhancement of GABA-mediated postsynaptic inhibition in cultured mammalian spinal cord neurons: a common mode of anticonvulsant action. *Brain Research* 1979, 167:323.

7. Mendelson WB, Martin JV, Wagner R: A calcium agonist potentiates hypnotic effects of flurazepam. *Sleep Research* 1986, 15:38.

8. Heyer EJ, Macdonald RL: Barbiturates reduce the duration of calcium-dependent action potentials of mouse spinal cord neurons in primary dissociated cell culture. *Neurology* 1981, 31:157.

9. Heyer EJ, Macdonald RL: Barbiturate reduction of calcium-dependent action potentials: correlation with anesthestic action. *Brain Research* 1982, 236:157.

10. Dailey JW: Sedative-hypnotic and anxiolytic drugs. In *Modern Pharmacology*, edn 4. Edited by Craig CR, Stitzel RE. Boston: Little, Brown & Co; 1994:369.

11. Greenblatt DJ, Harmatz JS, Shader RI: Clinical pharmacokinetics of anxiolytics and hypnotics in the elderly. Therapeutic considerations (Pt I) [review]. *Clin Pharmacokinet* 1991, 21:165.

12. McEvoy GK: AHFS Drug Information: American Hospital Formulary Service. Bethesda, Maryland: American Society of Hospital Pharmacists; 1993:2424.

13. Shephard TH: *Catalog of Teratogenic Agents*, edn 3. Baltimore: Johns Hopkins University Press; 1980.

14. Hartz SC, Heinonen OP, Shapiro S: Antenatal exposure to meprobamate and chlordiazepoxide in relation to malformations, mental development and childhood mortality. *N Engl J Med* 1975, 292:726.

15. Saxen I, Saxen L: Association between maternal intake of diazepam and oral clefts. *Lancet* 1975, 2:498.

16. Safra MJ, Oakley GP: Association between cleft lip with or without cleft palate and prenatal exposure to diazepam. *Lancet* 1975, 2:478.

17. Shannon M, Albers G, Burkhart K, et al.: Safety and efficacy of flumazenil in the reversal of benzodiazepine-induced conscious sedation. The Flumazenil Pediatric Study Group. *J Pediatr* 1997, 131:582.

18. Chudnofsky CR: Safety and efficacy of flumazenil in reversing conscious sedation in the emergency department. Emergency Medicine Conscious Sedation Study Group. *Acad Emerg Med* 1997, 4:944.

19. Delle Chiaie R, Pancheri P, Casachia M, et al.: Assessment of the efficacy of buspirone in patients affected by generalized anxiety disorder, shifting to buspirone from prior treatment with lorazepam: a placebo-controlled, double-blind study. *J Clin Psychopharmacol* 1995, 15:12.

APROBARBITAL
(Alurate Elixir)

Aprobarbital is a short-acting barbiturate. It is used primarily for routine sedation and short-term treatment of insomnia.

SPECIAL PRECAUTIONS

Physical and psychologic dependence and tolerance may occur with continued use of these agents. Use with extreme caution in patients with history of drug abuse and in those with a history of mental depression or suicidal tendencies.

Rapid IV administration may cause respiratory depression, apnea, laryngospasm, or vasodilation with fall in blood pressure. Parenteral solutions are highly alkaline; avoid perivascular extravasation and intraarterial injection. Any complaint concerning a limb warrants discontinuation of injection.

Use with caution in presence of acute or chronic pain. Paradoxic excitement may occur, and important symptoms may be masked. (However, use of barbiturates as sedatives postoperatively and as adjuncts to cancer chemotherapy is well established.)

Abrupt discontinuation may cause status epilepticus in patients with seizure disorders.

Barbiturates may increase vitamin D requirements.

Use with extreme caution in debilitated patients; those with severe hepatic impairment, pulmonary or cardiac disease, status asthmaticus, shock, or uremia or in the presence of fever, hyperthyroidism, diabetes mellitus, and severe anemia. Reactions may occur.

For prolonged therapy, perform periodic laboratory evaluation of organ systems (hematopoietic, renal, and hepatic).

Systemic effects of exogenous hydrocortisone and endogenous hydrocortisone (cortisol) may be diminished. Use with caution in patients with borderline hypoadrenal function, regardless of origin.

Some preparations contain tartrazine, which can cause allergic-type reactions in some patients.

SPECIAL GROUPS

Children: May cause irritability, excitability, inappropriate tearfulness, and aggression. Hyperkinetic states may be induced or aggravated and are related to drug sensitivity.

Elderly: May produce significant excitement, depression, and confusion.

Pregnancy: Can cause fetal damage. Advise patient of hazards.

Breast-feeding: Excreted in breast milk. Drowsiness in nursing infants has been reported. Use with caution.

Renal impairment: Contraindicated.

Hepatic impairment: Reduce dosage, and use with caution.

Do not use in patients demonstrating signs of hepatic coma.

DOSAGE

Adults: For sedative effect, 40 mg three times daily. For mild insomnia, 40 to 80 mg before bedtime. For pronounced insomnia, 80 to 160 mg before bedtime.

In Brief

INDICATIONS
Short-term sedation and sleep induction

CONTRAINDICATIONS
Barbiturate sensitivity, history of manifest or latent porphyria, marked hepatic impairment, use of large doses in patients who are nephritic or with severe respiratory distress, previous addiction to sedative-hypnotic group, acute or chronic pain

INTERACTIONS
Acetaminophen, anticoagulants (oral), antidepressants (tricyclic), β-adrenergic blockers, chloramphenicol, CNS depressants, contraceptives (oral, corticosteroids, digitoxin, doxycycline, estrogens, furosemide, griseofulvin, MAO inhibitors, metronidazole, phenmetrazine, phenytoin, quinidine, rifampin, theophylline, valproic acid

ADVERSE EFFECTS
Note: Categorized by organ system or type in decreasing order of frequency.
Cardiovascular: Bradycardia, hypotension, syncope
CNS: Somnolence, agitation, confusion, hyperkinesia, ataxia, vertigo, CNS depression, nervousness, psychiatric disturbance, lethargy, residual sedation (hangover effect), paradoxic excitement, abnormal thinking, delirium and stupor (excessive doses), headache and fever (chronic use)
GI: Nausea, vomiting, constipation, diarrhea, epigastric pain
Hematologic: Megaloblastic anemia (chronic use), blood dyscrasias (rare)
Hypersensitivity: Rash, angioneurotic edema, serum sickness, morbilliform rash and urticaria (patients with asthma), exfoliative dermatitis and Stevens-Johnson syndrome (rare, may prove fatal)
Local: Arterial spasm with resultant thrombosis and gangrene of an extremity (with inadvertent intraarterial injection); SC injection may produce tissue necrosis, pain (with inadvertent intraarterial injection); SC injection may produce tissue necrosis, pain, tenderness, redness; injection near or into a nerve may cause permanent neurologic deficit; thrombophlebitis after IV use and pain at injection site
Other: Pain syndrome suggestive of myalgic, neuralgic, or arthritic pain (rare); rickets and osteomalacia (rare, prolonged use)
Respiratory: Hypoventilation, apnea, respiratory depression, laryngospasm, bronchospasm, circulatory collapse

PHARMACOKINETICS AND PHARMACODYNAMICS
Duration of action: 6–8 h
Onset of action: 45–60 min
Peak Action: within 3 h following oral administration
Plasma half-life: 14–34 h
Bioavailability: well distributed to all tissues
Metabolism: hepatic
Excretion: in urine (25%–50% of dose unchanged)
Protein binding: increases directly as a function of lipid solubility
Renal impairment: contraindicated
Hepatic impairment: contraindicated when marked
Elderly: may be more susceptible to CNS effects

PROLONGED USE
Perform periodic laboratory evaluation of organ systems (including hematopoietic, renal, and hepatic systems). For treatment of insomnia, aprobarbital should not be administered for more than 2 wk.

(Continued on next page)

OVERDOSAGE

Toxic doses vary. Generally, a dose of 1 g will produce serious toxic symptoms in an adult. Fatality often occurs after ingestion of 2–10 g. Symptoms include CNS and respiratory depression (possibly progressing to Cheyne-Stokes respiration), areflexia, oliguria, tachycardia, hypotension, lowered body temperature, and coma. Typical shock syndrome also may occur. In extreme overdose, all electrical activity in the brain may cease, which will produce a "flat" EEG normally associated with clinical death; however, this should not be accepted as such. The effect is reversible unless hypoxic damage occurs. The possibility of barbiturate overdose should be considered even in situations appearing to involve trauma. Complications, such as pneumonia, pulmonary edema, cardiac arrhythmias, congestive heart failure, and renal failure, may occur. Uremia may increase CNS sensitivity to barbiturates if renal function is impaired. Hypoglycemia, head trauma, cerebrovascular accidents, convulsive states, and diabetic coma should be included in differential diagnosis.

Treatment is supportive. Adequate airway should be maintained, with respiratory assistance and oxygen therapy as necessary. Vital signs and fluid balance should be monitored. If patient is conscious and has not lost gag reflex, emesis may be induced using syrup of ipecac. After vomiting, 30 g of activated charcoal may be administered with water. If emesis is not possible, perform gastric lavage with patient face down and using a cuffed endotracheal tube. Again, activated charcoal may be left in the emptied stomach, and a saline cathartic may be administered. If renal function is normal, forced diuresis may aid in elimination. If the patient is anuric or in shock, hemodialysis may be helpful. Patient should be rolled from side to side every 30 min.

PATIENT INFORMATION

Do not increase dosage without contacting physician. Avoid tasks requiring alertness and dexterity. Do not consume alcohol; do not take other barbiturates or CNS depressants. Contact physician if any of the following occur: sore throat, fever, mouth sores, easy bruising or bleeding, nosebleed, or petechiae.

AVAILABILITY

Elixir—40 mg/5 mL (20% alcohol)

BUTABARBITAL SODIUM
(Butisol Sodium, Butalan, Sarisol)

This intermediate-acting barbiturate is used for routine sedation and to relieve anxiety.

SPECIAL PRECAUTIONS

Physical and psychological dependence and tolerance may occur with continued use of these agents. Use with extreme caution in patients with history of drug abuse and in those with a history of mental depression or suicidal tendencies.

Rapid IV administration may cause respiratory depression, apnea, laryngospasm, or vasodilation with fall in blood pressure. Parenteral solutions are highly alkaline; avoid perivascular extravasation and intraarterial injection. Any complaint concerning a limb warrants discontinuation of injection.

Use with caution in presence of acute or chronic pain. Paradoxic excitement may occur, and important symptoms may be masked. (However, use of barbiturates as sedatives postoperatively and as adjuncts to cancer chemotherapy is well established.)

Abrupt discontinuation may cause status epilepticus in patients with seizure disorders.

Barbiturates may increase vitamin D requirements.

Use with extreme caution in debilitated patients; those with severe hepatic impairment, pulmonary or cardiac disease, status asthmaticus, shock or uremia or in the presence of fever, hyperthyroidism, diabetes mellitus, and severe anemia. Reactions may occur.

For prolonged therapy, perform periodic laboratory evaluation of organ systems (hematopoietic, renal, and hepatic).

Systemic effects of exogenous hydrocortisone and endogenous hydrocortisone (cortisol) may be diminished. Use with caution in patients with borderline hypoadrenal function, regardless of origin.

Some preparations contain tartrazine, which can cause allergic-type reactions in some patients.

(Continued on next page)

In Brief

INDICATIONS

Sedative, hypnotic. Used for routine sedation and to relieve anxiety and provide sedation preoperatively. Effectiveness is lost after 2 wk of continued use for treatment of insomnia.

CONTRAINDICATIONS

Barbiturate sensitivity, history of manifest or latent porphyria, marked hepatic impairment, use of large doses in patients who are nephritic or with severe respiratory distress, previous addiction to sedative-hypnotic group, acute or chronic pain

INTERACTIONS

Acetaminophen, anticoagulants (oral), antidepressants (tricyclic), β-adrenergic blockers, chloramphenicol, CNS depressants, contraceptives (oral), corticosteroids, digitoxin, doxycycline, estrogens, furosemide, griseofulvin, MAO inhibitors, metronidazole, phenmetrazine, phenytoin, quinidine, rifampin, theophylline, valproic acid

ADVERSE EFFECTS

Note: Categorized by organ system or type in decreasing order of frequency.

Cardiovascular: Bradycardia, hypotension, syncope

CNS: Somnolence, agitation, confusion, hyperkinesia, ataxia, vertigo, CNS depression, nervousness, psychiatric disturbance, lethargy, residual sedation (hangover effect), paradoxical excitement, abnormal thinking, delirium and stupor (excessive doses), headache and fever (chronic use)

GI: Nausea, vomiting, constipation, diarrhea, epigastric pain

Hematologic: Megaloblastic anemia (chronic use), blood dyscrasias (rare)

Hypersensitivity: Rash, angioneurotic edema, serum sickness, morbilliform rash and urticaria (patients with asthma), exfoliative dermatitis and Stevens-Johnson syndrome (rare, may prove fatal)

Local: Arterial spasm with resultant thrombosis and gangrene of an extremity (with inadvertent intraarterial injection); SC injection may produce tissue necrosis, pain, tenderness, redness; injection near or into a nerve may cause permanent neurologic deficit; thrombophlebitis after IV use and pain at injection site

(Continued on next page)

BUTABARBITAL SODIUM
(CONTINUED)

SPECIAL GROUPS

Children: May cause irritability, excitability, inappropriate tearfulness, and aggression. Hyperkinetic states may be induced or aggravated and are related to drug sensitivity.

Elderly: May produce significant excitement, depression, and confusion.

Pregnancy: Can cause fetal damage. Advise patient of hazards.

Breast-feeding: Excreted in breast milk. Drowsiness in nursing infants has been reported. Use with caution.

Renal impairment: Use with extreme caution (phenobarbitol, mephobarbital, aprobarbital, and talbutal: contraindicated).

Hepatic impairment: Reduce dosage, and use with caution. Do not use in patients demonstrating signs of hepatic coma.

DOSAGE

Adults: For daytime sedation, 15 to 30 mg three to four times a day. For hypnotic effect at bedtime, 50 to 100 mg. For preoperative sedation, 50 to 100 mg 60 to 90 minutes prior to surgery.

Children: For preoperative sedation, 2 to 6 mg/kg, to a maximum of 100 mg. For daytime sedation, 7.5 to 30 mg, depending on age, weight, and effect desired. For hypnotic effect at bedtime, base dosage on age and weight.

ADVERSE EFFECTS (CONTINUED)

Other: Pain syndrome suggestive of myalgic, neuralgic, or arthritic pain (rare); rickets and osteomalacia (rare, prolonged use)

Respiratory: Hypoventilation, apnea, respiratory depression, laryngospasm, bronchospasm, circulatory collapse

PHARMACOKINETICS AND PHARMACODYNAMICS

Duration of action: 6–8 h
Onset of action: 45–60 min
Peak action: 3–4 h after oral administration
Plasma half-life: 66–140 h
Bioavailability: well distributed to all tissues
Metabolism: hepatic
Excretion: in urine
Protein binding: increases directly as a function of lipid solubility
Renal impairment: use with extreme caution
Hepatic impairment: contraindicated when marked
Elderly: may be more susceptible to CNS effects

PROLONGED USE

Perform periodic laboratory evaluation of organ systems (including hematopoietic, renal, and hepatic systems).

OVERDOSAGE

Toxic doses vary. Generally, a dose of 1 g will produce serious toxic symptoms in an adult. Fatality often may occur after ingestion of 2–10 g.

Symptoms include CNS and respiratory depression (possibly progressing to Cheyne-Stokes respiration), areflexia, oliguria, tachycardia, hypotension, lowered body temperature, and coma. Typical shock syndrome also may occur. In extreme overdose, all electrical activity in the brain may cease, which will produce a "flat" EEG normally associated with clinical death; however, this should not be accepted as such. The effect is reversible unless hypoxic damage occurs. The possibility of barbiturate overdose should be considered even in situations appearing to involve trauma. Complications, such as pneumonia, pulmonary edema, cardiac arrhythmias, congestive heart failure, and renal failure, may occur. Uremia may increase CNS sensitivity to barbiturates if renal function is impaired. Hypoglycemia, head trauma, cerebrovascular accidents, convulsive states, and diabetic coma should be included in differential diagnosis.

Treatment is supportive. Adequate airway should be maintained, with respiratory assistance and oxygen therapy as necessary. Vital signs and fluid balance should be monitored. If patient is conscious and has not lost gag reflex, emesis may be induced using syrup of ipecac. After vomiting, 30 g of activated charcoal may be administered with water. If emesis is not possible, perform gastric lavage with patient face down and using a cuffed endotracheal tube. Again, activated charcoal may be left in the emptied stomach, and a saline cathartic may be administered. If renal function is normal, forced diuresis may aid in elimination. If the patient is anuric or in shock, hemodialysis may be helpful. Patient should be rolled from side to side every 30 min.

PATIENT INFORMATION

Do not increase dosage without contacting physician. Avoid tasks requiring alertness and dexterity. Do not consume alcohol; do not take other barbiturates or CNS depressants. Contact physician if any of the following occur: sore throat, fever, mouth sores, easy bruising or bleeding, nosebleed, or petechiae.

AVAILABILITY

Tablets—15, 30, 50, and 100 mg
Capsules—15 and 30 mg
Elixir—30 mg/5 mL and 33.3 mg/5 mL

MEPHOBARBITAL
(Mebaral)

This drug is used for routine sedation and to manage patients with epilepsy at subhypnotic concentrations. Part of its pharmacologic action is through N-demethylation by the liver to form phenobarbital.

SPECIAL PRECAUTIONS

Use with caution in patients with myasthenia gravis and myxedema. Physical and psychological dependence and tolerance may occur with continued use of these agents. Use with extreme caution in patients with history of drug abuse and in those with a history of mental depression or suicidal tendencies.

Rapid IV administration may cause respiratory depression, apnea, laryngospasm, or vasodilation with fall in blood pressure. Parenteral solutions are highly alkaline; avoid perivascular extravasation and intraarterial injection. Any complaint concerning a limb warrants discontinuation of injection.

Use with caution in presence of acute or chronic pain. Paradoxical excitement may occur, and important symptoms may be masked. (However, use of barbiturates as sedatives postoperatively and as adjuncts to cancer chemotherapy is well established.)

Abrupt discontinuation may cause status epilepticus in patients with seizure disorders.

Barbiturates may increase vitamin D requirements.

Use with extreme caution in debilitated patients; those with severe hepatic impairment, pulmonary or cardiac disease, status asthmaticus, shock, or uremia or in the presence of fever, hyperthyroidism, diabetes mellitus, and severe anemia. Reactions may occur.

For prolonged therapy, perform periodic laboratory evaluation of organ systems (hematopoietic, renal, and hepatic).

Systemic effects of exogenous hydrocortisone and endogenous hydrocortisone (cortisol) may be diminished. Use with caution in patients with borderline hypoadrenal function, regardless of origin.

Some preparations contain tartrazine, which can cause allergic-type reactions in some patients.

SPECIAL GROUPS

Children: May cause irritability, excitability, inappropriate tearfulness, and aggression. Hyperkinetic states may be induced or aggravated and are related to drug sensitivity.

Elderly: May produce significant excitement, depression, and confusion.

Pregnancy: Can cause fetal damage. Advise patient of hazards.

Breast-feeding: Excreted in breast milk. Drowsiness in nursing infants has been reported. Use with caution.

Renal impairment: Use with extreme caution (phenobarbital, mephobarbital, aprobarbital, and talbutal: contraindicated).

Renal impairment: Contraindicated.

Hepatic impairment: Reduce dosage, and use with caution. Do not use in patients demonstrating signs of hepatic coma.

DOSAGE

Adults: Administer orally. For sedative effect, 32 to 100 mg three to four times a day. Optimum dose is 50 mg three to four times per day. For epilepsy, 400 to 600 mg/d. Take at bedtime if seizures usually occur at night and during the day if episodes are usually diurnal. Begin therapy with small doses, and increase gradually to determine optimum dosage.

Children: For sedative effect, 16 to 32 mg three to four times a day. For epilepsy less than 5 years old, 16 to 32 mg three to four times per day; more than 5 years old, 32 to 64 mg three to four times per day.

(Continued on next page)

In Brief

INDICATIONS
Sedative for the relief of anxiety, tension, and apprehension; anticonvulsant in the treatment of grand mal and petit mal epilepsy

CONTRAINDICATIONS
Barbiturates sensitivity, history of manifest or latent porphyria, marked hepatic impairment, use of large doses in patients who are nephritic or with severe respiratory distress, previous addiction to sedative-hypnotic group, acute or chronic pain

INTERACTIONS
Acetaminophen, anticoagulants (oral), antidepressants (tricyclic), β-adrenergic blockers, chloramphenicol, CNS depressants, contraceptives (oral), corticosteroids, digitoxin, doxycycline, estrogens, furosemide, griseofulvin, MAO inhibitors, metronidazole, phenmetrazine, phenytoin, quinidine, rifampin, theophylline, valproic acid

ADVERSE EFFECTS
Note: Categorized by organ system or type in decreasing order of frequency.

Cardiovascular: Bradycardia, hypotension, syncope

CNS: Somnolence, agitation, confusion, hyperkinesia, ataxia, vertigo, CNS depression, nervousness, psychiatric disturbance, lethargy, residual sedation (hangover effect), paradoxical excitement, abnormal thinking, delirium and stupor (excessive doses), headache and fever (chronic use)

GI: Nausea, vomiting, constipation, diarrhea, epigastric pain

Hematologic: Megaloblastic anemia (chronic use), blood dyscrasias (rare)

Hypersensitivity: Rash, angioneurotic edema, serum sickness, morbilliform rash and urticaria (patients with asthma), exfoliative dermatitis and Stevens-Johnson syndrome (rare, may prove fatal)

Local: Arterial spasm with resultant thrombosis and gangrene of an extremity (with inadvertent intraarterial injection); SC injection may produce tissue necrosis, pain, tenderness, redness; injection near or into a nerve may cause permanent neurologic deficit; thrombophlebitis after IV use and pain at injection site

Other: Pain syndrome suggestive of myalgic, neuralgic, or arthritic pain (rare); rickets and osteomalacia (rare, prolonged use)

Respiratory: Hypoventilation, apnea, respiratory depression, laryngospasm, bronchospasm, circulatory collapse

PHARMACOKINETICS AND PHARMACODYNAMICS
Duration of action: 10–12 h
Onset of action: ≥ 60 min
Plasma half-life: 11–67 h
Bioavailability: well distributed to all tissues
Metabolism: hepatic
Excretion: in urine
Protein binding: increases directly as a function of lipid solubility
Renal impairment: contraindicated
Hepatic impairment: contraindicated when marked
Elderly: may be more susceptible to CNS effects

PROLONGED USE
Perform periodic laboratory evaluation of organ systems (including hematopoietic, renal, and hepatic systems).

MEPHOBARBITAL *(CONTINUED)*

OVERDOSAGE

Toxic doses vary. Generally, a dose of 1 g will produce serious toxic symptoms in an adult. Fatality may often occur after ingestion of 2–10 g.

Symptoms include CNS and respiratory depression (possibly progressing to Cheyne-Stokes respiration), areflexia, oliguria, tachycardia, hypotension, lowered body temperature, and coma. Typical shock syndrome also may occur. In extreme overdose, all electrical activity in the brain may cease, which will produce a "flat" EEG normally associated with clinical death; however, this should not be accepted as such. The effect is reversible unless hypoxic damage occurs. The possibility of barbiturate overdose should be considered even in situations appearing to involve trauma. Complications, such as pneumonia, pulmonary edema, cardiac arrhythmias, congestive heart failure, and renal failure, may occur. Uremia may increase CNS sensitivity to barbiturates if renal function is impaired. Hypoglycemia, head trauma, cerebrovascular accidents, convulsive states, and diabetic coma should be included in differential diagnosis.

Treatment is supportive. Adequate airway should be maintained, with respiratory assistance and oxygen therapy as necessary. Vital signs and fluid balance should be monitored. If patient is conscious and has not lost gag reflex, emesis may be induced using syrup of ipecac. After vomiting, 30 g of activated charcoal may be administered with water. If emesis is not possible, perform gastric lavage with patient face down and using a cuffed endotracheal tube. Again, activated charcoal may be left in the emptied stomach, and a saline cathartic may be administered. If renal function is normal, forced diuresis may aid in elimination. If the patient is anuric or in shock, hemodialysis may be helpful. Patient should be rolled from side to side every 30 min.

PATIENT INFORMATION

Do not increase dosage without contacting physician. Avoid tasks requiring alertness and dexterity. Do not consume alcohol; do not take other barbiturates or CNS depressants. Contact physician if any of the following occur: sore throat, fever, mouth sores, easy bruising or bleeding, nosebleed, or petechiae.

AVAILABILITY

Tablets—32, 50, and 100 mg

TALBUTAL

(Lotusate)

Talbutal is used to treat insomnia.

SPECIAL PRECAUTIONS

Physical and psychological dependence and tolerance may occur with continued use of these agents. Use with extreme caution in patients with history of drug abuse and in those with a history of mental depression or suicidal tendencies.

Rapid IV administration may cause respiratory depression, apnea, laryngospasm, or vasodilation with fall in blood pressure. Parenteral solutions are highly alkaline; avoid perivascular extravasation and intraarterial injection. Any complaint concerning a limb warrants discontinuation of injection.

Use with caution in presence of acute or chronic pain. Paradoxical excitement may occur, and important symptoms may be masked. (However, use of barbiturates as sedatives postoperatively and as adjuncts to cancer chemotherapy is well established.)

Abrupt discontinuation may cause status epilepticus in patients with seizure disorders.

Barbiturates may increase vitamin D requirements.

Use with extreme caution in debilitated patients; those with severe hepatic impairment, pulmonary or cardiac disease, status asthmaticus, shock, or uremia or in the presence of fever, hyperthyroidism, diabetes mellitus, and severe anemia. Reactions may occur.

For prolonged therapy, perform periodic laboratory evaluation of organ systems (hematopoietic, renal, and hepatic).

Systemic effects of exogenous hydrocortisone and endogenous hydrocortisone (cortisol) may be diminished. Use with caution in patients with borderline hypoadrenal function, regardless of origin.

Some preparations contain tartrazine, which can cause allergic-type reactions in some patients.

In Brief

INDICATIONS

Hypnotic, short-term treatment of insomnia. Effectiveness is lost after 2 wk of continued use.

CONTRADICATIONS

Barbituate sensitivity, history of manifest or latent porphyria, marked hepatic impairment, use of large doses in patients who are nephritic or patients with severe respiratory distress, previous addiction to sedative-hypnotic group, acute or chronic pain

INTERACTIONS

Acetaminophen, anticoagulants (oral) antidepressants (tricyclic), β-adrenergic blockers, chloramphenicol, CNS depressants, contraceptives (oral), corticosteroids, digitoxin, doxycycline, estrogens, furosemide, griseofulvin, MAO inhibitors, metronidazole, phenmetrazine, phenytoin, quinidine, rifampin, theophylline, valproic acid

ADVERSE EFFECTS

Note: Categorized by organ system or type in decreasing order of frequency.

Cardiovascular: Bradycardia, hypotension, syncope

CNS: Somnolence, agitation, confusion, hyperkinesia, ataxia, vertigo, CNS depression, nervousness, psychiatric disturbance, lethargy, residual sedation (hangover effect), paradoxical excitement, abnormal thinking, delirium and stupor (excessive dose), headache and fever (chronic use)

GI: Nausea, vomiting, constipation, diarrhea, epigastric pain

Hematologic: Megaloblastic anemia (chronic use), blood dyscrasias (rare)

Hypersensitivity: Rash, angioneurotic edema, serum sickness, morbilliform rash and urticaria (patients with asthma), exfoliative dermatitis and Stevens-Johnson syndrome (rare, may prove fatal)

Local: Arterial spasm with resultant thrombosis and gangrene of an extremity (with inadvertent intraarterial injection); SC injection may produce tissue necrosis, pain, tenderness, redness; injection near or into a nerve may cause permanent neurologic deficit; thrombophlebitis after IV use at injection site

(Continued on next page)

(Continued on next page)

SPECIAL GROUPS

Renal impairment: Contraindicated.

Children: May cause irritability, excitability, inappropriate tearfulness, and aggression. Hyperkinetic states may be induced or aggravated and are related to drug sensitivity.

Elderly: May produce significant excitement, depression, and confusion.

Pregnancy: Can cause fetal damage. Advise patient of hazards.

Breast-feeding: Excreted in breast milk. Drowsiness in nursing infants has been reported. Use with caution.

Hepatic impairment: Reduce dosage, and use with caution. Do not use in patients demonstrating signs of hepatic coma.

DOSAGE

Adults: 120 mg 15 to 30 minutes before bedtime.

Children: Has not been established for hypnosis. For sedation, 6 mg/kg or 180 mg/m^2 daily administered in 3 divided doses. For treating anxiety, 2 to 6 mg/kg.

ADVERSE EFFECTS (CONTINUED)

Other: Pain syndrome suggestive of myalgic, neuralgic, or arthritic pain (rare); rickets and osteomalacia (rare, prolonged use)

Respiratory: Hypoventilation, apnea, respiratory depression, laryngospasm, bronchospasm, circulatory collapse

PHARMACOKINETICS AND PHARMACODYNAMICS

Duration of action: 6–8 h

Onset of action: 45–60 min

Peak action: 3–4 h after oral administration

Plasma half-life: 15 h

Bioavailability: well distributed to all tissues

Metabolism: hepatic

Excretion: in urine

Protein binding: increase directly as a function of lipid solubility

Renal impairment: contraindicated

Hepatic impairment: contraindicated when marked

Elderly: may be more susceptible to CNS effects

PROLONGED USE

Perform periodic laboratory evaluation of organ systems (including hematopoietic, renal, and hepatic systems).

OVERDOSAGE

Toxic doses vary. Generally, a dose of 1 g will produce serious toxic symptoms in an adult. Fatality often occurs after ingestion of 2–10 g.

Symptoms include CNS and respiratory depression (possibly progressing to Cheyne-Stokes respiration), areflexia, oliguria, tachycardia, hypotension, lowered body temperature, and coma. Typical shock syndrome also may occur. In extreme overdose, all electrical activity in the brain may cease, which will produce a "flat" EEG normally associated with clinical death; however, this should not be accepted as such. The effect is reversible unless hypoxic damage occurs. The possibility of barbiturate overdose should be considered even in situations appearing to involve trauma. Complications, such as pneumonia, pulmonary edema, cardiac arrhythmias, congestive heart failure, and renal failure, may occur. Uremia may increase CNS sensitivity to barbiturates if renal function is impaired. Hypoglycemia, head trauma, cerebrovascular accidents, convulsive states, and diabetic coma should be included in differential diagnosis.

Treatment is supportive. Adequate airway should be maintained, with respiratory assistance and oxygen therapy as necessary. Vital signs and fluid balance should be monitored. If patient is conscious and has not lost gag reflex, emesis may be induced using syrup of ipecac. After vomiting, 30 g of activated charcoal may be administered with water. If emesis is not possible, perform gastric lavage with patient face down and using a cuffed endotracheal tube. Again, activated charcoal may be left in the emptied stomach, and a saline cathartic may be administered. If renal function is normal, forced diuresis may aid in elimination. If the patient is anuric or in shock, hemodialysis may be helpful. Patient should be rolled from side to side every 30 min.

PATIENT INFORMATION

Do not increase dosage without contacting physician. Avoid tasks requiring alertness and dexterity. Do not consume alcohol; do not take other barbiturates or CNS depressants. Contact physician if any of the following occur: sore throat, fever, mouth sores, easy bruising or bleeding, nosebleed, or petechiae.

AVAILABILITY

Tablets—120 mg

PHENOBARBITAL

(Solfoton, Phenobarbital Elixir, Polytress),

PHENOBARBITAL SODIUM

(Phenobarbital Sodium Injection, Luminal Sodium)

All of the barbiturates are substituted pyrimidine derivatives. They are derived from barbituric acid, which has no therapeutic efficacy. Phenobarbitital is a sedative-hypnotic, anticonvulsant, and part of the therapy of drug withdrawal. Its pharmacologic action may be through its effect on $GABA_A$ channels, although this simplified view has been questioned.

DOSAGE

Adults: *Oral*—For daytime sedation, 30 to 120 mg/d in two to three divided doses. For hypnotic effect, 100 to 320 mg. For anticonvulsant effect, the usual oral dosage is 100 to 300 mg/d. The drug frequently is given at bedtime. There is no advantage in dividing the daily dosage because of the long half-life of phenobarbital. *Parenteral*—Usual dosage range is 100 to 300 mg. Do not exceed 600 mg/d; observe for toxicity effects. For sedation, 100 to 130 mg IM or IV. For preoperative medication, 130 to 200 mg IM.

Elderly or debilitated patients: May require significant dosage reduction.

Children: *Oral*—For preoperative sedation, 1 to 3 mg/kg. For anticonvulsant effect (phenobarbital sodium), 3 to 5 mg/kg or 125 mg/m^2 daily. *Parenteral*—For sedative effect, 2 mg/kg or 60 mg/m^2 IM three times a day. For preoperative medication, 16 to 100 mg IM. For postoperative medication, 8 to 30 mg IM.

Renal impairment: Contraindicated.

In Brief

INDICATIONS
Oral: Sedative for preanesthetic use; hypnotic for short-term treatment of insomnia

Parenteral: Sedative to treat anxiety or tension states, hyperthyroidism, essential hypertension, nausea and vomiting of functional origin, motion sickness, acute labyrinthritis, pylorospasm in infants, and cardiac failure; adjunct in the treatment of hemorrhage from the respiratory or GI tract

ADVERSE EFFECTS
Hematologic: Megaloblastic anemia (chronic use)

AVAILABILITY
Tablets—8, 32, 65, and 100 mg
Capsules—16 mg
Elixir—15 mg and 20 mg/5 mL
Injection—30, 60, 65, and 130 mg/mL
Powder for injection in 120-mg amps

AMOBARBITAL (AMYTAL), AMOBARBITAL SODIUM

This drug is used for the short-term treatment of insomnia and to control status epilepticus. When used with neuroradiographic procedures, it has locally anesthetized a brain area to determine function, as for localization of language.

SPECIAL PRECAUTIONS

Physical and psychological dependence and tolerance may occur with continued use of these agents. Use with extreme caution in patients with history of drug abuse and in those with a history of mental depression or suicidal tendencies.

Rapid IV administration may cause respiratory depression, apnea, laryngospasm, or vasodilation with fall in blood pressure. Parenteral solutions are highly alkaline; avoid perivascular extravasation and intraarterial injection. Any complaint concerning a limb warrants discontinuation of injection.

Use with caution in presence of acute or chronic pain. Paradoxical excitement may occur, and important symptoms may be masked. (However, use of barbiturates as sedatives postoperatively and as adjuncts to cancer chemotherapy is well established.)

Abrupt discontinuation may cause status epilepticus in patients with seizure disorders.

Barbiturates may increase vitamin D requirements.

Use with extreme caution in debilitated patients; those with severe hepatic impairment, pulmonary or cardiac disease, status asthmaticus, shock, or uremia or in the presence of fever, hyperthyroidism, diabetes mellitus, and severe anemia. Reactions may occur.

For prolonged therapy, perform periodic laboratory evaluation of organ systems (hematopoietic, renal, and hepatic).

Systemic effects of exogenous hydrocortisone and endogenous hydrocortisone (cortisol) may be diminished. Use with caution in patients with borderline hypoadrenal function, regardless of origin.

Some preparations contain tartrazine, which can cause allergic-type reactions in some patients.

In Brief

INDICATIONS
Oral: Sedation, relief of anxiety (minimum doses), hypnotic effects, preanesthetic medication; control of convulsive disorders
Parenteral: Management of catatonic and negativistic reactions, manic reactions, and epileptiform seizures; useful in narcoanalysis and narcotherapy; diagnostic aid in schizophrenia; control of convulsive seizures, such as those due to chorea, eclampsia, meningitis, tetanus, procaine or cocaine reactions, or from poisoning from such drugs as strychnine or picrotoxin

CONTRAINDICATIONS
Barbiturate sensitivity, history of manifest or latent porphyria, marked hepatic impairment, use of large doses in patients who are nephritic or in patients with severe respiratory distress, previous addiction to sedative-hypnotic group, acute or chronic pain

INTERACTIONS
Acetaminophen, anticoagulants (oral), antidepressants (tricyclic), β-adrenergic blockers, chloramphenicol, CNS depressants, contraceptives (oral), corticosteroids, digitoxin, doxycycline, estrogens, furosemide, griseofulvin, MAO inhibitors, metronidazole, phenmetrazine, phenytoin, quinidine, rifampin, theophylline, valproic acid

ADVERSE EFFECTS
Note: Categorized by organ system or type in decreasing order of frequency.
Cardiovascular: Bradycardia, hypotension, syncope
CNS: Somnolence, agitation, confusion, hyperkinesia, ataxia, vertigo, CNS depression, nervousness, psychiatric disturbance, lethargy, residual sedation (hangover effect), paradoxical excitement, abnormal thinking, delirium and stupor (excessive doses), headache and fever (chronic use)
GI: Nausea, vomiting, constipation, diarrhea, epigastric pain
Hematologic: Megaloblastic anemia (chronic use), blood dyscrasias (rare)
Hypersensitivity: Rash, angioneurotic edema, serum sickness, morbilliform rash and urticaria (patients with asthma), exfoliative dermatitis and Stevens-Johnson syndrome (rare, may prove fatal)
Local: Arterial spasm with resultant thrombosis and gangrene of an extremity (with inadvertent intraarterial injection); SC injection may produce tissue necrosis, pain, tenderness, redness; injection near or into a nerve may cause permanent neurologic deficit; thrombophlebitis after IV use and pain at injection site
Other: Pain syndrome suggestive of myalgic, neuralgic, or arthritic pain (rare); rickets and osteomalacia (rare, prolonged use)
Respiratory: Hypoventilation, apnea, respiratory depression, laryngospasm, bronchospasm, circulatory collapse

PHARMACOKINETICS AND PHARMACODYNAMICS
Duration of action: 6–8 h
Onset of action: 45–60 min
Plasma half-life: 16–40 h
Bioavailability: well distriputed to all tissues
Metabolism: hepatic
Excretion: in urine
Protein binding: increases directly as a function of lipid solubility
Renal impairment: use with extreme caution
Hepatic impairment: contraindicated when marked
Elderly: may be more susceptible to CNS effects

PROLONGED USE
Perform periodic laboratory evaluation of organ systems (including hematopoietic, renal, and hepatic systems).

(Continued on next page)

AMOBARBITAL, AMOBARBITAL SODIUM *(CONTINUED)*

DOSAGE

Adults: Dosage must be individualized. For daytime sedation, dosage range is 15 to 120 mg two to four times a day; however, usual dosage is 30 to 50 mg two to three times a day. For hypnotic effect, 100 to 200 mg; larger doses may be used occasionally. For insomnia, 65 to 200 mg (as sodium) at bedtime. For preanesthetic sedation, 200 mg (as sodium) 1 to 2 hours prior to surgery. For labor, initial dose is 200 to 400 mg (as sodium); additional doses of 200 to 400 mg may be given at 1- to 3-hour intervals for a total not exceeding 1 g. Maximum IM dose should not exceed 500 mg. Do not use a volume greater than 5 mL, regardless of drug concentration, at any one site. Average IM dose range is 65 to 500 mg. Solutions of 20% may be used so that a small volume can deliver a high dose. Superficial IM or SC injections may cause pain, sterile abscesses, or sloughs. Do not exceed the IV rate of 1 mL/min. When 10% solution is used, faster rates of administration may cause serious respiratory depression.

Children: Children may tolerate comparatively larger IV doses than adults owing to their higher metabolic rate. A child 6 to 12 years old may ordinarily be given 65 to 500 mg; final dosage is determined by patient response to slow administration of medication.

OVERDOSAGE

Toxic doses vary. Generally, a dose of 1 g will produce serious toxic symptoms in an adult. Fatality may often occur after ingestion of 2–10 g.

Symptoms include CNS and respiratory depression (possibly progressing to Cheyne-Stokes respiration), areflexia, oliguria, tachycardia, hypotension, lowered body temperature, and coma. Typical shock syndrome also may occur. In extreme overdose, all electrical activity in the brain may cease, which will produce a "flat" EEG normally associated with clinical death; however, this should not be accepted as such. The effect is reversible unless hypoxic damage occurs. The possibility of barbiturate overdose should be considered even in situations appearing to involve trauma. Complications, such as pneumonia, pulmonary edema, cardiac arrhythmias, congestive heart failure, and renal failure, may occur. Uremia may increase CNS sensitivity to barbiturates if renal function is impaired. Hypoglycemia, head trauma, cerebrovascular accidents, convulsive states, and diabetic coma should be included in differential diagnosis.

Treatment is supportive. Adequate airway should be maintained, with respiratory assistance and oxygen therapy as necessary. Vital signs and fluid balance should be monitored. If patient is conscious and has not lost gag reflex, emesis may be induced using syrup of ipecac. After vomiting, 30 g of activated charcoal may be administered with water. If emesis is not possible, perform gastric lavage with patient face down and using a cuffed endotracheal tube. Again, activated charcoal may be left in the emptied stomach, and a saline cathartic may be administered. If renal function is normal, forced diuresis may aid in elimination. If the patient is anuric or in shock, hemodialysis may be helpful. Patient should be rolled from side to side every 30 min.

PATIENT INFORMATION

Do not increase dosage without contacting physician. Avoid tasks requiring alertness and dexterity. Do not consume alcohol; do not take other barbiturates or CNS depressants. Contact physician if any of the following occur: sore throat, fever, mouth sores, easy bruising or bleeding, nosebleed, or petechiae.

AVAILABILITY

Capsules—65 and 200 mg
Tablets—30, 50, and 100 mg
Powder for injection—250- and 500-mg vials

PENTOBARBITAL, PENTOBARBITAL SODIUM

(Nembutal Sodium)

Pentobarbital is used for the short-term treatment of insomnia, to control status epilepticus, to treat withdrawal from other hypnotics, and to induce coma in the management of cerebral ischemia and increased intracranial pressure.

SPECIAL PRECAUTIONS

Physical and psychological dependence and tolerance may occur with continued use of these agents. Use with extreme caution in patients with a history of mental depression or suicidal tendencies.

Rapid IV administration may cause respiratory depression, apnea, laryngospasm, or vasodilation with fall in blood pressure. Parenteral solutions are highly alkaline; avoid perivascular extravasation and intraarterial injection. Any complaint concerning a limb warrants discontinuation of injection.

Use with caution in presence of acute or chronic pain. Paradoxical excitement may occur, and important symptoms may be masked. (However, use of barbiturates as sedatives postoperatively and as adjuncts to cancer chemotherapy is well established.)

Abrupt discontinuation may cause status epilepticus in patients with seizure disorders.

Barbiturates may increase vitamin D requirements.

Use with extreme caution in debilitated patients; those with severe hepatic impairment, pulmonary or cardiac disease, status asthmaticus, shock, or uremia or in the presence of fever, hyperthyroidism, diabetes mellitus, and severe anemia. Reactions may occur.

For prolonged therapy, perform periodic laboratory evaluation of organ systems (hematopoietic, renal, and hepatic).

Systemic effects of exogenous hydrocortisone and endogenous hydrocortisone (cortisol) may be diminished. Use with caution in patients with borderline hypoadrenal function, regardless of origin.

Some preparations contain tartrazine, which can cause allergic-type reactions in some patients.

SPECIAL GROUPS

Children: May cause irritability, excitability, inappropriate tearfulness, and aggression. Hyperkinetic states may be induced or aggravated and are related to drug sensitivity.

Elderly: May produce significant excitement, depression, and confusion.

Pregnancy: Can cause fetal damage. Advise patient of hazards.

Breast-feeding: Excreted in breast milk. Drowsiness in nursing infants has been reported. Use with caution.

Renal impairment: Use with extreme caution (phenobarbital, mephobarbital, aprobarbital, and talbutal: contraindicated).

Hepatic impairment: Reduce dosage, and use with caution. Do not use in patients demonstrating signs of hepatic coma.

In Brief

INDICATIONS

Oral: Sedative or a hypnotic for the short-term treatment of insomnia; preanesthetic medication.

Rectal: Sedation when oral or parenteral routes are not possible or desirable; hypnotic for short-term treatment of insomnia.

Parenteral: Sedative; preanesthetic; anticonvulsant

CONTRAINDICATIONS

Barbiturate sensitivity, history of manifest or latent porphyria, marked hepatic impairment, use of large doses in patients who are nephritic or in patients with severe respiratory distress, previous addiction to sedative-hypnotic group, acute or chronic pain

INTERACTIONS

Acetaminophen, anticoagulants (oral), antidepressants (tricyclic), β-adrenergic blockers, chloramphenicol, CNS depressants, contraceptives (oral), corticosteroids, digitoxin, doxycycline, estrogens, furosemide, griseofuvin, MAO inhibitors, metronidazole, phenmetrazine, phenytoin, quinidine, rifampin, theophylline, valproic acid

ADVERSE EFFECTS

Note: Categorized by organ system or type in decreasing order of frequency.

Cardiovascular: Bradycardia, hypotension, syncope

CNS: Somnolence, agitation, confusion, hyperkinesia, ataxia, vertigo, CNS depression, nervousness, psychiatric disturbance, lethargy, residual sedation (hangover effect), paradoxical excitement, abnormal thinking, delirium and stupor (excessive doses), headache and fever (chronic use)

GI: Nausea, vomiting, constipation, diarrhea, epigastric pain

Hematologic: Megaloblastic anemia (chronic use), blood dyscrasias (rare)

Hypersensitivity: Rash, angioneurotic edema, serum sickness, morbilliform rash and urticaria (patients with asthma), exfoliative dermatitis and Stevens-Johnson syndrome (rare, may prove fatal)

Local: Arterial spasm with resultant thrombosis and gangrene of an extremity (with inadvertent intraarterial injection); SC injection may produce tissue necrosis, pain, tenderness, redness; injection near or into a nerve may cause permanent neurologic deficit; thrombophlebitis after IV use and pain at injection site

Other: Pain syndrome suggestive of myalgic, neuralgic, or arthritic pain (rare); rickets and osteomalacia (rare, prolonged use)

Respiratory: Hypoventilation, apnea, respiratory depression, larygospasm, bronchospasm, circulatory collapse

PHARMACOKINETICS AND PHARMACODYNAMICS

Duration of action: 3–4 h

Onset of action: 10–15 min

Peak action: 30–60 min following oral administration

Plasma half-life: 15–50 h

Bioavailability: rapidly distributed to all tissues

Metabolism: hepatic

Excretion: in urine

Protein binding: high

Renal impairment: use with extreme caution

Hepatic impairment: contraindicated when marked

Elderly: may be more susceptible to CNS effects

PROLONGED USE

Perform periodic laboratory evaluation of organ systems (including hematopoietic, renal, and hepatic systems).

(Continued on next page)

PENTOBARBITAL, PENTOBARBITAL SODIUM
(CONTINUED)

DOSAGE

Adults: *Oral*—For daytime sedation, 20 mg three to four times a day. For hypnotic effect at bedtime, 100 to 200 mg orally or 120 to 200 mg. *Rectal*—Do not divide suppositories.

Parenteral—Pentobarbital solutions are very alkaline. Use extreme caution to avoid perivascular extravasation or intraarterial injection. Restrict IV use to conditions in which other routes are not possible, including an unconscious patient or when rapid action is essential. Slow IV injection is imperative; observe patients carefully during administration. Do not exceed rate of 50 mg/min. Clinical response is basis for dosage determination; weight and age also may influence amount required. Give an initial dose of 100 mg for a 70-kg adult. Wait at least 1 minute to determine full effect. Small increments may be given, if necessary, to a total of 200 to 500 mg for normal adults. Keep dosages to a minimum in convulsive states to avoid compounding ensuing depressive states. Inject slowly with regard to time required for drug to cross the blood–brain barrier. IM injection should not exceed a volume of 5 mL at any one site due to possibility for irritation.

Calculate dosage on basis of age, weight, and patient condition. Usual adult dosage is 150 to 200 mg.

Elderly: Calculate dosage on basis of age, weight, and patient condition.

Children: *Oral*—For preoperative sedation, 2 to 6 mg/kg per day; maximum is 100 mg. For hypnotic effect, base dosage on age and weight. *Rectal*—Do not divide suppositories. 12 to 14 years old, 60 or 120 mg; 5 to 12 years old, 60 mg; 1 to 4 years old, 30 or 60 mg; 2 months to 1 year old, 30 mg. *Parenteral*—Usual children's dose is 25 to 80 mg or 2 to 6 mg/kg as a single IM injection; do not exceed 100 mg. Calculate dosage based on age, weight, and patient condition.

OVERDOSAGE

Toxic doses vary. Generally, a dose of 1 g will produce serious toxic symptoms in an adult. Fatality may often occur after ingestion of 2–10 g.

Symptoms include CNS and respiratory depression (possibly progressing to Cheyne-Stokes respiration), areflexia, oliguria, tachycardia, hypotension, lowered body temperature, and coma. Typical shock syndrome also may occur. In extreme overdose, all electrical activity in the brain may cease, which will produce a "flat" EEG normally associated with clinical death; however, this should not be accepted as such. The effect is reversible unless hypoxic damage occurs. The possibility of barbiturate overdose should be considered even in situations appearing to involve trauma. Complications, such as pneumonia, pulmonary edema, cardiac arrhythmias, congestive heart failure, and renal failure, may occur. Uremia may increase CNS sensitivity to barbiturates if renal function is impaired. Hypoglycemia, head trauma, cerebroascular accidents, convulsive states, and diabetic coma should be included in differential diagnosis.

Treatment is supportive. Adaquate airway should be maintained, with respiratory assistance and oxygen therapy as necessary. Vital signs and fluid balance should be monitored. If patient is conscious and has not lost gag reflex, emesis may be induced using syrup of ipecac. After vomiting, 30 g of activated charcoal may be administered with water. If emesis is not possible, perform gastric lavage with patient face down and using a cuffed endotracheal tube. Again, activated charcoal may be left in the emptied stomach, and a saline cathartic may be administered. If renal function is normal, forced diuresis may aid in elimination. If the patient is anuric or in shock, hemodialysis may be helpful. Patient should be rolled from side to side every 30 min.

PATIENT INFORMATION

Do not increase dosage without contacting physician. Avoid tasks requiring alertness and dexterity. Do not consume alcohol; do not take other barbiturates or CNS depressants. Contact physician if any of the following occur: sore throat, fever, mouth sores, easy bruising or bleeding, nosebleed, or petechiae.

AVAILABILITY

Capsules—50 and 100 mg
Elixir—18.2 mg pentobarbital (equivalent to 20 mg pentobarbital sodium) per 5 mL
Suppositories—30, 60, 120, and 200 mg
Injection—50 mg/mL

SECOBARBITAL, SECOBARBITAL SODIUM
(Seconal)

Secobarbital is used for the short-term treatment of insomnia and to control status epilepticus.

SPECIAL PRECAUTIONS

Physical and psychological dependence and tolerance may occur with continued use of these agents. Use with extreme caution in patients with history of drug abuse and in those with a history of mental depression or suicidal tendencies.

Rapid IV administration may cause respiratory depression, apnea, laryngospasm, or vasodilation with fall in blood pressure. Parenteral solutions are highly alkaline; avoid perivascular extravasation and intraarterial injection. Any complaint concerning a limb warrants discontinuation of injection.

Use with caution in presence of acute or chronic pain. Paradoxical excitement may occur, and important symptoms may be masked. (However, use of barbiturates as sedatives postoperatively and as adjuncts to cancer chemotherapy is well established.)

Abrupt discontinuation may cause status epilepticus in patients with seizure disorders.

Barbiturates may increase vitamin D requirements.

Use with extreme caution in debilitated patients; those with severe hepatic impairment, pulmonary or cardiac disease, status asthmaticus, shock, or uremia or in the presence of fever, hyperthyroidism, diabetes mellitus, and severe anemia. Reactions may occur.

For prolonged therapy, perform periodic laboratory evaluation of organ systems (hematopoietic, renal, and hepatic).

Systemic effects of exogenous hydrocortisone and endogenous hydrocortisone (cortisol) may be diminished. Use with caution in patients with borderline hypoadrenal function, regardless of origin.

Some preparations contain tartrazine, which can cause allergic-type reactions in some patients.

SPECIAL GROUPS

Children: May cause irritability, excitability, inappropriate tearfulness, and aggression.
Hyperkinetic states may be induced or aggravated and are related to drug sensitivity.
Elderly: May produce significant excitement, depression, and confusion.
Pregnancy: Can cause fetal damage. Advise patient of hazards.
Breast-feeding: Excreted in breast milk. Drowsiness in nursing infants has been reported. Use with caution.
Renal impairment: Use with extreme caution (phenobarbital, mephobarbital, aprobarbital, and talbutal: contraindicated).
Hepatic impairment: Reduce dosage, and use with caution.
Do not use in patients demonstrating signs of hepatic coma.

In Brief

INDICATIONS

Oral: Hypnotic, short-term treatment of insomnia; preanesthetic
Rectal: Intermittent sedative and hypnotic when indicated
Parenteral: Intermittent use as a sedative, hypnotic, or preanesthetic

CONTRAINDICATIONS

Parenteral route is contraindicated during obstetric delivery. Barbiturate sensitivity, history of manifest or latent porphyria, marked hepatic impairment, use of large doses in patients who are nephritic or in patients with severe respiratory distress, previous addiction to sedative-hypnotic group, acute or chronic pain

INTERACTIONS

Acetaminophen, anticoagulants (oral), antidepressants (tricyclic), β-adrenergic blockers, chloramphenicol, CNS depressants, contraceptives (oral), corticosteroids, digitoxin, doxycycline, estrogens, furosemide, griseofulvin, MAO inhibitors, metronidazole, phenmetrazine, phenytoin, quinidine, rifampin, theophylline, valproic acid

ADVERSE EFFECTS

Note: Categorized by organ system or type in decreasing order of frequency.
Cardiovascular: Bradycardia, hypotension, syncope
CNS: Somnolence, agitation, confusion, hyperkinesia, ataxia, vertigo, CNS depression, nervousness, psychiatric disturbance, lethargy, residual sedation (hangover effect), paradoxical excitement, abnormal thinking, delirium and stupor (excessive doses), headache and fever (chronic use)
GI: Nausea, vomiting, constipation, diarrhea, epigastric pain
Hematologic: Megaloblastic anemia (chronic use), blood dyscrasias (rare)
Hypersensitivity: Rash, angioneurotic edema, serum sickness, morbilliform rash and urticaria (patients with asthma), exfoliative dermatitis and Stevens-Johnson syndrome (rare, may prove fatal)
Local: Arterial spasm with resultant thrombosis and gangrene of an extremity (with inadvertent intraarterial injection); SC injection may produce tissue necrosis, pain, tenderness, redness; injection near or into a nerve may cause permanent neurologic deficit; thrombophlebitis after IV use and pain at injection site
Other: Pain syndrome suggestive of myalgic, neuralgic, or arthritic pain (rare); rickets and osteomalacia (rare, prolonged use)
Respiratory: Hypoventilation, apnea, respiratory depression, laryngospasm, bronchospasm, circulatory collapse

PHARMACOKINETICS AND PHARMACODYNAMICS

Duration of action: short, 3–4 h
Onset of action: short, 10–15 min
Peak action: 2–4 h after oral administration
Plasma half-life: 15–40 h
Bioavailability: rapidly distributed to all tissues
Metabolism: hepatic
Excretion: urine
Protein binding: high
Renal impairment: use with extreme caution
Hepatic impairment: contraindicated when marked
Elderly: may be more susceptible to CNS effects

PROLONGED USE

Perform periodic laboratory evaluation of organ systems (including hematopoietic, renal, and hepatic systems).

(Continued on next page)

SECOBARBITAL, SECOBARBITAL SODIUM (CONTINUED)

DOSAGE

Adults: *Oral*—For preoperative sedation, 200 to 300 mg 1 to 2 hours prior to surgery. For hypnotic effect at bedtime, 100 mg. *Parenteral*—For hypnotic effect at bedtime, 100 to 200 mg IM. For anesthetic procedures, administer at an IV rate of no more than 50 mg per 15-seconds; discontinue as soon as desired effect is achieved. Total dosage in excess of 250 mg is not recommended. If hypnosis is inadequate after 250 mg, add a small amount of meperidine. When used as an adjunct to spinal or regional anesthesia, a minimum of 50 to 100 mg is necessary. For dentistry, give 2.2 mg/kg to a maximum of 100 mg, 10 to 15 minutes before start of procedure. IM administration is recommended rather than IV. Effects should persist for 3 to 4 hours. For light sedation, use 1.1 to 1.6 mg/kg. For patients receiving nerve blocks, 100 to 150 mg may be given IV. The patient will awaken in 15 minutes and can be discharged in the company of another person after 30 min. If nitrous oxide is used, use secobarbital as above (anesthetic procedures). For control of convulsions in tetanus, give an initial dose of 5.5 mg/kg. Repeat every 3 to 4 hours, as necessary. Do not exceed the rate of 50 mg per 15-seconds with IV injections.

Children: *Oral*—For preoperative sedation, 50 to 100 mg up to a maximum of 100 mg. *Rectal (injectable solution)*—For premedication before ear, nose, and throat procedures; dilute solution with lukewarm water to a concentration of 1% to 1.5%, and administer after a cleansing enema. Children weighing less than 40 kg may receive up to 5 mg/kg; researchers recommend that larger children receive only 4 mg/kg. Atropine may be given. Hypnosis occurs in 15 to 20 minutes after rectal administration. Observe patients during this period. *Parenteral*—For dentistry, use same dose as adults (2.2 mg/kg).

OVERDOSAGE

Toxic doses vary. Generally, a dose of 1 g will produce serious toxic symptoms in an adult. Fatality may often occur after ingestion of 2–10 g.

Symptoms include CNS and respiratory depression (possibly progressing to Cheyne-Stokes respiration), areflexia, oliguria, tachycardia, hypotension, lowered body temperature, and coma. Typical shock syndrome also may occur. In extreme overdose, all electrical activity in the brain may cease, which will produce a "flat" EEG normally associated with clinical death; however, this should not be accepted as such. The effect is reversible unless hypoxic damage occurs. The possibility of barbiturate overdose should be considered even in situations appearing to involve trauma. Complications, such as pneumonia, pulmonary edema, cardiac arrhythmias, congestive heart failure, and renal failure, may occur. Uremia may increase CNS sensitivity to barbiturates if renal function is impaired. Hypoglycemia, head trauma, cerebrovascular accidents, convulsive states, and diabetic coma should be included in differential diagnosis.

Treatment is supportive. Adequate airway should be maintained, with respiratory assistance and oxygen therapy as necessary. Vital signs and fluid balance should be monitored. If patient is conscious and has not lost gag reflex, emesis may be induced using syrup of ipecac. After vomiting, 30 g of activated charcoal may be administered with water. If emesis is not possible, perform gastric lavage with patient face down and using a cuffed endotracheal tube. Again, activated charcoal may be left in the emptied stomach, and a saline cathartic may be administered. If renal function is normal, forced diuresis may aid in elimination. If the patient is anuric or in shock, hemodialysis may be helpful. Patient should be rolled from side to side every 30 min.

PATIENT INFORMATION

Do not increase dosage without contacting physician. Avoid tasks requiring alertness and dexterity. Do not consume alcohol; do not take other barbiturates or CNS depressants. Contact physician if any of the following occur: sore throat, fever, mouth sores, easy bruising or bleeding, nosebleed, or petechiae.

AVAILABILITY

Capsules—50 and 100 mg
Tablets—100 mg
Rectal injection—50 mg/mL
Injection—50 mg/mL

METHOHEXITAL SODIUM

(Brevital)

This drug is used primarily as an induction agent for general anesthesia. Its pharmacologic action is terminated by redistribution. It is frequently used for sedation during electroconvulsive therapy because it does not suppress the seizure focus.

DOSAGE

Note: Preanesthetic medication is recommended in most cases. Methohexital may be used with any of the recognized preanesthetic agents, but phenothiazines are less acceptable than the combination of an opiate and a belladonna derivative.

Adults: Dosage must be individualized. A 1% solution is recommended for induction of anesthesia and for maintenance by intermittent injection. Usual dosage range is 5 to 12 mL of a 1% solution (50–120 mg). This dose will allow for 5 to 7 minutes of anesthesia. Rate of injection is not fixed but is usually about 1 mL of the 1% solution (10 mg) in 5 seconds. If intermittent injection of a 1% solution is used for maintenance, additional amounts of about 2 to 4 mL (20–40 mg) will be necessary about every 4 to 7 minutes. Some anesthesiologists prefer the continuous drip method of maintenance with a 0.2% solution. Rate of flow should be individualized. As guidance, a rate of 1 drop/second may be used. This preparation is not compatible with lactated Ringer injection.

For 1% solution (10 mg/mL), the solution in the vial will be yellow when the first dilution is made. After it is diluted further to make a 1% solution, it should be clear and colorless; if it is not, do not use. Use the following table to prepare a 1% solution:

Dosage Form	Amount of Diluent
500-mg vial	50 mL
2.5-g vial	250 mL
2.5-g ampule	15 mL to ampule; dilute to 250 mL
5.0-g vial	500 mL
5.0-g ampule	30 mL to ampule; dilute to 500 mL

For continuous drip anesthesia, prepare a 0.2% solution by adding 500 mg to 250 mL diluent. Use 5% dextrose or isotonic (0.9%) sodium chloride instead of distilled water for this dilution to avoid extreme hypotonicity.

Note: Methohexital is not compatible with acid solutions (eg, atropine sulfate, metocurine iodide, succinylcholine chloride). Solutions are not compatible with silicone; avoid contact with rubber stoppers or parts of disposable syringes that have been treated with silicone.

Children: Safety and efficacy has not been established.

In Brief

INDICATIONS

Induction of anesthesia, supplementation of other anesthetic agents, IV anesthesia for short surgical procedures with minimal painful stimuli, induction of hypnotic state

AVAILABILITY

Powder for injection—500 mg in 50-mL vials; 500 mg in 50-mL vials with diluent; 2.5-g ampuls; 2.5 g in 250-mL vials; 5-g ampuls; 5 g in 500-mL vials

Injection—250-, 400-, and 500-mg syringes; 500-mg and 1-g vials with diluent; 1 mg/mL in 10-mL vials; 2 mg/mL in 2- and 5-mL amps and syringes; 500 mg in 20-mL syringes

Rectal suspension—400 mg/g of suspension (with mineral oil and dimethyldioctadecylammonium bentonite)

THIOPENTAL SODIUM
(Pentothal)

This drug is used primarily as an induction agent for general anesthesia. Its pharmacologic action is terminated by redistribution. It also can be used to terminate seizures if the physician is prepared to secure the airway.

DOSAGE

Adults: *Parenteral*—Administer by IV route only. Individual patient response is too varied for a fixed dosage to be established. Dosage titration is necessary, using age, gender, and weight as guidelines. For test dose, inject 25 to 75 mg, and observe for tolerance and sensitivity for at least 60 seconds. For anesthesia, moderately slow induction can be achieved in the average adult patient by injecting 50 to 75 mg (2–3 mL of a 2.5% solution) at intervals of 20 to 40 seconds, depending on patient response. After anesthesia is established, additional injections of 25 to 50 mg may be given whenever the patient moves. To minimize respiratory depression, slow injection is indicated. *Note:* When used as the only anesthetic agent, the objective level of anesthesia may be maintained by injection of small repeated doses as necessary or by using a continuous IV drip in a 0.2% or 0.4% concentration.

For convulsive states following anesthesia (inhalation or local) or other causes, give 75 to 125 mg (3–5 mL of a 2.5% solution) as soon as possible after the convulsions start.

Convulsions following the use of local anesthesia may require 125 to 250 mg given over 10 minutes.

Rectal suspension—Follow instructions carefully for filling dispenser; extrude a small amount before setting the stop device at the desired dose for rectal instillation. Extrusion may occasionally be difficult and may require considerable pressure on the syringe plunger, sometimes causing the stop device to break or slip and resulting in an overdose. If overdose occurs during administration, evacuate rectum immediately. Do not give further medication until degree of absorption is evaluated. For preanesthetic sedation, average dose is 1 g/34 kg or about 30 mg/kg.

For basal narcosis, give up to 1 g/22.5 kg to normally active adults or children. This dose is equivalent to a dose of 44 mg/kg and is the safe upper limit of dosage. Use a lower dosage in patients who are inactive or debilitated. Do not exceed total dosage of 1 to 1.5 g for children weighing 34 kg or more or 3 to 4 g for adults weighing 90 kg or more. A cleansing enema usually is not required, unless there are unusual circumstances, such as fecal impaction. The small volume used does not usually induce defecation; therefore, strapping of the buttocks is not necessary.

Children: *See* Adults dosage information.

In Brief

INDICATIONS

IV—Control of convulsive states; use in neurosurgical patients with increased intracranial pressure if adequate ventilation is provided; narcoanalysis and narcosynthesis in psychiatric orders; *Rectal suspension*—when preanesthetic sedation or basal narcosis by the rectal route is desired; may be used as the sole agent in selected, brief, minor procedures when muscular relaxation and analgesia are not required.

Induction of anesthesia; supplementation of other anesthetic agents; IV anesthesia for short surgical procedures with minimal painful stimuli; induction of hypnotic state

CHLORAZEPATE
(Tranxene)

Chlorazepate is a benzodiazepine used for the treatment of agitation caused by acute alcohol withdrawal, for the treatment of anxiety as part of anxiety disorders, for the short-term relief of symptoms of anxiety, and as an adjunct in the management of seizure disorders.

CHLORDIAZEPOXIDE
(Librium, Libritabs, Limbitrol)

This benzodiazepine is used for the management of anxiety disorders or for the short-term relief of anxiety, and for the management of agitation associated with acute alcohol withdrawal.

DOSAGE

Adults: *Oral*—Dosage must be individualized. For mild to moderate anxiety, 5 to 10 mg three to four times a day. For severe anxiety, 20 to 25 mg three to four times a day. For preoperative anxiety, on days preceding surgery, 5 to 10 mg three to four times a day. For acute alcohol withdrawal, 50 to 100 mg, followed with repeat doses as necessary, up to 300 mg/d. Parenteral form is generally used first. Reduce dose to maintenance levels as soon as possible. *Parenteral*—Prepare solution immediately before injection. Reconstitute only with special diluent that is provided (do not use diluent if opaque or hazy). If solution must be made with physiologic saline or sterile water for injection, do not administer IM because of pain on injection. Discard any unused solution. For control of acute symptoms (subsequent dosing should be oral), do not exceed 300 mg in a 6-hour period. For acute alcohol withdrawal, give initial dose of 50 to 100 mg IM or IV, repeated in 2 to 4 hours if necessary. For acute or severe anxiety, give initial dose of 50 to 100 mg IM or IV; follow with 25 to 50 mg three to four times a day if necessary. For preoperative tension and anxiety, 50 to 100 mg IM 1 hour before surgery.
Elderly (or debilitated patients): *Oral*—5 mg two to four times a day. *Parenteral*—Use lower adult doses (25–50 mg).
Children: Give initial dose of 5 mg two to four times a day; some children may require an increase to 10 mg two to three times a day. Not recommended for use in children younger than 6 years. An alternative dosage for children older than 6 years is 0.5 mg/kg/day every 6 to 8 hours.
Parenteral—Not recommended for use in children younger than 12 years. Use lower adult doses (25–50 mg) for children older than 12 years.

In Brief

INDICATIONS
Management of anxiety disorders; short-term relief of symptoms of anxiety; treatment of symptoms of acute alcohol withdrawal; relief of preoperative anxiety

AVAILABILITY
Capsules—5, 10, and 25 mg
Tablets—2, 5, 10, and 25 mg
Powder for injection—100 mg (as HCl) per amp

DIAZEPAM

(Valium)

This benzodiazepine is one of the first used therapeutically for sedation and hypnotic action. It is used to treat anxiety and provide light sedation and anterograde amnesia. It is also used as an anticonvulsant, especially for treatment of status epilepticus, as an agent for treatment of withdrawal, and as an adjuvant for relief of skeletal muscle spasms. Diazepam is classified primarily as an antianxiety agent.

DOSAGE

Adults: *Oral tablets and oral solution*—Dosage must be individualized and increased gradually to minimize incidence of adverse effects. Solution must be mixed with a liquid or semisolid food (water, juice, pudding, applesauce). For management of anxiety disorders and relief of symptoms of anxiety (depending on severity), 2 to 10 mg two to four times a day. For acute alcohol withdrawal, 10 mg three to four times for first 24 hours, reducing dose 5 mg three to four times a day, as necessary. For adjunct in skeletal muscle spasms, 2 to 10 mg three to four times a day. For adjunct in convulsive disorders, 2 to 10 mg two to four times a day. *Oral (sustained-release)*—Dosage must be individualized; do not crush or chew tablets. One 15-mg sustained-release capsule may be used whenever oral diazepam 5 mg three times a day is appropriate. This form is recommended for elderly patients, debilitated patients, and children. For management of anxiety disorders and relief of symptoms of anxiety, 15 to 30 mg/d, according to severity of symptoms. For adjunct in skeletal muscle spasm, 15 to 30 mg/d. *Parenteral*—Dosage must be individualized. Usual dose is 2 to 20 mg IM or IV, according to indication and severity. Some conditions may require larger doses (eg, tetanus). Injection may be repeated in 1 hour in acute conditions; however, an interval of three to four hours is usually effective. Use lower doses if other sedatives are also being given. For sedation or muscle relaxation, 2 to 10 mg/dose every three to four hours as necessary. *Note:* When administering IV, use appropriate procedures to reduce risk of venous thrombosis, phlebitis, local irritation, swelling, or vascular impairment.
Elderly or debilitated patients: Initial dose is 2 to 2.5 mg one to two times a day, increasing gradually as necessary, if tolerated. *Parenteral*—Use lower doses (2–5 mg) and more gradual increases (when necessary).
Children: Initial dose is 1 to 2.5 mg three to four times a day, increasing gradually as necessary, if tolerated. Do not use in children younger than 6 months. For sedation and muscle relaxation, give 0.12–0.8 mg/kg/24 h in divided doses three to four times a day. *Parenteral*—For maximum clinical effect with minimal doses and to reduce incidence of dangerous adverse effects, administer slowly over a period of 3 minutes. Do not exceed 0.25 mg/kg. Dose may be repeated after an interval of 15 to 30 minutes. Use appropriate adjunctive therapy if no relief occurs after third dose. Equipment for respiratory assistance should be ready. For moderate anxiety, 2 to 5 mg IM or IV, repeated in 3 to 4 hours if necessary. For severe anxiety, 5 to 10 mg IM or IV, repeated in 3 to 4 hours if necessary. For acute alcohol withdrawal, initially give 10 mg IM or IV, then 5 to 10 mg in 3 to 4 hours if necessary. For endoscopic procedures, use IV; titrate dosage to desired sedative response, such as slurred speech. Give slowly just before start of procedure. Narcotic dosage should be reduced by at least one third and may sometimes be omitted. If IV route cannot be used, IM 5 to 10 mg about 30 minutes before

(Continued on next page)

In Brief

INDICATIONS

FDA-approved: Management of anxiety disorders; short-term relief of symptoms of anxiety; treatment of symptoms of acute alcohol withdrawal impending on acute delirium tremens and hallucinosis; as an adjunct for the relief of skeletal muscle spasms caused by reflex spasm from local pathology. *Parenteral*—As an adjunct in status epilepticus and severe recurrent convulsive seizures (oral form may also be used in convulsive seizures); preoperative relief of anxiety and tension
Off-label: Treatment of panic attacks

AVAILABILITY

Capsules (sustained-release)—15 mg
Tablets—2, 5, and 10 mg
Oral solution—5 mg/mL and 5 mg/5 mL
Injection—5 mg/mL

DOSAGE *(CONTINUED)*

surgery is acceptable. For muscle spasm, give initial dose of 5 to 10 mg IM or IV, then 5 to 10 mg in 3 to 4 hours if necessary (tetanus may require higher doses). For status epilepticus and severe recurrent convulsive seizures, IV route is preferable, used slowly. Use IM route if IV is not possible. Give initial dose of 5 to 10 mg and repeat at 10 to 15 minutes intervals if necessary to a maximum of 30 mg total. Therapy may be repeated in 2 to 4 hours; a dose of 0.2 to 0.5 mg/kg every 15 to 30 minutes for 2 to 3 doses (maximum dose, 30 mg) has been recommended. Use extreme caution in patients with chronic lung disease or unstable cardiovascular status.

For infants older than 30 days and children younger than 5 years, inject 0.2 to 0.5 mg slowly every 2 to 5 minutes up to a maximum of 5 mg; 0.2 to 0.5 mg/kg/dose every 15 to 30 minutes for 2 to 3 doses (maximum dose 5 mg) has also been recommended. For neonates, 0.5 to 1 mg/kg/dose every 15 to 30 minutes for 2 to 3 doses has been suggested.

For children 5 years old and older, inject 1 mg every 2 to 5 minutes up to a maximum of 10 mg. Repeat in 2 to 4 hours if necessary. EEG monitoring of seizure may be helpful. A dose of 0.2 to 0.5 mg/kg/dose every 15 to 30 min for 2 to 3 doses (maximum dose 10 mg) has also been recommended.

As preoperative medication, 10 mg IM before surgery; if atropine, scopolamine, or other premedications are also desired, use separate syringes.

For cardioversion, 5 to 15 mg IV, 5 to 10 minutes before procedure. For tetanus in infants older than 30 days old, give 1 to 2 mg IM or IV slowly, and repeat dose every 3 to 4 hours as needed. For tetanus in children older than 5 years, 5 to 10 mg repeated every 3 to 4 hours may be necessary.

For sedation or muscle relaxation, 0.04 to 0.2 mg/kg/dose every 2 to 4 hours, to a maximum of 0.6 mg/kg within 8 hours.

ESTAZOLAM
(ProSom)

This benzodiazepine is used as a hypnotic agent in the short-term treatment of insomnia.

SPECIAL PRECAUTIONS

Monitor periodic blood counts, urinalysis, and blood chemistry analysis. EEG changes may occur, generally low-voltage fast activity, and are of no known significance.

Use with caution in patients with impaired respiratory function. Respiratory depression and sleep apnea have occurred with benzodiazepine use. Monitor patients closely.

May cause physical dependence. Withdrawal symptoms have occurred with sudden discontinuation in patients receiving high doses over prolonged periods. Use with caution in patients known to be at greater susceptibility for addictive effects. If withdrawal of drug is necessary, do so gradually.

Use with caution in patients who are depressed or in those who demonstrate evidence of latent depression or suicidal tendencies. Symptoms of depression may be intensified; protective measures may be necessary.

Anterograde amnesia and paradoxical reactions have occurred with use of therapeutic amounts of benzodiazepines (may be most common with triazolam).

Rebound sleep disorder may occur after sudden discontinuation of benzodiazepines. This condition is less likely to occur in drugs with longer half-lives (estazolam, flurazepam, quazepam).

Nocturnal sleep disturbance may occur on the first or second evening (or both) after discontinuation.

Whereas agents with short half-lives (temazepam, triazolam) appear to cause early-morning insomnia more frequently than do drugs with intermediate or long half-lives, the latter appear to cause daytime drowsiness more frequently.

(Continued on next page)

In Brief

INDICATIONS
Treatment of insomnia

CONTRAINDICATIONS
Allergy or hypersensitivity to benzodiazepines; pregnancy

INTERACTIONS
Alcohol, CNS depressants, cimetidine, contraceptives (oral), digoxin, disulfiram, isoniazid, neuromuscular blocking agents, phenytoin, probenecid, rifampin, smoking, theophyllines

ADVERSE EFFECTS
Note: Categorized by organ system in decreasing order of frequency.
Cardiovascular: Palpitations, chest pain, tachycardia, hypotension (rare)
CNS: Headache, nervousness, talkativeness, apprehension, irritability, confusion, euphoria, relaxed feeling, weakness, tremor, inability to concentrate, coordination impairment, memory impairment, depression, nightmares, insomnia, paresthesia, restlessness, tiredness, dyesthesia, hallucinations, horizontal nystagmus and paradoxical reactions, dizziness, drowsiness, lightheadedness, ataxia, severe sedation, lethargy, disorientation, coma (in overdose)
Dermatologic: Dermatitis, allergy, sweating, flushes, pruritus, skin rash (rare)
GI: Heartburn, nausea, vomiting, diarrhea, constipation, GI pain, anorexia, taste alterations, dry mouth, excessive salivation (rare), death from hepatic failure in a patient also receiving diuretics, jaundice, glossitis
Miscellaneous: Body pain, joint pain, tinnitus, GU effects, cramps, congestion, leukopenia, granulocytopenia, blurred vision, burning eyes, faintness, visual disturbances, shortness of breath, apnea, slurred speech (rare)

PHARMACOKINETICS AND PHARMACODYNAMICS
Duration of action: considerable variation in plasma concentrations; bioavailability in humans has not been established
Peak action: to peak plasma concentration, 2 h
Plasma half-life: 10–24 h
Bioavailability: completely and rapidly absorbed within 1 h of administration
Metabolism: hepatic, extensive (does not form active long-acting metabolite)

(Continued on next page)

ESTAZOLAM (CONTINUED)

SPECIAL GROUPS

Pregnancy: Not recommended.
Children: Do not use in children younger than 18 years (except flurazepam, < 15 y).
Elderly: Risk is increased for oversedation and CNS effects; use lowest dose possible.
Breast-feeding: Excreted in breast milk; safety not established.
Renal impairment: Use with caution.
Hepatic impairment: Use with caution.

DOSAGE

Adults: Give 1 mg at bedtime; some patients may require 2 mg for adequate effect.
Children: Not recommended for use in children younger than 18 years.
Elderly: If completely healthy, 1 mg at bedtime. Increase dose with caution. In patients who are of low weight or debilitated, try 0.5 mg as a starting dose.
Renal impairment: Use with caution.

PHARMACOKINETICS AND PHARMACODYNAMICS
(CONTINUED)

Excretion: < 5% unchanged in urine
Protein binding: 93%
Renal impairment: use with caution
Hepatic impairment: use with caution; metabolism reduced
Elderly: may be more susceptible to oversedation and CNS effects; use lowest dose

PROLONGED USE

Not intended for prolonged administration.

OVERDOSAGE

Symptoms include somnolence, confusion, reduced or absent reflexes, respiratory depression, apnea, hypotension, impaired coordination, slurred speech, seizures, and coma (ultimately). Fatalities have occurred with benzodiazepines alone and in combination with alcohol.

Treatment should include monitoring of respiration, pulse, and blood pressure; general supportive care; administration of IV fluids; and maintenance of airway. Gastric lavage is useful. Hemodialysis and forced diuresis are of little benefit. IV pressor agents may be required for treatment of hypotension; give IV fluids to bring on diuresis. Do not use barbiturates to treat excitement states. The possibility of multiple drugs being ingested must be considered.

PATIENT INFORMATION

Do not use alcohol or other CNS depressants; do not exceed prescribed dosage. Nocturnal sleep may be disturbed for one or two nights following discontinuation. If pregnancy occurs, is planned, or is already present, inform physician immediately. Use caution when performing tasks requiring alertness and dexterity; may cause drowsiness or dizziness.

AVAILABILITY

Tablets—1 and 2 mg

FLURAZEPAM HYDROCHLORIDE

(Dalmane)

This benzodiazepine is a hypnotic agent for the treatment of insomnia for up to 4 weeks.

SPECIAL PRECAUTIONS

Use with caution in patients with impaired respiratory function. Respiratory depression and sleep apnea have occurred with benzodiazepine use. Monitor patients closely.

May cause physical dependence. Withdrawal symptoms have occurred with sudden discontinuation in patients receiving high doses over prolonged periods. Use with caution in patients known to be at greater susceptibility for addictive effects. If withdrawal of drug is necessary, do so gradually.

Use with caution in patients who are depressed or in those who demonstrate evidence of latent depression or suicidal tendencies. Symptoms of depression may be intensified; protective measures may be necessary.

In Brief

INDICATIONS
Treatment of insomnia

CONTRAINDICATIONS
Allergy and hypersensitivity to benzodiazepines; pregnancy

INTERACTIONS
Alcohol, CNS depressants, cimetidine, contraceptives (oral), digoxin, disulfiram, isoniazid, neuromuscular blocking agents, phenytoin, probenecid, rifampin, smoking, theophyllines

ADVERSE EFFECTS
Laboratory test interactions: Elevated AST, ALT, total and direct bilirubin, and alkaline phosphatase
Note: Categorized by organ system in decreasing order of frequency.
Cardiovascular: Palpitations, chest pain, tachycardia, hypotension (rare)

(Continued on next page)

(Continued on next page)

SPECIAL PRECAUTIONS (CONTINUED)

Anterograde amnesia and paradoxical reactions have occurred with use of therapeutic amounts of benzodiazepines (may be most common with triazolam).

Rebound sleep disorder may occur after sudden discontinuation of benzodiazepines. This condition is less likely to occur in drugs with longer half-lives (estazolam, flurazepam, quazepam).

Nocturnal sleep disturbance may occur on the first or second evening (or both) after discontinuation.

Whereas agents with short half-lives (temazepam, triazolam) appear to cause early-morning insomnia more frequently than do drugs with intermediate or long half-lives, the latter appear to cause daytime drowsiness more frequently.

SPECIAL GROUPS

Children: Do not use in children younger than 15 years.
Elderly: Risk is increased for oversedation and CNS effects; use lowest dose possible.
Pregnancy: Contraindicated (FDA Category X).
Breast-feeding: Excreted in breast milk; safety not established.
Renal impairment: Use with caution.
Hepatic impairment: Use with caution.

DOSAGE

Adults: Dosage must be individualized. Usual dose is 30 mg before bedtime; 15 mg may be adequate in some patients.
Children: Not recommended for children younger than 15 years of age.
Elderly or debilitated patients: Begin with 15 mg and determine dosage according to individual response.
Renal impairment: Use with caution.

ADVERSE EFFECTS (CONTINUED)

CNS: Headache, nervousness, talkativeness, apprehension, irritability, confusion, euphoria, relaxed feeling, weakness, tremor, inability to concentrate, coordination impairment, memory impairment, depression, nightmares, insomnia, paresthesia, restlessness, tiredness, dysesthesia, hallucinations, horizontal nystagmus and paradoxical reactions, dizziness, drowsiness, lightheadedness, ataxia, severe sedation, lethargy, disorientation, coma (in overdose)
Dermatologic: Dermatitis, allergy, sweating, flushes, pruritus, skin rash (rare)
GI: Heartburn, nausea, vomiting, diarrhea, constipation, GI pain, anorexia, taste alterations, dry mouth, excessive salivation (rare), death from hepatic failure in a patient also receiving diuretics, jaundice, glossitis
Miscellaneous: Body pain, joint pain, tinnitus, GU effects, cramps, congestion, leukopenia, granulocytopenia, blurred vision, burning eyes, faintness, visual disturbances, shortness of breath, apnea, slurred speech (rare)

PHARMACOKINETICS AND PHARMACODYNAMICS

Peak action: to peak plasma concentration, 0.5–1 h; 1–3 h (N-desalkylfulrazepam, active metabolite)
Plasma half-life: 47–100 h (N-desalkylfulrazepam, active metabolite)
Bioavailability: completely and rapidly absorbed within 1 h of administration
Metabolism: hepatic, extensive to active metabolite, N-desalkylfulrazepam
Excretion: < 1% unchanged in urine
Protein binding: 97%
Renal impairment: use with caution
Hepatic impairment: use with caution; metabolism reduced
Elderly: may be more susceptible to oversedation and CNS effects; use lowest dose

PROLONGED USE

Not intended for prolonged administration.

OVERDOSAGE

Symptoms include somnolence, confusion, reduced or absent reflexes, respiratory depression, apnea, hypotension, impaired coordination, slurred speech, seizures, and coma (ultimately). Fatalities have occurred with benzodiazepines alone and in combination with alcohol.

Treatment should include monitoring of respiration, pulse, and blood pressure; general supportive care; administration of IV fluids; and maintenance of airway. Gastric lavage is useful. Hemodialysis and forced diuresis are of little benefit. IV pressor agents may be required for treatment of hypotension; give IV fluids to bring on diuresis. Do not use barbiturates to treat excitement states. The possibility of multiple drugs being ingested must be considered.

PATIENT INFORMATION

Do not use alcohol or other CNS depressants; do not exceed prescribed dosage. Nocturnal sleep may be disturbed for one or two nights following discontinuation. If pregnancy occurs, is planned, or is already present, inform physician immediately. Use caution when performing tasks requiring alertness and dexterity; may cause drowsiness or dizziness.

AVAILABILITY

Capsules—15 and 30 mg

HALAZEPAM

(Paxipam)

This benzodiazepine is used for the treatment of anxiety disorders or for the short-term relief of symptoms of anxiety.

DOSAGE

Adults: Dosage must be individualized and increased gradually to reduce risk of adverse effects. Usual dose is 20–40 mg 3–4 times a day. Optimal dosage range is from 80–160 mg/d. If adverse effects occur with initial dose, reduce subsequent doses.
Elderly or debilitated patients: 20 mg once or twice a day. Individualize dosage carefully.
Children: Safety and efficacy in children younger than 18 years has not been established.

In Brief

INDICATIONS
Management of anxiety disorders; short-term relief of symptoms of anxiety

AVAILABILITY
Tablets—20 and 40 mg

LORAZEPAM

(Ativan)

This benzodiazepine is used for the management of anxiety disorders or for the short-term relief of anxiety and for the production of antegrade amnesia.

DOSAGE

Adults: Dosage must be individualized and increased gradually to minimize incidence of adverse effects. If higher doses are indicated, increase evening dose before daytime doses. *Oral*—General dose is 2 to 6 mg/d (ranges from 1–10 mg/d) in divided doses; largest dose should be taken before bedtime. For anxiety, initial dose is 2 to 3 mg/d given in divided doses two to three times a day. For insomnia due to anxiety or transient situational stress, 2 to 4 mg at bedtime. *Parenteral*—IM, usual dose is 0.05 mg/kg up to a maximum of 4 mg. For optimum effect, give at least 2 hours before surgery. Inject undiluted, deep into muscle mass.
IV, usual initial dose is 2 mg total or 0.044 mg/kg, whichever is smallest. Sedation should occur with this dose in most adults; do not exceed this dose in patients older than 50 years. If a greater lack of recall is desired, doses as high as 0.05 mg/kg up to a total of 4 mg may be used. For optimum effect, give 15 to 20 minutes before surgery.
Note: Lorazepam must be diluted with an equal volume of compatible solution (sterile water for injection, sodium chloride injection, or 5% dextrose injection) immediately before IV use. Inject directly into vein or into the tubing of an existing IV infusion. Do not exceed a rate of 2 mg/min. Equipment for airway maintenance should be readily available.
Elderly or debilitated patients: Give an initial dose of 1 to 2 mg/d in divided doses; largest dose should be taken before bedtime.
Children: *Parenteral*—Use not recommended.

In Brief

INDICATIONS
FDA-approved: Management of anxiety disorders; short-term relief of anxiety or anxiety associated with depressive symptoms
Off-label: Management of status epilepticus; relief of chemotherapy-induced nausea and vomiting; treatment of acute alcohol withdrawal syndrome; treatment of psychogenic catatonia
Parenteral: Preanesthetic use in adults, for sedation, relief of anxiety, and an amnesia-like effect for surgical events. *Oral:* Treatment of insomnia.

AVAILABILITY
Tablets—0.5, 1, and 2 mg
Concentrated oral solution—2 mg/mL
Injection—2 and 4 mg/mL

MIDAZOLAM HYDROCHLORIDE

(Versed)

This benzodiazepine is structurally different in that it has an imidazole ring fused at positions 1 and 2 of the benzodiazepine ring. This substitution makes it water soluble, especially at acidic pH. At physiologic pH, it becomes more lipophilic. It is frequently used for sedation and inducing amnesia, especially associated with induction of anesthesia or monitored anesthesia care. It is used for short-term treatment of insomnia, sedation without general anesthesia, treatment of acute agitation, and the acute treatment of seizures (this use has not been fully determined).

SPECIAL PRECAUTIONS

IV midazolam is associated with respiratory depression and respiratory arrest, particularly when used for conscious sedation. This effect has resulted in death and hypoxic encephalopathy in cases in which it was not promptly recognized and effectively treated. Administer IV only in a hospital setting, with appropriate support equipment and staff present. Monitor respiratory and cardiac function continuously. Do not exceed doses of 2.5 mg (1 mg is initial dose). Do not give any dose as a bolus; give over period of at least 2 minutes and allow for additional 2 minutes for sedative effect to occur.

Dosages must be individualized. Resuscitative equipment must be readily available at all times, and continuous monitoring of patients is essential.

Serious cardiorespiratory adverse effects have occurred; use with caution in all patients. Do not give to patients who are in shock or coma or who are in acute alcohol intoxication with depression of vital signs. Use particular care in patients with uncompensated acute illness, eg, severe fluid or electrolyte imbalance.

Extreme caution is necessary to avoid intraarterial injection; hazards of this route are unknown. Avoid extravasation.

Hazardous tasks or tasks requiring alertness and dexterity must not be attempted by patients receiving midazolam until its effects have subsided or until the day after anesthesia and surgery (whichever is longer).

Patients at higher risk for adverse effects include elderly patients, debilitated patients, those with COPD, those with chronic renal impairment or failure, and those with CHF. Dosage requirements decrease with age.

Midazolam does not protect against increase in intracranial pressure or circulatory effects following administration of succinylcholine or pancuronium or associated with endotracheal intubation under light general anesthesia.

SPECIAL GROUPS

Children: Safety and efficacy not established for use in children younger than 18 years.
Elderly: At higher risk for adverse effects; dosage requirements decrease with increasing age.
Pregnancy: Increased risk of congenital malformations. Advise patient of risk.
Breast-feeding: Not known whether excreted. Use with caution.
Renal impairment: Use with caution; lower dosage recommended.
Hepatic impairment: Use with caution. The drug is metabolized extensively in the liver.

In Brief

INDICATIONS

IM: Preoperative sedation and impairment of memory of perioperative events
IV: Conscious sedation before short diagnostic or endoscopic procedures, alone or with a narcotic; induction of general anesthesia before administration of other anesthetic agents; as a supplement to nitrous oxide and oxygen (balanced anesthesia) for short surgical procedures

CONTRAINDICATIONS

Allergy or hypersensitivity to benzodiazepines; acute narrow-angle glaucoma
Note: Use in open-angle glaucoma only if patient is receiving appropriate therapy.

INTERACTIONS

Alcohol, barbiturates, CNS depressants (other), anesthetics (inhalation), narcotics, thiopental

ADVERSE EFFECTS

Most serious—Cardiorespiratory events and paradoxical reactions. *Most frequent*—Fluctuations in vital signs (including decreased tidal volume or respiratory rate decrease and apnea); headache, pain at injection site, muscle stiffness (IM); hiccoughs, nausea, vomiting, oversedation, headache, coughing, drowsiness, injection site irritation (IV). *Note:* The following adverse effects occurred generally with IV route. *Less frequent*—Laryngospasm, bronchospasm, dyspnea, hyperventilation, wheezing, shallow respirations, airway obstruction, tachypnea, bigeminy, premature ventricular contractions, vasovagal episode, tachycardia, nodal rhythm, acid taste, excessive salivation, retching, retrograde amnesia, euphoria, confusion, argumentativeness, nervousness, restlessness, delirium, prolonged emergency from anesthesia, insomnia, tonic-clonic movements, muscle tremor, involuntary or athetoid movements, ataxia, dizziness, dysphoria, slurred speech, dysphonia, paresthesia, blurred vision, diplopia, nystagmus, pinpoint pupils, blocked ears, hives, burning sensation, cold sensation, rash, pruritus, lethargy, chills, weakness, toothache, faint feeling, hematoma

PHARMACOKINETICS AND PHARMACODYNAMICS

Duration of action: plasma concentration declines in a biphasic manner; the terminal phase is 1–4 h.
Onset of action: 15 min (IM); 3–5 min (IV)
Peak action: 30–60 min; peak plasma concentrations, 45 min
Plasma half-life: elimination, 1.8–6.4 h (mean, 3 h)
Bioavailability: > 90% (IM)
Metabolism: rapid, to 1-hydroxymethyl midazolam (conjugated)
Excretion: < 0.03% unchanged in urine
Protein binding: 97%
Renal impairment: use with caution
Hepatic impairment: use with caution
Elderly: lower doses necessary

(Continued on next page)

MIDAZOLAM HYDROCHLORIDE
(CONTINUED)

DOSAGE

Adults: Dosage must be individualized. Administer slowly, and monitor continuously. Excessive doses or rapid or single bolus IV doses may cause respiratory depression or arrest. Midazolam is three to four times as potent as diazepam.

IM—Give midazolam slowly for conscious sedation. For induction of general anesthesia, give initial dose over 20 to 30 seconds. Avoid intraarterial injection or extravasation. For preoperative sedation and reduction of memory of perioperative events, give 0.07 to 0.08 mg/kg (about 5 mg for an average adult) IM, 1 hour before surgery.

IV—For conscious sedation before short diagnostic or endoscopic procedures (use alone or with a narcotic; use with topical anesthetic for oral procedures and narcotic for bronchoscopic procedures), 1 mg/mL by slow IV injection; dilute the 1- and 5-mg/mL formulations with 0.9% sodium chloride or 5% dextrose in water. If narcotic premedication or other CNS depressants are used, midazolam dose should be reduced by 30%.

For maintenance, give in increments of 25% of initial dose by slow titration only if a thorough clinical evaluation clearly indicates need for further sedation.

For induction of general anesthesia, before use of other anesthetics, IV, individual response varies, especially if narcotic premedication is not used. Dosage should be titrated to desired clinical effect according to patient's age and clinical status. Usual adult dose is 0.3 to 0.35 mg/kg over 20 to 30 seconds, allowing 2 minutes for effect.

Elderly or debilitated patients: In all cases, lower doses are necessary. Adjust dosage according to age or according to type and amount of premedication used.

Children: Safety and efficacy not established for use in children younger than 18 years.

Renal impairment: Use lower dosage.

PROLONGED USE

Not for prolonged use.

OVERDOSAGE

Symptoms include sedation, somnolence, confusion, coordination and reflex impairment, coma, and adverse effects on vital signs. Treatment includes monitoring of respiratory and cardiac function, pulse, and blood pressure and use of supportive measures. Maintain airway and support ventilation. IV infusion should be instituted. Hypotension should be treated with IV fluid therapy, repositioning, and judicious use of vasopressors and other measures. The value of peritoneal dialysis, forced diuresis, or hemodialysis is not known.

AVAILABILITY

Injection—1 mg (as HCl) per mL (with 1% benzyl alcohol and EDTA); 5 mg (as HCl) per mL (with 1% benzyl alcohol and EDTA)

OXAZEPAM

(Serax)

This benzodiazepine is used for the management of agitation associated with acute alcohol withdrawal and the management of anxiety disorders or the short-term relief of symptoms of anxiety or anxiety associated with depressive symptoms.

DOSAGE

Adults: Dosage must be individualized. For mild to moderate anxiety (with associated tension, irritability, agitation, or related symptoms of functional origin or secondary to organic disease), give 10 to 15 mg three to four times a day.

For severe anxiety syndromes or agitation or anxiety associated with depression, 15 to 30 mg three to four times a day.

For treatment of alcoholics with acute inebriation, tremulousness, or anxiety on withdrawal, 15 to 30 mg three to four times a day.

Elderly or debilitated patients: For anxiety, tension, irritability, and agitation, give initial dose of 10 mg three to four times a day; dosage may cautiously be increased to 15 mg three to four times a day, if necessary.

Children: Dosage not established.

Renal impairment: Use with caution.

In Brief

INDICATIONS

Management of anxiety disorders; short-term relief of symptoms of anxiety; treatment of anxiety associated with depression; management of anxiety, tension, agitation, and irritability in elderly patients; treatment of symptoms of alcohol withdrawal

AVAILABILITY

Capsules—10, 15, and 30 mg
Tablets—15 mg

PRAZEPAM
(Centrax)

Prazepam is a benzodiazepine that is used for the management of anxiety disorders or the short-term relief of symptoms of anxiety.

DOSAGE

Adults: Dosage must be individualized. Usual dosage is 30 mg/d given in divided doses. Dosage should be adjusted gradually, within the range of 20 to 60 mg/d according to patient response.
Elderly or debilitated patients: Start with a dose of 10 to 15 mg/d given in divided doses.
Children: Safety and efficacy in children younger than 18 years has not been established.

In Brief

INDICATIONS
Management of anxiety disorders; short-term relief of symptoms of anxiety

AVAILABILITY
Capsules—5, 10, and 20 mg
Tablets—5 and 10 mg

QUAZEPAM
(Doral)

This benzodiazepine is used as a hypnotic agent for the short-term treatment of insomnia. It is rapidly well absorbed from the GI tract.

SPECIAL PRECAUTIONS

Use with caution in patients with impaired respiratory function. Respiratory depression and sleep apnea have occurred with benzodiazepine use. Monitor patients closely.

May cause physical dependence. Withdrawal symptoms have occurred with sudden discontinuation in patients receiving high doses over prolonged periods. Use with caution in patients known to be at greater susceptibility for addictive effects. If withdrawal of drug is necessary, do so gradually.

Use with caution in patients who are depressed or in those who demonstrate evidence of latent depression or suicidal tendencies. Symptoms of depression may be intensified; protective measures may be necessary.

Anterograde amnesia and paradoxical reactions have occurred with use of therapeutic amounts of benzodiazepines (may be most common with triazolam).

Rebound sleep disorder may occur after sudden discontinuation of benzodiazepines. This condition is less likely to occur in drugs with longer half-lives (estazolam, flurazepam, quazepam).

Nocturnal sleep disturbance may occur on the first or second evening (or both) after discontinuation.

Whereas agents with short half-lives (temazepam, triazolam) appear to cause early-morning insomnia more frequently than do drugs with intermediate or long half-lives, the latter appear to cause daytime drowsiness more frequently.

In Brief

INDICATIONS
Treatment of insomnia

CONTRAINDICATIONS
Allergy or hypersensitivity to benzodiazepines; established or suspected sleep apnea; pregnancy

INTERACTIONS
Alcohol, CNS depressants, cimetidine, contraceptives (oral), digoxin, disulfiram, isoniazid, neuromuscular blocking agents, phenytoin, probenecid, rifampin, smoking, theophyllines

ADVERSE EFFECTS
Note: Categorized by organ system in decreasing order of frequency.
Cardiovascular: Palpitations, chest pain, tachycardia, hypotension (rare)
CNS: Headache, nervousness, talkativeness, apprehension, irritability, confusion, euphoria, relaxed feeling, weakness, tremor, inability to concentrate, coordination impairment, memory impairment, depression, nightmares, insomnia, paresthesia, restlessness, tiredness, dysesthesia, hallucinations, horizontal nystagmus and paradoxical reactions, dizziness, drowsiness, lightheadedness, ataxia, severe sedation, lethargy, disorientation, coma (in overdose)
Dermatologic: Dermatitis, allergy, sweating, flushes, pruritus, skin rash (rare)
GI: Heartburn, nausea, vomiting, diarrhea, constipation, GI pain, anorexia, taste alterations, dry mouth, excessive salivation (rare), death from hepatic failure in a patient also receiving diuretics, jaundice, glossitis
Miscellaneous: Body pain, joint pain, tinnitus, GU effects, cramps, congestion, leukopenia, granulocytopenia, blurred vision, burning eyes, faintness, visual disturbances, shortness of breath, apnea, slurred speech (rare)

PHARMACOKINETICS AND PHARMACODYNAMICS
Peak action: to peak plasma concentration, 2 h
Plasma half-life: 39 h
Bioavailability: completely and rapidly absorbed within 1 h of administration

(Continued on next page)

(Continued on next page)

QUAZEPAM (CONTINUED)

SPECIAL GROUPS

Breast-feeding: Not recommended.
Children: Do not use in children younger than 18 years (except flurazepam, < 15 y).
Elderly: Risk is increased for oversedation and CNS effects; use lowest dose possible.
Pregnancy: Contraindicated (FDA Category X).
Renal impairment: Use with caution.
Hepatic impairment: Use with caution.

DOSAGE

Adults: Start with 15 mg and determine dosage according to individual response; some patients may be treated adequately with 7.5 mg.
Children: Not recommended for use in children younger than 18 years.
Elderly or debilitated patients: Try to reduce nightly dose after the first or second night of treatment.
Renal impairment: Use with caution.

PHARMACOKINETICS AND PHARMACODYNAMICS (CONTINUED)

Metabolism: hepatic, extensive to active metabolite, 2-oxoquazepam (further metabolized to N-desalkyl-2-oxoquazepam, which is identical to N-desalkylflurazepam)
Excretion: trace amounts excreted unchanged in urine
Protein binding: > 95%
Renal impairment: use with caution
Hepatic impairment: use with caution; metabolism reduced
Elderly: may be more susceptible to oversedation and CNS effects; use lowest dose

PROLONGED USE

Not intended for prolonged administration.

OVERDOSAGE

Symptoms include somnolence, confusion, reduced or absent reflexes, respiratory depression, apnea, hypotension, impaired coordination, slurred speech, seizures, and coma (ultimately). Fatalities have occurred with benzodiazepines alone and in combination with alcohol.

Treatment should include monitoring of respiration, pulse, and blood pressure; general supportive care; administration of IV fluids; and maintenance of airway. Gastric lavage is useful. Hemodialysis and forced diuresis are of little benefit. IV pressor agents may be required for treatment of hypotension; give IV fluids to bring on diuresis. Do not use barbiturates to treat excitement states. The possibility of multiple drugs being ingested must be considered.

PATIENT INFORMATION

Do not use alcohol or other CNS depressants; do not exceed prescribed dosage. Nocturnal sleep may be disturbed for one or two nights following discontinuation. If pregnancy occurs, is planned, or is already present, inform physician immediately. Use caution when performing tasks requiring alertness and dexterity; may cause drowsiness or dizziness.

AVAILABILITY

Tablets—7.5 and 15 mg

TEMAZEPAM
(Restoril)

This benzodiazepine is used as a hypnotic agent for the short-term treatment of insomnia for periods of up to 5 weeks.

SPECIAL PRECAUTIONS

Use with caution in patients with impaired respiratory function. Respiratory depression and sleep apnea have occurred with benzodiazepine use. Monitor patients closely.

May cause physical dependence. Withdrawal symptoms have occurred with sudden discontinuation in patients receiving high doses over prolonged periods. Use with caution in patients known to be at greater susceptibility for addictive effects. If withdrawal of drug is necessary, do so gradually.

Use with caution in patients who are depressed or in those who demonstrate evidence of latent depression or suicidal tendencies. Symptoms of depression may be intensified; protective measures may be necessary.

Anterograde amnesia and paradoxical reactions have occurred with use of therapeutic amounts of benzodiazepines (may be most common with triazolam).

Rebound sleep disorder may occur after sudden discontinuation of benzodiazepines. This condition is less likely to occur in drugs with longer half-lives (estazolam, flurazepam, quazepam).

Nocturnal sleep disturbance may occur on the first or second evening (or both) after discontinuation.

Whereas agents with short half-lives (temazepam, triazolam) appear to cause early-morning insomnia more frequently than do drugs with intermediate or long half-lives, the latter appear to cause daytime drowsiness more frequently.

SPECIAL GROUPS

Children: Do not use in children younger than 18 years (except flurazepam, < 15 y).
Elderly: Risk is increased for oversedation and CNS effects; use lowest dose possible.
Pregnancy: Contraindicated (FDA Category X).
Breast-feeding: Excreted in breast milk; safety not established.
Renal impairment: Use with caution.
Hepatic impairment: Use with caution.

In Brief

INDICATIONS
Treatment of insomnia

CONTRAINDICATIONS
Allergy and hypersensitivity to benzodiazepines; pregnancy

INTERACTIONS
Alcohol, CNS depressants, cimetidine, contraceptives (oral), digoxin, disulfiram, isoniazid, neuromuscular blocking agents, phenytoin, probenecid, rifampin, smoking, theophyllines

ADVERSE EFFECTS
Note: Categorized by organ system in decreasing order of frequency.
Cardiovascular: Palpitations, chest pain, tachycardia, hypotension (rare)
CNS: Headache, nervousness, talkativeness, apprehension, irritability, confusion, euphoria, relaxed feeling, weakness, tremor, inability to concentrate, coordination impairment, memory impairment, depression, nightmares, insomnia, paresthesia, restlessness, tiredness, dysesthesia, hallucinations, horizontal nystagmus and paradoxical reactions, dizziness, drowsiness, lightheadedness, ataxia, severe sedation, lethargy, disorientation, coma (in overdose)
Dermatologic: Dermatitis, allergy, sweating, flushes, pruritus, skin rash (rare)
GI: Heartburn, nausea, vomiting, diarrhea, constipation, GI pain, anorexia, taste alterations, dry mouth, excessive salivation (rare), death from hepatic failure in a patient also receiving diuretics, jaundice, glossitis
Miscellaneous: Body pain, joint pain, tinnitus, GU effects, cramps, congestion, leukopenia, granulocytopenia, blurred vision, burning eyes, faintness, visual disturbances, shortness of breath, apnea, slurred speech (rare)

PHARMACOKINETICS AND PHARMACODYNAMICS
Peak action: to peak plasma concentration, 2–4 h
Plasma half-life: 9.5–12.4 h
Bioavailability: completely and rapidly absorbed within 1 h of administration
Metabolism: hepatic, extensive (does not form active long-acting metabolite)
Excretion: < 1.5% unchanged in urine
Protein binding: 96%
Renal impairment: use with caution
Hepatic impairment: use with caution; metabolism reduced
Elderly: may be more susceptible to oversedation and CNS effects; use lowest dose

PROLONGED USE
Not intended for prolonged administration.

OVERDOSAGE
Symptoms include somnolence, confusion, reduced or absent reflexes, respiratory depression, apnea, hypotension, impaired coordination, slurred speech, seizures, and coma (ultimately). Fatalities have occurred with benzodiazepines alone and in combination with alcohol.

Treatment should include monitoring of respiration, pulse, and blood pressure; general supportive care; administration of IV fluids; and maintenance of airway. Gastric lavage is useful. Hemodialysis and forced diuresis are of little benefit. IV pressor agents may be required for treatment of hypotension; give IV fluids to bring on diuresis. Do not use barbiturates to treat excitement states. The possibility of multiple drugs being ingested must be considered.

(Continued on next page)

TEMAZEPAM (CONTINUED)

DOSAGE

Adults: Dosage must be individualized. Usual dose is 15 to 30 mg before bedtime.

Children: Not recommended for use in children younger than 18 years.

Elderly or debilitated patients: Begin with a dose of 15 mg and determine dosage according to individual response.

Renal impairment: Use with caution.

PATIENT INFORMATION

Do not use alcohol or other CNS depressants; do not exceed prescribed dosage. Nocturnal sleep may be disturbed for one or two nights following discontinuation. If pregnancy occurs, is planned, or is already present, inform physician immediately. Use caution when performing tasks requiring alertness and dexterity; may cause drowsiness or dizziness.

AVAILABILITY

Capsules—15 and 30 mg

TRIAZOLAM

(Halcion)

This benzodiazepine is used as a hypnotic agent in the short-term treatment of insomnia generally for periods of 7 to 10 days. Anterograde amnesia and other behavioral effects (eg, confusion, bizarre or abnormal behavior, agitation, hallucinations) may occur more frequently with triazolam than with other benzodiazepines, especially at doses exceeding 0.25 mg or in elderly patients.

SPECIAL PRECAUTIONS

Monitor periodic blood counts, urinalysis, and blood chemistry analysis. EEG changes may occur, generally low-voltage fast activity, and are of no known significance.

Use with caution in patients with impaired respiratory function. Respiratory depression and sleep apnea have occurred with benzodiazepine use. Monitor patients closely.

May cause physical dependence. Withdrawal symptoms have occurred with sudden discontinuation in patients receiving high doses over prolonged periods. Use with caution in patients known to be at greater susceptibility for addictive effects. If withdrawal of drug is necessary, do so gradually.

Use with caution in patients who are depressed or in those who demonstrate evidence of latent depression or suicidal tendencies. Symptoms of depression may be intensified; protective measures may be necessary.

Anterograde amnesia and paradoxical reactions have occurred with use of therapeutic amounts of benzodiazepines (may be most common with triazolam).

Rebound sleep disorder may occur after sudden discontinuation of benzodiazepines. This condition is less likely to occur in drugs with longer half-lives (estazolam, flurazepam, quazepam).

Nocturnal sleep disturbance may occur on the first or second evening (or both) after discontinuation.

Whereas agents with short half-lives (temazepam, triazolam) appear to cause early-morning insomnia more frequently than do drugs with intermediate or long half-lives, the latter appear to cause daytime drowsiness more frequently.

In Brief

INDICATIONS

Treatment of insomnia

CONTRAINDICATIONS

Allergy and hypersensitivity to benzodiazepines; pregnancy

INTERACTIONS

Alcohol, CNS depressants, cimetidine, contraceptives (oral), digoxin, disulfiram, isoniazid, macrolides, neuromuscular blocking agents, phenytoin, probenecid, rifampin, smoking, theophyllines

ADVERSE EFFECTS

Note: Categorized by organ system in decreasing order of frequency.

Cardiovascular: Palpitations, chest pain, tachycardia, hypotension (rare)

CNS: Headache, nervousness, talkativeness, apprehension, irritability, confusion, euphoria, relaxed feeling, weakness, tremor, inability to concentrate, coordination impairment, memory impairment, depression, dreaming or nightmares, insomnia, paresthesia, restlessness, tiredness, dysesthesia, hallucinations, horizontal nystagmus and paradoxical reactions, dizziness, drowsiness, lightheadedness, ataxia, severe sedation, lethargy, disorientation, coma (in overdose)

Dermatologic: Dermatitis, allergy, sweating, flushes, pruritus, skin rash (rare)

GI: Heartburn, nausea, vomiting, diarrhea, constipation, GI pain, anorexia, taste alterations, dry mouth, excessive salivation (rare), death from hepatic failure in patient also receiving diuretics, jaundice, glossitis

Miscellaneous: Body pain, joint pain, tinnitus, GU effects, cramps, congestion, leukopenia, granulocytopenia, blurred vision, burning eyes, faintness, visual disturbances, shortness of breath, apnea, slurred speech (rare)

PHARMACOKINETICS AND PHARMACODYNAMICS

Peak action: to peak plasma concentration, 0.5–2h.

Plasma half-life: 1.5–5.5 h

Bioavailability: completely and rapidly absorbed within 1 h of administration

Metabolism: hepatic, extensive (does not form active long-acting metabolite)

Excretion: < 2% unchanged in urine

Protein binding: 78%–89%

Renal impairment: use with caution

Hepatic impairment: use with caution; metabolism reduced

Elderly: may be more susceptible to oversedation and CNS effects; use lowest dose

(Continued on next page)

SPECIAL GROUPS

Breast-feeding: Not recommended.
Children: Do not use in children younger than 18 years (except flurazepam, < 15 y).
Elderly: Risk is increased for oversedation and CNS effects; use lowest dose possible.
Pregnancy: Contraindicated (FDA Category X).
Renal impairment: Use with caution.
Hepatic impairment: Use with caution.

DOSAGE

Adults: Give 0.125 to 0.5 mg before bedtime.
Children: Not recommended for use in children younger than 18 years.
Elderly or debilitated patients: Begin with 0.125 mg and determine dosage according to individual response.
Renal impairment: Use with caution.

PROLONGED USE

Not intended for prolonged administration.

OVERDOSAGE

Symptoms include somnolence, confusion, reduced or absent reflexes, respiratory depression, apnea, hypotension, impaired coordination, slurred speech, seizures, and coma (ultimately). Fatalities have occurred with benzodiazepines alone and in combination with alcohol.

Treatment should include monitoring of respiration, pulse, and blood pressure; general supportive care; administration of IV fluids; and maintenance of airway. Gastric lavage is useful. Hemodialysis and forced diuresis are of little benefit. IV pressor agents may be required for treatment of hypotension; give IV fluids to bring on diuresis. Do not use barbiturates to treat excitement states. The possibility of multiple drugs being ingested must be considered.

PATIENT INFORMATION

Patients must be advised not to take triazolam when a full night's sleep and clearance of the drug from the body are not possible before they would again need to be functionally active.

AVAILABILITY

Tablets—0.125 and 0.25 mg

BUSPIRONE HYDROCHLORIDE

(BuSpar)

Buspirone hydrochloride is an antianxiety drug that is chemically and pharmacologically unrelated to the benzodiazepines, barbiturates, or other sedative-anxiety drugs. Buspirone does not have anticonvulsant or muscle-relaxant properties; significant sedation has not been observed.

SPECIAL PRECAUTIONS

Administration of buspirone to a patient taking an MAO inhibitor may pose a hazard.

Because buspirone has no established antipsychotic activity, it should not be used in place of appropriate antipsychotic treatment.

Studies indicate that buspirone is less sedating than are other anxiolytics and that it does not produce significant functional impairment; however, patients should be cautioned about driving until they are reasonably certain that buspirone treatment does not affect them adversely.

Although formal studies of the interaction of buspirone with alcohol indicate that buspirone does not increase alcohol-induced impairment, patients should avoid concomitant use of alcohol and buspirone.

In Brief

INDICATIONS

FDA-approved: No information found for use as sedative-hypnotic. The following indications were cited: management of anxiety disorders or short-term relief of symptoms of anxiety.
Off-label: Buspirone may be effective in treating patients with a number of disorders, such as depression in patients who have had limited response to SSRIs; social phobia; premenstrual syndrome; coping with reducing alcohol consumption; agitation associated with dementia; aiding in the cessation of smoking; or SSRI-induced sexual dysfunction.

CONTRAINDICATIONS

Patients with known hypersensitivity to buspirone hydrochloride

INTERACTIONS

MAO inhibitors, haloperidol, propranolol, phenytoin, warfarin, phenobarbital, digoxin

ADVERSE EFFECTS

Most common: Lightheadedness, dizziness, nausea, headache, nervousness, excitement
Other: Drowsiness, insomnia, decreased concentration, excitement, anger or hostility, confusion, depression, blurred vision, nausea, dry mouth, abdominal or gastric distress, diarrhea, constipation, vomiting, musculoskeletal aches or pains, numbness, paresthesia, incoordination, tremor, skin rash, fatigue, weakness, sweating, clamminess

(Continued on next page)

BUSPIRONE HYDROCHLORIDE (CONTINUED)

SPECIAL PRECAUTIONS (CONTINUED)

Before starting therapy with buspirone, withdraw patients gradually from prior treatment. This may be necessary because buspirone does not exhibit cross-tolerance with benzodiazepines and other sedative-hypnotics. Therefore, rebound or withdrawal symptoms may occur, depending in part on the type of drug used for prior treatment and its effective half-life of elimination. Several studies support an overlap regimen when switching from benzodiazepines to buspirone.

Because buspirone can bind to central dopamine receptors, its potential to cause acute and chronic changes in dopamine-mediated neurologic function (eg, dystonia, pseudoparkinsonism, akathisia, and tardive dyskinesia) is a concern, even though controlled studies have failed to identify significant neuroleptic activity.

SPECIAL GROUPS

Children: Safety and efficacy of buspirone in patients younger than 18 years have not been established, although some think it may be useful in this population.

Elderly: Buspirone has not been systematically evaluated in older patients; however, several hundred elderly patients have participated in clinical studies, and no unusual adverse age-related phenomena have been identified.

Pregnancy: Category B drug. No adequate and well-controlled studies in pregnant women have been conducted. Use only if clearly needed. The effect on labor and delivery in women also is unknown.

Breast-feeding: The extent of excretion and its metabolites in human breast milk are unknown. Avoid use in nursing women if clinically possible.

Renal impairment: Administration to patients with severe renal impairment cannot be recommended; this does not preclude administration to patients with mild renal dysfunction.

Hepatic impairment: Administration to patients with severe hepatic impairment cannot be recommended; this does not preclude administration to patients with mild hepatic dysfunction.

DOSAGE

Adults: Use with caution in patients with mild kidney or liver disease; use in patients with severe hepatic or renal impairment is not recommended. Initial dose is 15 mg daily (or 7.5 mg two times per day). To achieve optimum therapeutic response, increase the dose 5 mg/d in intervals of 2 to 3 days as needed. Do not exceed 60 mg/d. Divided doses of 20 to 30 mg/d have been used.

Elderly: Consider lower starting doses, although the target dose range is the same (30 mg/d to 60 mg/d).

Children: Not recommended for patients younger than 18 years.

PHARMACOKINETICS AND PHARMACODYNAMICS

Peak action: 40–90 min

Plasma half-life: 2–3 h (range, 2–11 h)

Bioavailability: although completely absorbed, systemic bioavailability is low (about 4%) because of great first-pass metabolism

Metabolism: rapidly absorbed and undergoes extensive first-pass metabolism; metabolized primarily by oxidation, producing several hydroxylated derivatives and active metabolite 1-pyrimidinyl piperazine

Excretion: eliminated by kidneys and excreted in urine (29%–63%) as metabolites and in feces (18%–38%)

Effect of food: food may decrease rate of absorption but increase the bioavailability by decreasing first-pass metabolism

Protein binding: 95% bound to plasma proteins

Renal impairment: renal pharmacokinetics related to buspirone have not been determined

Hepatic impairment: hepatic kinetics related to buspirone have not been determined

PROLONGED USE

Effectiveness for more than 3–4 wk has not been demonstrated in controlled trials; however, patients have been treated for several months without ill effect, and some may require long-term therapy if used for extended periods, periodically reassess usefulness of drug therapy

OVERDOSAGE

In clinical pharmacology trials, doses as high as 375 mg/d were administered to healthy male volunteers. As this dose was approached, nausea, vomiting, dizziness, drowsiness, miosis, and gastric distress occurred. No deaths have been reported either with deliberate or accidental overdose.

General symptomatic and supportive measures should be used, along with immediate gastric lavage. Respiration, pulse, and blood pressure should be monitored. No specific antidote buspirone is known, and dialyzability of buspirone has not been determined.

PATIENT INFORMATION

Patients should inform physician about any prescription or nonprescription drugs they are taking or are planning to take during buspirone therapy. Patients should inform physicians if they are pregnant, plan to become pregnant, or become pregnant during therapy. Likewise, patients should inform physician if they are breast-feeding. Driving a car should be avoided until patients experience how the medication affects them.

AVAILABILITY

Tablets—5 and 10 mg in 100s, 500s, and UD 100s
Dividose—15-mg tablet in 60s and 180s

CHLORAL HYDRATE
(Noctec)

This chloral derivative has been used as a hypnotic to treat insomnia. It is effective for short-term use for inducing and maintaining sleep, but by the end of 2 weeks, it loses much of its effectiveness. Newer agents, primarily benzodiazepines, have replaced this drug.

SPECIAL PRECAUTIONS

Patients should be advised to use caution when performing tasks requiring alertness and dexterity.

Do not use larger doses in patients with heart disease, esophagitis, gastritis, or gastric or duodenal ulcers.

Potential for addiction and abuse exists, especially with prolonged use of large doses. Tolerance and psychological dependence may develop as soon as the second week of continued administration. Symptoms of addiction may include slurred speech, incoordination, tremulousness, and nystagmus; also observed from excessive intake are drowsiness, lethargy, and hangover.

May cause irritation to skin and mucous membranes; gastric necrosis has occurred with ingestion of intoxicating amounts.

Some formulations may contain tartrazine, which can cause allergic-type reactions in some individuals; this is more common in patients sensitive to aspirin.

SPECIAL GROUPS

Children: Safe for use.
Pregnancy: Safety not established.
Breast-feeding: Excreted in breast milk; may cause sedation in nursing infant.
Renal impairment: Contraindicated in significant impairment.
Hepatic impairment: Contraindicated in significant impairment.

DOSAGE

Adults: For hypnotic effect, 500 mg to 1 g 15 to 30 minutes before bedtime or 30 minutes before surgery. For sedative effect, 250 mg twice daily after meals.
Children: For hypnotic effect, 500 mg/kg per day up to 1 g per single dose; also may be given in divided doses.
For sedative effect, 25 mg/kg per day up to 500 mg per single dose; also may be given in divided doses.
For dental sedation, doses higher than those suggested by the manufacturer are generally used; doses of 75 mg/kg, supplemented with nitrous oxide, may provide better sedation than the lower dose with no change in vital signs and no adverse effects.

In Brief

INDICATIONS

Nocturnal sedation, preoperative sedation to reduce anxiety and bring on sleep without depressing respiratory function or cough reflex; postoperative care and control of pain as an adjunct to opiates and analgesics; preventing or suppressing alcohol withdrawal symptoms (rectal).
Also effective as a hypnotic for short-term use only; after 2 wk of use, effectiveness is reduced.

CONTRAINDICATIONS

Allergy, hypersensitivity, or idiosyncrasy to chloral derivatives; significant renal or hepatic impairment; severe cardiac disease; gastritis

INTERACTIONS

Alcohol, anticoagulants (oral), CNS depressants, furosemide, hydantoins
Laboratory test interactions: May interfere with copper sulfate test for glycosuria; confirm such diagnosis with glucose oxidase test. Also may affect fluorometric tests for urine catecholamines; do not give medications for 48 h prior to testing. May alter urinary 17-hydroxycorticosteroid determinations when using the Reddy, Jenkins, and Thorn procedure.

ADVERSE EFFECTS

Most frequent: Drowsiness, dizziness
Frequent: Somnambulism, disorientation, incoherence, hangover (large doses; abrupt withdrawal), excitement, delirium, ataxia, mental confusion, nightmares, headache
Less frequent: Paranoid behavior, leukopenia, eosinophilia, rashes, GI irritation, nausea and vomiting, flatulence, diarrhea, unpleasant taste in mouth
Rare: Hallucinations, idiosyncratic syndrome, ketonuria

PHARMACOKINETICS AND PHARMACODYNAMICS

Duration of action: 1–4 h
Onset of action: about 30 min
Plasma half-life: trichloroethanol, 7–10 h
Bioavailability: readily absorbed
Metabolism: rapid, to active metabolite trichloroethanol; converted in liver and kidney to trichloroacetic acid (inactive)
Excretion: in urine and bile
Effect of food: no significant effect
Protein binding: 35%–41%; trichloroacetic acid, 71%–88%
Renal impairment: contraindicated in significant impairment
Hepatic impairment: contraindicated in significant impairment

PROLONGED USE

Not intended for prolonged use.

(Continued on next page)

CHLORAL HYDRATE
(CONTINUED)

OVERDOSAGE

Symptoms include stupor; coma; pinpoint pupils; hypotension; slow, rapid, or shallow respiration; hypothermia; areflexia; muscle flaccidity; nausea; vomiting. Excessive doses may cause esophagitis, gastritis, hemorrhagic gastritis, gastric necrosis, enteritis, hepatic damage, renal damage, cardiac damage. Amounts > 2 g can produce toxicity; however, death has occurred following doses of 1.25 and 3 g. Treatment includes gastric lavage or induction of vomiting; activated charcoal may follow to prevent drug absorption. Give general supportive care. Hemodialysis (aids in clearance of trichloroethanol) and hemoperfusion may be of benefit, but peritoneal dialysis is not.

PATIENT INFORMATION

May cause GI upset. Take medication whole with a full glass of water or other liquid; take syrup in half glass of water, juice, or ginger ale. Use caution when performing tasks requiring alertness and dexterity; may cause drowsiness or dizziness. Avoid alcohol and other CNS depressants.

AVAILABILITY

Capsules—250 and 500 mg
Syrup—250 mg/5 mL and 500 mg/5 mL
Suppositories—324, 500, and 648 mg

PARALDEHYDE

(Paral)

This aldehyde has been used to treat status epilepticus and for sedation in the treatment of delirium tremens. It has major side effects that preclude its use routinely.

SPECIAL PRECAUTIONS

Dilution is essential before administration; paraldehyde is irritating to mucous membranes, and esophagitis, gastritis, and proctitis have occurred.

May cause strong, unpleasant breath for as long as 24 hours after ingestion.

May be addictive; sudden withdrawal, especially after chronic use, should be avoided.

SPECIAL GROUPS

Children: Safety and efficacy not established.
Pregnancy: Use only if benefit outweighs risk. Do not use in labor; may cause respiratory depression in neonate.
Breast-feeding: Problems not documented; consider benefit versus risk.
Hepatic impairment: Contraindicated.

DOSAGE

Adults: *Oral*—For hypnosis, give 4 to 8 mL in milk or iced fruit juice to improve taste and odor. For delerium tremens, 10 to 35 mL may be required. *Rectal*—Dissolve in oil as a retention enema, mixing 10 to 20 mL with one or two parts of olive oil or isotonic sodium chloride solution to avoid rectal irritation.
For sedation, give 5 to 10 mg orally or rectally.
Children: For hypnosis, 0.3 mL/kg orally or rectally. For sedation, 0.15 mL/kg orally or rectally. Although children's dosage exists, safety has not been established.

In Brief

INDICATIONS

Used as a sedative and a hypnotic, to quiet patients, and to bring on sleep during delerium tremens and other psychiatric states characterized by excitement

CONTRAINDICATIONS

Allergy or hypersensitivity; bronchopulmonary disease; hepatic impairment; gastroenteritis

INTERACTIONS

Disulfiram

ADVERSE EFFECTS

Frequent: Strong, unpleasant breath odor
Prolonged use: Drug dependency resembling alcoholism (withdrawal may cause delirium tremens and hallucinations; several cases of metabolic acidosis have occurred with uncertain etiology); jaundice

PHARMACOKINETICS AND PHARMACODYNAMICS

Duration of action: 8–12 h
Onset of action: 10–15 min
Peak action: peak concentration, 30–60 min with oral form
Plasma half-life: 3.4–9.8 h
Bioavailability: rapidly absorbed after oral administration
Metabolism: 70%–80% hepatic
Excretion: exhalation (11%–25%) and negligible amounts in urine
Hepatic impairment: increased excretion through lungs; elimination rate decreased

PROLONGED USE

Drug dependence resembling alcoholism may occur; do not discontinue drug suddenly.

(Continued on next page)

OVERDOSAGE

Symptoms may include unconsciousness, coma, rapid or labored breathing, pulmonary hemorrhage, edema, throat or stomach or rectum irritation, nausea, vomiting, esophagitis, hemorrhagic gastritis, hepatitis, renal damage, agitation, pseudoketosis, hyperacetaldehydemia, and right heart dilation. Primary effect of toxicity is metabolic acidosis, which should be treated with IV sodium bicarbonate or sodium lactate. Death has occurred after 25 mL oral or 12 mL rectal. Treatment includes intensive support therapy. Respiratory function, acidosis correction, and hepatic protection are essential. Gastric lavage is not appropriate because this agent is absorbed rapidly following administration. Hemodialysis or peritoneal dialysis may be necessary to treat acidosis and support renal function.

PATIENT INFORMATION

May cause GI upset; take with food, or mix with milk or fruit juice. Avoid alcohol and other CNS depressants. Use caution when performing activities requiring alertness and dexterity; may cause drowsiness and dizziness. Throw away any unused drug after bottle has been opened. Do not use if liquid is brown or has a strong, vinegar-like odor.

AVAILABILITY

Liquid (oral or rectal)—1 g/mL in 30-mL bottles

ZOLPIDEM TARTRATE

(Ambien)

This imidazopyridine is a new agent used to treat insomnia. Unlike the benzodiazepines, it has little or no myorelaxant, anticonvulsant, or anxiolytic properties.

SPECIAL PRECAUTIONS

Hypnotics should be limited to 7 to 10 days of use only; if such agents are needed for more than 2 to 3 weeks, reevaluate the patient. Do not prescribe more than a 1-month supply.

Sleep disturbances may be the presenting symptom of a physical or psychiatric disorder; therefore, initial treatment should proceed only after a thorough examination of the patient.

Abnormal thinking and behavior changes are associated with sedative and hypnotic drug use. These changes may include decreased inhibition and other similar effects produced by alcohol and other CNS depressants; bizarre behavior; agitation; hallucinations; depersonalization; amnesia; and worsening of depression (including suicidal thoughts).

Adverse effects are generally dose related; use lowest possible effective dose (particularly in elderly patients).

Zolpidem causes CNS depressant effects, which are additive when this drug is combined with alcohol (and other CNS depressants). Advise patients of risk of performing activities requiring alertness and dexterity.

Avoid abrupt discontinuation; withdrawal symptoms may occur. This drug is carcinogenic in rats.

Use with caution in patients with respiratory function impairment.

SPECIAL GROUPS

Children: Safety and efficacy not established in children younger than 18 years.
Elderly: Monitor closely and use lowest possible dose; risk is increased for adverse effects.
Pregnancy: Human studies not performed; use only when absolutely necessary.
Breast-feeding: Excreted in breast milk; avoid nursing.
Renal impairment: No dosage adjustment necessary; however, close monitoring is recommended.
Hepatic impairment: Modified dosage is necessary.

(Continued on next page)

In Brief

INDICATIONS
Short-term treatment of insomnia

CONTRAINDICATIONS
None

INTERACTIONS
Alcohol, CNS depressants

ADVERSE EFFECTS
Most frequent: Headache, drowsiness
Frequent: Nausea, dizziness, dyspepsia, abdominal pain, upper respiratory infection, sinusitis, pharyngitis, dry mouth, constipation, back pain, flu-like symptoms, lethargy, drugged feeling, lightheadedness, depression, arthralgia
Less frequent: Diarrhea, myalgia, abnormal dreams, amnesia, anxiety, anorexia, vomiting, rhinitis, infection, palpitation, rash, urinary tract infection, fatigue

PHARMACOKINETICS AND PHARMACODYNAMICS
Onset of action: rapid
Peak action: 1.6 h
Plasma half-life: 2.6
Bioavailability: rapid absorption from the GI tract
Metabolism: to two primary metabolites
Excretion: renal
Effect of food: decreases bioavailability and C_{max}
Protein binding: 92.5%
Renal impairment: no significant changes in pharmacokinetics; not dialyzable in end-stage renal failure
Hepatic impairment: half-life prolonged
Elderly: half-life, bioavailability, and C_{max} increased

PROLONGED USE
Not recommended for prolonged use.

OVERDOSAGE
Results of overdose have included symptoms ranging from somnolence to light coma; one case of cardiovascular compromise and one of respiratory compromise were reported. Full recovery has been made in patients ingesting overdoses of up to 400 mg. Overdosage involving multiple CNS depressants (including zolpidem) have caused more serious symptoms, including fatalities. Treatment includes

(Continued on next page)

ZOLPIDEM TARTRATE
(CONTINUED)

DOSAGE

Adults: Dosage must be individualized. Usual dose is 10 mg immediately before bedtime.
Elderly or debilitated patients: Use initial dose of 5 mg.
Children: Safety not established.
Hepatic impairment: Use initial dose of 5 mg.

OVERDOSAGE (CONTINUED)

general supportive and symptomatic therapy. Use immediate gastric lavage when appropriate. Give IV fluids if necessary. Monitor hypotension and CNS depression, using medical intervention if necessary. Withhold sedative agents after zolpidem overdose, even if excitation occurs. Zolpidem is not dialyzable. In one study, flumazenil reversed sedative-hypnotic effects of zolpidem; however, it did not affect the pharmacokinetics.

PATIENT INFORMATION

Do not use alcohol or other CNS depressants during zolpidem therapy. Use caution when performing activities requiring alertness and dexterity; may cause drowsiness and dizziness.

AVAILABILITY

Tablets—5 and 10 mg

GLUTETHIMIDE
(Doriden)

This piperidine derivative is used as a hypnotic agent in the short-term treatment of insomnia, generally for 3 to 7 days.

SPECIAL PRECAUTIONS

Advise patient to use caution when performing tasks requiring alertness and dexterity; may cause drowsiness and dizziness.
This drug causes physical and psychological dependence; evaluate patient carefully prior to prescribing drug. Prescribe 1-week supply only; reevaluate patient. If dependence occurs, reduce dose gradually.

SPECIAL GROUPS

Children: Not recommended. Safety and efficacy not established.
Pregnancy: Use only if clearly indicated; potential for harm to fetus not known.
Breast-feeding: Potential for serious adverse effects to infant; decide whether to discontinue nursing or discontinue drug.
Renal impairment: Contraindicated.
Hepatic impairment: Contraindicated in patients with porphyria.

DOSAGE

Adults: Dosage must be individualized. Usual dose is 250 to 500 mg taken at bedtime.
Children: Not recommended.
Elderly or debilitated patients: Do not exceed initial daily dosage of 500 mg at bedtime to avoid oversedation.
Renal impairment: Contraindicated.

In Brief

INDICATIONS

FDA-approved: Short-term relief of insomnia (3–7 d). Not intended for chronic use. If further treatment is necessary, an interval of at least 1 wk should elapse before retreatment. Nondrug therapy should be attempted for patients with chronic insomnia.

CONTRAINDICATIONS

Allergy or hypersensitivity to glutethimide; porphyria

INTERACTIONS

Alcohol, CNS depressants, anticoagulants (oral), charcoal

ADVERSE EFFECTS

Frequent: Rash, nausea, drowsiness
Less frequent: Vertigo, headache, depression, dizziness, ataxia, confusion, edema, indigestion, nocturnal diaphoresis, dry mouth, euphoria, memory impairment, tinnitus, slurred speech
Rare: Paradoxical excitation, blurred vision, acute hypersensitivity, porphyria, blood dyscrasias

PHARMACOKINETICS AND PHARMACODYNAMICS

Duration of action: irregularly absorbed from GI tract
Onset of action: irregularly absorbed from GI tract
Peak action: peak plasma concentration, 1–6 h
Plasma half-life: 10–12 h
Bioavailability: erratically absorbed from GI tract
Metabolism: glutethimide is a racemate; both isomers are hydroxylated and then conjugated with glucuronic acid; the glucuronides pass into enterohepatic circulation and then are excreted
Excretion: in urine, < 2% unchanged
Protein binding: 50%
Renal impairment: contraindicated
Hepatic impairment: contraindicated in patients with porphyria; almost completely metabolized in the liver

PROLONGED USE

Not intended for prolonged use.

(Continued on next page)

OVERDOSAGE

Symptoms are dose dependent and indistinguishable from barbiturate intoxication. Treatment should include cardiopulmonary support (including plasma volume expanders and vasopressor agents if necessary), monitoring of vital signs, gastric lavage in the conscious patient, maintained urinary output in prolonged coma, dialysis/hemoperfusion in grade III or grade IV coma (or when renal function is impaired or shut down or in life-threatening situations with serious systemic complications), alternative use of charcoal hemoperfusion (simpler and more effective than hemodialysis).

Note: This drug is highly lipid soluble. Even after significant amounts have been removed, blood level rebound due to release from fat storage can cause coma to persist or recur. Continue drug extraction procedures for a minimum of 2 h after patient regains consciousness.

PATIENT INFORMATION

Avoid alcohol and other CNS depressants. Use caution when performing task requiring alertness and dexterity; may cause drowsiness or dizziness.

AVAILABILITY

Tablets—250 and 500 mg

METHYPRYLON

(Noludar)

This is a piperidine derivative used to treat insomnia.

SPECIAL PRECAUTIONS

Can cause physical and psychological dependence; withdrawal symptoms mimic those of barbiturate withdrawal and should be treated as such. Use with caution in patients who are likely to be more susceptible to addiction.

Do not exceed 400 mg/d total dosage; no benefit is derived from higher doses.

Advise patients of potential to cause drowsiness and dizziness and of need to use caution while driving or performing other tasks requiring alertness and dexterity.

Perform blood counts periodically if this drug is used repeatedly or over a prolonged period.

Porphyria may be exacerbated; use with caution in patients at risk. Stimulates hepatic microsomal enzyme system.

SPECIAL GROUPS

Children: Safety and efficacy not established in children younger than 12 years.
Elderly: Age-related renal or hepatic impairment more likely; use caution when dosing; may be more susceptible to toxic effects.
Pregnancy: Adequate studies not performed. Use only when benefit is greater than risk.
Breast-feeding: Not known whether excreted; use with caution.
Renal impairment: Use with caution.
Hepatic impairment: Use with caution.

DOSAGE

Adults: Dosage must be individualized. Usual dose is 200 to 400 mg administered before bedtime.
Children (older than 12 years): Initiate treatment with 50 mg at bedtime, increasing to 200 mg if necessary. Effective dosage varies greatly.

In Brief

INDICATIONS

FDA-approved: For short-term use as a hypnotic (effective for at least 7 d)

CONTRAINDICATIONS

Allergy or hypersensitivity to methyprylon

INTERACTIONS

Alcohol, CNS depressants

ADVERSE EFFECTS

Most frequent: Morning drowsiness, dizziness, headache, vertigo
Frequent: Hypotension, nausea, confusion (particularly in elderly patients), nightmares
Less frequent: Hangover effect, rash, EEG changes, pyrexia, syncope, paradoxical excitation, anxiety, depression, blurred vision, diarrhea, constipation, allergic reactions, acute brain syndrome, hallucinations

PHARMACOKINETICS AND PHARMACODYNAMICS

Duration of action: 5–8 h
Onset of action: 45 min
Peak action: 1–2 h, peak plasma concentrations
Plasma half-life: 4 h; longer with intoxication
Bioavailability: rapidly absorbed after oral administration
Metabolism: dehydrogenation with subsequent oxidation to form the alcohol and corresponding acid and oxidation to produce 6-oxymethyprylon
Excretion: < 1% recovered in urine tract; 23% as metabolites in 72 h
Protein binding: 60%
Renal impairment: use with caution
Hepatic impairment: use with caution
Elderly: may have age-related renal and hepatic impairment; may be more susceptible to toxic effects

(Continued on next page)

METHYPRYLON (CONTINUED)

PROLONGED USE
Monitor blood counts. Observe carefully for signs of drug dependence.

OVERDOSAGE
Symptoms include somnolence, confusion, coma, shock, constricted pupils, respiratory depression, hypotension, tachycardia, edema, and hepatic dysfunction. Drug concentrations in blood associated with severe toxicity range from 3–6 mg/dL. Range for fatalities is 5.3–114 mg/dL. One fatality has occurred from the digestion of 6 g. Treatment includes monitoring of respiration, pulse, and blood pressure. General supportive measures are recommended, as is immediate gastric lavage (use caution to avoid pulmonary aspiration). Give

IV fluids as appropriate; use norepinephrine or metaraminol to treat hypotension. When supportive measure are not adequate, hemodialysis may be beneficial. In cases of severe excitation and convulsions (rare), barbiturates may be used with extreme caution.

PATIENT INFORMATION
Do not exceed prescribed dosage. Do not take more than 400 mg/d. May cause dependency; do not discontinue medication suddenly. Use caution when performing tasks requiring alertness and dexterity; may cause drowsiness or dizziness. Avoid alcohol and other CNS depressants.

AVAILABILITY
Capsules—300 mg
Tablets—200 mg

MEPROBAMATE
(Equanil, Mitocon)

This is one of the first drugs used for treatment of anxiety disorders or for the short-term relief of symptoms of anxiety.

SPECIAL PRECAUTIONS
Physical and psychological dependence may occur. Use with caution in patients at risk for substance abuse or for suicidal tendencies. Supervise amounts prescribed and dosage carefully, dispensing small amounts each time.

Abrupt withdrawal may produce adverse symptoms. If prolonged dosage has been used, decrease dose gradually over a period of 1 to 2 weeks.

Hypersensitivity may occur after the first to fourth doses in patients with no known previous exposure or sensitivity. If effects occur, discontinue drug and treat supportively. Also consider allergy to excipients.

Use with caution in patients with epilepsy; may precipitate seizures.

Advise patients of potential for medication to cause drowsiness or dizziness; caution should be observed when performing tasks requiring alertness and dexterity.

SPECIAL GROUPS
Children: Do not use in children younger than 6 years. The 600-mg tablet is not for use in children.
Elderly: Use lowest effective dose to avoid oversedation.
Pregnancy: Increased risk of congenital malformation during first trimester. Use with extreme caution, if at all, during pregnancy. Advise patients of risk and consider possibility of pregnancy in women of childbearing age before start of therapy.
Breast-feeding: Excreted in breast milk. Effects of drug on infant are not known.
Renal impairment: Use with caution to avoid accumulation.
Hepatic impairment: Use with caution to avoid accumulation.

(Continued on next page)

In Brief

INDICATIONS
Management of anxiety disorders; short-term relief of symptoms of anxiety.
Note: Anxiety associated with everyday life usually does not necessitate treatment with an anxiolytic. Effectiveness in long-term use (> 4 mo) has not been evaluated by systematic clinical studies. Usefulness of drug in patients should be assessed per individual at periodic intervals.

CONTRAINDICATIONS
Allergy or hypersensitivity; acute intermittent porphyria; idiosyncratic reactions to meprobamate or related compounds

INTERACTIONS
Alcohol

ADVERSE EFFECTS
Frequent: Drowsiness, ataxia, dizziness, slurred speech, headache, nausea
Less frequent: Vertigo, weakness, impairment of vision, euphoria, overstimulation, paradoxical excitement, fast EEG activity, palpitations, diarrhea, tachycardia, arrhythmias, transient ECG changes, rash, exacerbation of porphyric symptoms, paresthesias
Rare: Hypersensitivity, agranulocytosis and aplastic anemia, thrombocytopenic purpura, syncope and hypotensive crises (one fatality)

PHARMACOKINETICS AND PHARMACODYNAMICS
Onset of action: < 1 h
Peak action: 1–3 h
Plasma half-life: 6–17 h (24–48 h in long-term administration)
Bioavailability: well absorbed from GI tract
Metabolism: hepatic, 80%–92%
Excretion: renal, 90%; < 10% in feces
Protein binding: 20% of drug is bound to plasma proteins, *in vitro*
Renal impairment: use with caution to avoid accumulation
Hepatic impairment: use with caution to avoid accumulation
Elderly: use lowest effective dose

PROLONGED USE
Effectiveness of long-term use (> 4 mo) has not been systematically evaluated in clinical studies.

DOSAGE

Adults: Usual dosage is 1.2 to 1.6 g/d in three to four divided doses. Do not exceed 2.4 g/d. *Sustained-release*—400 to 800 mg in the morning and at bedtime.
Children (6–12 y): 100 to 200 mg two to three times a day. *Sustained-release*—200 mg in the morning and at bedtime.
Elderly or debilitated patients: Use lowest effective dose.
Renal impairment: Use with caution to avoid accumulation.

OVERDOSAGE

Symptoms of acute intoxication include drowsiness, lethargy, stupor, ataxia, coma, shock, vasomotor and respiratory collapse, and death. Cardiovascular effects may include arrhythmias, tachycardia, bradycardia, and reduced venous return. Hypotension, profound and persistent, occurs and can manifest unexpectedly in mildly comatose patients. Airway obstruction problems may result from excessive oronasal secretions or relaxation of the pharyngeal wall. Treatment is supportive and symptomatic. Gastric lavage is of value only immediately after ingestion owing to rapid absorption. Gastroscopy may be indicated; ingestion of large amounts may result in drug conglomerates in the stomach. Continue gastric lavage. Relapse and death occurring after initial recovery have been attributed to incomplete gastric emptying and delayed absorption. Frequent evaluation of vital signs is essential. Hypotension may occur rapidly and become persistent unless blood volume is expanded. Avoid fluid overload because fatal pulmonary edema has occurred. Respiratory assistance should be provided as needed. Use caution in treatment of convulsions because of combined effects of agents on CNS depression. If patient's coordination deteriorates despite assisted respiration, forced diuresis and pressor agents should be attempted and then followed by hemodialysis. Meprobamate is dialyzable. Hemoperfusion (resin or charcoal) is more effective than is hemodialysis; it may reduce the half-life more than threefold.

AVAILABILITY

Tablets—200, 400, and 600 mg
Capsules (sustained-release)—200 and 400 mg

ETHCHLORVYNOL

(Placidyl)

This tertiary acetylenic alcohol is used to treat short-term, simple insomnia for up to 1 week.

SPECIAL PRECAUTIONS

May cause physical and psychological dependence; use with caution in patients with mental depression or suicidal tendencies and in those who have known or suspected potential for drug dependency.

Withdrawal symptoms similar to barbiturate withdrawal may occur.

Advise patient of drug's potential to cause drowsiness or dizziness and of need for caution while driving or performing other tasks requiring alertness and dexterity.

Patients who experience paradoxical or unpredictable behavior with alcohol or barbiturates also may experience such effects with ethchlorvynol.

Do not use to manage insomnia if pain is present. Use only if insomnia persists after pain has been relieved with analgesics.

Some preparations contain tartrazine, which can cause a hypersensitivity reaction in some patients. Reactions are more frequent in patients with aspirin sensitivity.

In Brief

INDICATIONS

FDA-approved: Short-term hypnotic treatment (for up to 1 wk in management of insomnia). Use for retreatment only after drug-free intervals of at least 1 wk and only after further evaluation of patient.

CONTRAINDICATIONS

Allergy or hypersensitivity to ethchlorvynol (or tartrazine in preparation); porphyria

INTERACTIONS

Alcohol, CNS depressants

ADVERSE EFFECTS

Most frequent: Dizziness, GI upset, aftertaste
Frequent: Transient giddiness and ataxia (rapid absorption), hypotension, nausea, mild hangover effect
Less frequent: Vomiting, syncope without marked hypotension, mild stimulation, facial numbness, rash, urticaria, blurred vision
Rare: Cholestatic jaundice, profound muscular weakness, thrombocytopenia, fatal immune thrombocytopenia (one case)

PHARMACOKINETICS AND PHARMACODYNAMICS

Duration of action: 5 h
Onset of action: 15–60 min
Peak action: 2 h
Plasma half-life: 10–12 h
Bioavailability: rapidly absorbed from GI tract; 90% of drug destroyed in liver; tissue localization is extensive, especially in adipose tissue
Metabolism: hepatic?

(Continued on next page)

(Continued on next page)

ETHCHLORVYNOL (CONTINUED)

SPECIAL GROUPS

Children: Not recommended. Safety and efficacy not established.
Elderly: Use lowest dose possible.
Pregnancy: Not recommended for use during first and second trimesters; use during third trimester may produce CNS depression and transient symptoms of withdrawal in the newborn. This drug is associated with a high percentage of stillbirths and a low survival rate of offspring in rats. Use only if benefit outweighs risk.
Breast-feeding: Not known whether excreted in breast milk. Due to potential for serious adverse effects in infant, decision must be made to discontinue nursing or discontinue drug.
Renal impairment: Use with caution.
Hepatic impairment: Use with caution.

DOSAGE

Adults: For hypnotic effect, 500 mg at bedtime; if response is inadequate or if patient is changing from a barbiturate to a nonbarbiturate, 750 mg may be used. Do not prescribe for more than 1 week. Use smallest possible dose in patients who are elderly or debilitated.
For severe insomnia, up to 1000 mg may be given as a single dose at bedtime.
For supplemental doses in cases of insomnia characterized by untimely awakening in early-morning hour, use 200 mg to bring on sleep in patients who have already received initial bedtime dose of 500 to 750 mg.
Children: Not recommended; safety not established.
Renal impairment: No dosage information found; use with caution.

PHARMACOKINETICS AND PHARMACODYNAMICS (CONTINUED)

Excretion: 33% in 24 h, primarily as metabolites
Effect of food: may reduce some adverse effects
Renal impairment: use with caution
Hepatic impairment: use with caution
Elderly: may be more susceptible to effects; use lowest dose possible

PROLONGED USE

Not intended for prolonged use.

OVERDOSAGE

Symptoms include prolonged, deep coma; severe respiratory depression; hypothermia; hypotension; relative bradycardia; and nystagmus and bradycardia. The range for fatal blood concentrations ranges from 20–50 µg/mL; however, because large amounts of the drug are taken up by adipose tissue, this is an unreliable parameter for overdose. Treatment includes gastric emptying (gastric lavage in the unconscious patient). Administer supportive care, with an emphasis on pulmonary and blood gas monitoring. Hemoperfusion using the Amberlite column technique (XAD-4 resin) is most effective in management of acute overdoses. Hemodialysis and peritoneal dialysis (with aqueous oil and dialysates) are helpful. Hemoperfusion with charcoal also has been effective, as is forced diuresis and high urinary output.

PATIENT INFORMATION

Avoid alcohol and other CNS depressants. Do not take more than prescribed. Take with food to decrease symptoms of giddiness, ataxia, or GI upset. May cause dependency; do not discontinue medication suddenly. Use caution when performing tasks requiring alertness and dexterity; may cause drowsiness or dizziness.

AVAILABILITY

Capsules—200, 500, and 750 mg

PROPIOMAZINE HYDROCHLORIDE

(Largon)

This tertiary acetylenic alcohol has been used for its sedative and antiemetic effects in surgery and obstetrics. As a preanesthetic, it reduces the doses of opiate analgesic required.

SPECIAL PRECAUTIONS

Neuroleptic malignant syndrome, a potentially fatal symptom complex, has been associated with antipsychotic drug use.

For IV injection, only use veins or vessels that have no previous damage (eg, from multiple injections or trauma). Chemical irritation may be severe; carefully avoid extravasation.

Advise patient of drug's potential to cause drowsiness or dizziness and of need for caution while driving or performing other tasks requiring alertness and dexterity.

In Brief

INDICATIONS

Sedative to relieve restlessness and apprehension, preoperatively or during surgery.
Analgesic adjunct for relief of restlessness and apprehension during labor.

CONTRAINDICATIONS

Allergy or hypersensitivity to propiomazine; intraarterial injection

INTERACTIONS

CNS depressants

ADVERSE EFFECTS

Frequent: Moderate elevation in blood pressure (desirable in many cases), dry mouth
Rare: Hypotension, autonomic reactions, tachycardia, neuroleptic malignant syndrome

(Continued on next page)

SPECIAL GROUPS

Children: Safe for use.
Pregnancy: Do not use in first trimester of pregnancy.

DOSAGE

Adults: *IM or IV*—For preoperative medication, 20 mg propiomazine with 50 mg meperidine; some patients may need as much as 40 mg propiomazine for sufficient sedation. Belladonna alkaloids may be added as necessary.

For sedation during surgery with local, nerve block, or spinal anesthesia, 10 to 20 mg.

For obstetrics, 20 mg will bring on sedation and relieve apprehension in early stages of labor; some patients may need up to 40 mg. After labor is established, give 20 to 40 mg of propiomazine with 25 to 75 mg of meperidine (average, 50 mg). Amnesic agents can be administered as necessary. It is rarely necessary to repeat doses during normal labor if average doses have been used initially. Additional doses may be given at 3-hour intervals.

Children: For use as a sedative the night before surgery or for preanesthetic and postoperative medication, in children less than 27 kg, calculate dosage on basis of 0.55 to 1.1 mg/kg. Higher doses should be used as necessary only in very excitable, nervous children. The following guidelines are provided:

Age, y	Single Dose, mg
2–4	10
4–6	15
6–12	25

PHARMACOKINETICS AND PHARMACODYNAMICS

Peak action: 1–3 h (peak serum concentrations after IM administration)
Plasma half-life: 7.7 ± 3.9 (IV) and 10.8 ± 1.9 (IM)
Bioavailability: 60%
Metabolism: not known; it probably is metabolized in the liver
Excretion: probably excreted in the urine and the bile like other phenothiazines

PROLONGED USE

Not intended for prolonged use.

OVERDOSAGE

As in other phenothiazines, overdosage may produce convulsive seizures, severe extrapyramidal symptoms, and CNS depression varying from hypotension to coma

AVAILABILITY

Injection—20 mg/mL

DIPHENHYDRAMINE
(Benadryl, Sominex, others)

This antihistamine compound has multiple uses: antitussive, antinausea, antivertigo, antiparkinsonism. It is also used for its sedative side effects to treat insomnia.

SPECIAL PRECAUTIONS

Advise patients to use caution when performing tasks requiring alertness and dexterity; may cause drowsiness and dizziness.

Not intended for use for longer than 2 weeks. Contact physician if insomnia persists for longer than 2 weeks.

Use with caution in patients with predisposition to urinary retention, history of bronchial asthma, increased intraocular pressure, hyperthyroidism, cardiovascular disease, or hypertension.

Antihistamines have varying degrees of atropine-like effects.

In Brief

INDICATIONS
Relief of insomnia

CONTRAINDICATIONS
Allergy or hypersensitivity; asthma; glaucoma or prostate gland enlargement (except under advice of a physician); stenosing peptic ulcer; bladder neck obstruction; pyloroduodenal obstruction; MAO inhibitor therapy; neonates or premature infants; nursing mothers

INTERACTIONS
Alcohol, CNS depressants (other), azole antifungals, macrolide antibiotics, MAO inhibitors

(Continued on next page)

DIPHENYDRAMINE *(CONTINUED)*

SPECIAL PRECAUTIONS *(CONTINUED)*

Photosensitivity may occur; advise patients to use protective measures such as sunscreen, clothing, and reduce exposure time.
Some products may contain sulfites, which can cause allergic-type reactions in some individuals.

SPECIAL GROUPS

Children: Do not use in children younger than 12 years.
Elderly: Increased risk for CNS effects; dosage reduction may be necessary.
Pregnancy: Contact physician before using this product.
Breast-feeding: Contact physician before using this product.
Renal impairment: Metabolites are excreted in urine.
Hepatic impairment: Use with caution.

DOSAGE

Adults: Give 50 mg before bedtime. Do not exceed 100 mg in 24 hours.
Children: Do not use in children younger than 12 years.

ADVERSE EFFECTS

Most frequent: Drowsiness (transient), sedation, dizziness, faintness, disturbed coordination, epigastric distress, anorexia, urinary frequency
Frequent: Postural hypotension, palpitations, lassitude, increased appetite or weight gain, early menses, decreased libido, tingling, heaviness of hands
Less frequent: Peripheral, angioneurotic, and laryngeal edema; dermatitis; asthma; lupus erythematosus–like syndrome; urticaria; photosensitivity; bradycardia; tachycardia; extrasystoles; increase or decrease in blood pressure; ECG changes; restlessness; excitation; tremor; vomiting; diarrhea; constipation; thickening of bronchial secretions; chest tightness; wheezing; dry mouth, nose, and throat; respiratory depression
Rare: Thrombocytopenic purpura, obstructive jaundice, stomatitis, high or prolonged glucose tolerance curves

PHARMACOKINETICS AND PHARMACODYNAMICS

Duration of action: 4–6 h
Onset of action: 15–30 min
Peak action: 1–2 h
Plasma half-life: IV, 8.5 h; PO, 9 h
Bioavailability: not extensively studied
Metabolism: hepatic
Excretion: in urine as antihistamine metabolites and small amounts of unchanged drug
Effect of food: not extensively studied
Protein binding: not extensively studied
Renal impairment: little renal excretion
Hepatic impairment: not extensively studied
Elderly: not extensively studied

PROLONGED USE

Not intended for use > 2 wk.

OVERDOSAGE

Symptoms vary from CNS depression to stimulation.

PATIENT INFORMATION

Avoid alcohol and other CNS depressants. Use caution when performing tasks requiring alertness and dexterity. Contact physician if insomnia persists > 2 wk. Avoid prolonged exposure to natural or artificial sunlight; use protective sunscreen and clothing.

AVAILABILITY

Tablets—25 and 50 mg, 25 mg (with 500 mg acetaminophen), 38 mg (with 500 mg acetaminophen)
Capsules—50 mg

DOXYLAMINE SUCCINATE

(Nitetime Sleep-Aid, Sleep 2-Nite, Unisom)

This antihistamine compound is used for its sedative effects for the short-term treatment of insomnia.

SPECIAL PRECAUTIONS

Advise patients to use caution when performing tasks requiring alertness and dexterity; may cause drowsiness and dizziness.

Not intended for use for longer than 2 weeks.

Use with caution in patients with predisposition to urinary retention, history of bronchial asthma, increased intraocular pressure, hyperthyroidism, cardiovascular disease, or hypertension.

Antihistamines have varying degrees of atropine-like effects.

Photosensitivity may occur; advise patients to use protective measures such as sunscreen, clothing, and reduced exposure time.

Some products may contain sulfites, which can cause allergic-type reactions in some individuals.

SPECIAL GROUPS

Children: Do not use in children younger than 12 years of age.
Elderly: Increased risk for CNS effects; dosage reduction may be necessary.
Pregnancy: Do not take if pregnant.
Breast-feeding: Do not use.
Hepatic impairment: Use with caution.

DOSAGE

Adults: Give 25 mg before bedtime. Do not exceed 100 mg in 24 hours.
Children: Do not use in children younger than 12 years of age.

In Brief

INDICATIONS
Relief of insomnia

CONTRAINDICATIONS
Allergy or hypersensitivity, asthma, glaucoma or prostate gland enlargement (except under advice of a physician), stenosing peptic ulcer, bladder neck obstruction, pyloroduodenal obstruction, MAO inhibitory therapy, neonates or premature infants, nursing mothers

INTERACTIONS
Alcohol, CNS depressants (other), azole antifungals, macrolide antibiotics, MAO inhibitors

ADVERSE EFFECTS
Most frequent: Drowsiness (transient), sedation, dizziness, faintness, disturbed coordination, epigastric distress, anorexia, urinary frequency
Frequent: Postural hypotension, palpitations, lassitude, increased appetite or weight gain, early menses, decreased libido, tingling, heaviness of hands
Less frequent: Anticholinergic effects; peripheral, angioneurotic, and laryngeal edema; dermatitis; asthma; lupus erythematosus–like syndrome; urticaria; photosensitivity; bradycardia; tachycardia; extrasystoles; increase or decrease in blood pressure; ECG changes; restlessness; excitation; tremor; vomiting; diarrhea; constipation; thickening of bronchial sections; chest tightness; wheezing; dry mouth, nose, or throat; respiratory depression
Rare: Thrombocytopenic purpura, obstructive jaundice, stomatitis, high or prolonged glucose tolerance curves

PHARMACOKINETICS AND PHARMACODYNAMICS
Duration of action: 4–6 h
Onset of action: 15–30 min
Peak action: 1–2 h
Metabolism: hepatic
Excretion: in urine as antihistamine metabolites and small amounts of unchanged drug

PROLONGED USE
Not intended for use > 2 wk.

OVERDOSAGE
Symptoms vary from CNS depression to stimulation

PATIENT INFORMATION
Avoid alcohol and other CNS depressants. Use caution when performing tasks requiring alertness and dexterity. Contact physician if insomnia persists > 2 wk. Avoid prolonged exposure to natural or artificial sunlight; use protective sunscreen and clothing.

AVAILABILITY
Tablets—25 mg
Unisom dual-relief tablets consist of acetaminophen and diphenhydramine; Unisom, only doxylamine succinate and 2-α-(2-dimethylaminoethoxy α-methylbenzyl) pyridine succinate

Antipsychotic Agents

Rajiv Tandon

DESCRIPTION OF CLASS

Antipsychotic drugs are primarily used to treat signs and symptoms of psychosis. Their beneficial effects on psychotic symptoms are observed in a range of conditions ranging from schizophrenia, psychotic depression, psychotic mania, and paranoia to various substance-induced psychotic disorders, psychoses secondary to various medical and neurologic disorders, and delirium. Antipsychotics were previously referred to as *major tranquilizers* and *neuroleptics*; however, both these terms are misnomers because they reflect unessential properties of many members of this class of medications that are separate from their antipsychotic effect. Because all compounds in this class cause sedation to varying extents, they were previously considered to be *major tranquilizers*; this led to the erroneous impression that their antipsychotic effects were secondary to or otherwise related to their sedative effects. The older or conventional antipsychotics all consistently caused extrapyramidal side effects leading to their being referred to as *neuroleptics*, but the introduction of clozapine and other atypical antipsychotics has demonstrated that it is possible to have antipsychotic efficacy without producing these neurologic adverse effects. In fact, these newer agents are considered atypical because they separate the antipsychotic therapeutic effect from the extrapyramidal side effect. Consequently, this class of medications should collectively be referred to as *antipsychotics*.

Antipsychotics are primarily used to treat psychotic symptoms in a variety of diagnostic settings. In addition to acute treatment, they are used in maintenance treatment to prevent psychotic relapses in schizophrenia and occasionally in other psychotic disorders. These medications are also frequently employed to treat agitation and marked mood instability in a variety of settings, even in the absence of psychotic symptoms. Although such use was previously discouraged because of the significant adverse effects associated with neuroleptics and the availability of alternative medications in other classes with a better benefit-to-risk ratio, the current widespread availability of many atypical antipsychotic medications with a better adverse-effect profile might make such use less unreasonable.

Currently available antipsychotics represent ten different broad chemical classes: benzisoxazols, butryophenones, dibenzodiazepines, dibenzothiazepines, dibenzoxazepines, dihydroindolones, diphenyl-butylpiperidines, phenothiazines, thienobenzodiazepines, and thioxanthenes. The only diphenylbutylpiperidine available in the United States is pimozide, which has only been approved for use in

Tourette's syndrome and is, therefore, not included in this review. The phenothiazine class is subdivided into three subclasses: aliphatic, piperidine, and piperazine. Whereas aliphatic and piperidine phenothiazines are low-potency typical antipsychotics, piperazine phenothiazines are high-potency typical antipsychotics (Table 5-1) (*see* discussion below). Similarly, thioxanthenes also have aliphatic and piperazine subclasses, which are low- and high-potency, respectively.

These different classes vary in adverse-effect profile but are generally equivalent in efficacy based on group comparisons of overall response rate [1]. The spectrum of therapeutic activity may differ, however, between typical and atypical antipsychotic agents, although such differences in therapeutic activity are confounded by differences in side effects. Clozapine is the only drug to date that has convincingly demonstrated superior efficacy in patients who have failed to respond adequately to conventional antipsychotics [2]. However, because its use causes an increased risk of agranulocytosis, it is not considered a first-line medication, and its use is generally reserved for treatment-refractory psychotic patients. Fluphenazine and haloperidol

Table 5-1. Antipsychotic Drugs Available in the United States: Typical Dosages and Estimated Relative Potency

Generic Name	Clinical Class*	Relative Potency†	Usual Range of Total Daily Dose, *mg/d*‡ Acute	Maintenance
Phenothiazines				
Aliphatic				
Chlorpromazine	A	100	300–1000	100–600
Triflupromazine	A	25	60–150	20–100
Piperazine				
Fluphenazine	B	2	5–30	2–20
Acetophenazine	B	20	60–100	40–80
Perphenazine	B	10	16–64	8–24
Prochlorperazine	B	15	60–150	20–60
Trifluoperazine	B	5	10–60	5–30
Piperidine				
Mesoridazine	A	50	100–400	50–200
Thioridazine	A	100	200–800	100–400
Thioxanthenes				
Chlorprothixene	A	80	200–600	50–300
Thiothixene	B	5	10–60	5–30
Butyrophenones				
Haloperidol	B	2	5–30	2–20
Dihydroindolones				
Molindone	B	10	40–200	10–60
Dibenzoxazepines				
Loxapine	B	10	30–200	10–60
Dibenzodiazepines				
Clozapine	C	50	300–900	200–500
Benzisoxazols				
Risperidone	D	1	2–8	1–6
Thienobenzodiazepines				
Olanzapine	D	2	10–20	??
Dibenzothiazepines				
Quetiapine	D	80	200–750	??
Long-acting injectable preparations				
Fluphenazine decanoate	B			6–50§
Haloperidol decanoate	B			50–200¶

*For clinical class, A—low-potency conventional antipsychotic B—high-potency conventional antipsychotic; C—clozapine; D—atypical antipsychotic other than clozapine.
†Milligram dose of drug whose effect is equivalent to 100 mg of chlorpromazine. These are approximate estimates of relative potency. It should be noted that relative potency may not be the same in the higher dosage ranges as it is in the lower.
‡Dosage may vary with individual responses to the antipsychotic agent employed.
§Prolixin decanoate may be given at intervals of up to 2–4 weeks. Dosage requirements vary widely.
¶Haloperidol decanoate may be given every 4 weeks. Dosage requirements vary widely.

are available as long-acting injectable preparations. Fluphenazine and haloperidol depot preparations are effective in 2- to 4-week and monthly dosing, respectively; these are particularly helpful in addressing the problem of noncompliance. Pimozide does have antipsychotic efficacy, but as previously mentioned, has an approved indication only for Tourette's syndrome. Benzodiazepines and mood stabilizers such as lithium and various anticonvulsants are also occasionally utilized adjunctively with antipsychotics in the treatment of psychoses, but these agents are not considered antipsychotics themselves [3,4].

From a clinical standpoint, antipsychotics are classifiable into four broad groups (*see* Table 5-1): 1) low-potency typical antipsychotics (relative potency > 25; *ie*, more than 25 mg of drug needed for effect equivalent to 100 mg of chlorpromazine; high-milligram daily dose); 2) high-potency typical antipsychotics (relative potency < 20; *ie*, less than 20 mg of drug needed for effect equivalent to 100 mg of chlorpromazine; low milligram daily dose); 3) clozapine; and 4) other atypical antipsychotics. Clozapine and other atypical antipsychotics are characterized by antipsychotic efficacy equal to that of the typical antipsychotics but have a significantly lower propensity to cause extrapyramidal side effects. Additionally, clozapine possesses the property of being effective in about half the psychotic patients refractory to conventional antipsychotics; it is presently unclear as to whether other atypical antipsychotics possess this property of clozapine. Low-potency typical antipsychotics tend to be more sedating than high potency typical antipsychotics and more likely to cause postural hypotension but less likely to cause extrapyramidal side effects.

EFFICACY AND USE

Psychotic disorders are characterized by a variable array of signs and symptoms, such as delusions, hallucinations, disorganized speech or behavior, excitement, and aggressiveness [5]. Although the cause may vary, antipsychotic medications can generally help with these symptoms. Schizophrenia is the most clear-cut indication for antipsychotic drugs, but these agents are also useful in the treatment of mania, delusional disorder, psychosis and behavioral disturbances associated with organic mental disorders or developmental disorders, and psychotic depression.

In general, antipsychotic drugs are initiated during an acute psychotic episode. Prior drug response appears to be the best guide in the selection of a particular antipsychotic agent for a given patient. Consequently, a detailed medication history is essential. When choosing between different antipsychotics, it is also necessary to evaluate the distinct side-effect profiles of the medications in the four clinical groups and the differences in adverse-effect profiles between medications in the same class, taking into consideration the side effects to which a particular patient is most vulnerable (or has previously developed).

When patients are too agitated or otherwise uncooperative to take medication orally, many antipsychotics can be administered intramuscularly. This route provides more rapid absorption, more consistent bioavailability, and more rapid onset of action (within 30 minutes). It is not usually necessary to continue intramuscular dosing beyond the first day or so, and oral medication should be initiated as soon as is feasible. Numerous studies have failed to find any real advantage for continued or high-dose parenteral medication over oral medication in rate of response or degree of therapeutic response [6]. Many antipsychotic agents can ultimately be given at bedtime (or with a larger proportion at bedtime), thereby reducing some daytime adverse effects such as sedation.

Although dosage requirements and time course of response can vary considerably between different patients, there is usually little to be gained by using mega-doses of antipsychotic drugs (*eg*, > 800 to 1000 mg/d of chlorpromazine or > 15 to 20 mg/d of

fluphenazine or haloperidol) because the incidence of adverse effects increases without any additional therapeutic benefit. Although some therapeutic effects of antipsychotic drugs (particularly in controlling agitation or aggressive behavior) can be seen in the first 24 to 48 hours, it can often take several weeks for the drugs to produce marked improvement, and progressive improvement can occur over a period of months. As a general rule, about 50% of the improvement occurs in the first 3 to 4 weeks of treatment, and the absence of any improvement within 4 to 6 weeks generally predicts that no improvement is likely to occur if the treatment is continued. This time frame can be doubled for clozapine.

Extrapyramidal (parkinsonian) side effects are experienced to some degree by the majority of patients receiving high-potency typical antipsychotic agents and by a significant number of patients receiving low-potency typical antipsychotic agents. The decision to use prophylactic antiparkinsonian medication should be based on clinical judgment (*eg*, involving past history), but clinicians should be sensitive to the ways in which extrapyramidal side effects can manifest themselves [7]. Antiparkinsonian drugs are usually oral anticholinergic agents, such as benztropine and trihexyphenidyl, and their use is associated with peripheral (dry mouth, blurred vision, urinary retention) and central (cognitive dysfunction) anticholinergic side effects. Atypical antipsychotics are significantly less likely to cause extrapyramidal side effects, and this advantage also results in several "secondary" benefits in the treatment of psychotic disorders (Fig. 5-1). However, extrapyramidal side effects can occur with increasing doses of some atypical antipsychotics (various available typical and atypical antipsychotic agents are compared with regard to this and other attributes in Table 5-2). It is critically important to utilize atypical agents in a way that is not associated with extrapyramidal side effects.

Once the episode is controlled, maintenance treatment should be considered and is almost always indicated in schizophrenia [8]. Among patients with schizophrenia, the risk of psychotic relapse within 1 year following drug discontinuation averages 75% in contrast to 20% on continued medication. For other psychotic conditions, indications for maintenance treatment are less well established, and alternative treatments should be considered.

Dosages required for maintenance treatment are generally lower than those required for acute treatment. Tardive dyskinesia is a syndrome of abnormal involuntary movements associated with long-term administration of antipsychotic medication. The risk appears to be higher in the elderly, in patients who demonstrate substantial vulnerability to early-occurring parkinsonian side effects, and in patients with recurrent depression [9]. The incidence of tardive dyskinesia in adult populations appears to be approximately 4% to 5% per year of cumulative antipsychotic drug treatment; the incidence in the elderly is about five times higher. Most cases are mild and not progressive, but severe, disabling forms of this syndrome can occur, and every attempt should be made to minimize the risk by using the lowest effective dosage of medication. Atypical antipsychotics appear to be associated with a significantly lower risk of tardive dyskinesia; although this is clearly proven for clozapine, emerging data suggest a similar lower occurrence with other atypical antipsychotics as well. Several studies have attempted to assess the effectiveness of targeted or intermittent medication strategies (*ie*, to use drugs only when a patient begins to relapse). However, the results have been largely discouraging, and continuous low-dose antipsychotic treatment is optimal for maintenance treatment of schizophrenia. A variety of other treatment modalities (*eg*, social skills training, family therapy, vocational rehabilitation) can also be helpful in reducing risk of relapse and improving quality of life when provided along with antipsychotic medication.

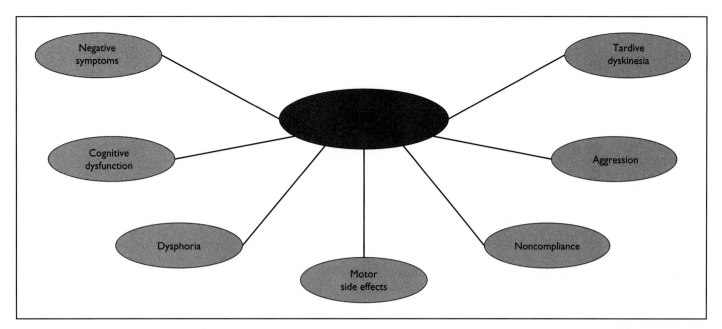

FIGURE 5-1

Therapeutic benefits related to the extrapyramidal–side-effects (EPS) advantage of the atypical antipsychotic agents. (*Adapted from* Jibson and Tandon [12].)

Table 5-2. Side-Effect Profile of the Atypical Antipsychotic Agents

	Chlorpromazine	Thioridazine	Haloperidol	Clozapine	Risperidone	Olanzapine	Quetiapine
EPS	++	+	+++	0	±	0	0
Dose-related EPS	++	++	+++	0	++	±	0
TD	+++	+++	+++	0	??	??	??
Prolactin elevation	++	++	+++	0	++	±	±
Agranulocytosis	±	±	±	++	±	±	±
Anticholinergic	++	+++	±	+++	±	++	±
AST or ALT elevation	+	+	+	+	±	+	±
Hypotension	+++	+++	+	+++	+	+	+ to ++
Sedation	+++	+++	+	+++	+	+ to ++	+ to ++
Seizures	+	+	±	++	±	±	±
Weight gain	+	+	+	+++	++	++ to +++	++

0—absent; ±—minimal; +—mild; ++—moderate; +++—severe.
ALT—alanine aminotransferase; AST—aspartate; EPS—extrapyramidal side effects; TD—tardive dyskinesia.

MODE OF ACTION

The pathophysiology of schizophrenia and other psychotic disorders has not been established [10]. However, the development of antipsychotic medications has been influenced by the dopamine hypothesis, which suggests that certain dopamine pathways are overactive in schizophrenia. Although compelling evidence of such dopamine hyperactivity is not yet available, it should be noted that all currently available antipsychotic drugs block dopamine receptors. The antagonism of dopamine in different brain regions can contribute to variable clinical effects. It is assumed that whereas therapeutic effects occur in the mesolimbic-mesocortical dopamine pathways, dopamine-receptor blockade in the striatum produces extrapyramidal side effects and tardive dyskinesia. In addition, dopamine-receptor blockade in the tuberoinfundibular pathway produces persistent hyperprolactinemia that is associated with amenorrhea, sexual dysfunction, gynecomastia, and galactorrhea. The extent to which particular dopamine pathways and particular dopamine receptor subtypes are involved in antipsychotic drug effects remains speculative, and further knowledge depends on the development and testing of more specific compounds. The rich pharmacologic profile of clozapine along with its unique therapeutic profile (particularly its distinctive efficacy in the treatment of psychotic symptoms refractory to conventional antipsychotics) have led to the suggestion that neuropharmacologic properties other than dopamine D_2 blockade may contribute to antipsychotic efficacy [11].

The serotonin- $(5HT_{2A})$ antagonist property of all currently available and soon-to-be-available atypical antipsychotics likely contributes to their lower propensity to cause extrapyramidal side effects and probably to other related "secondary" benefits. Varying effects at other receptors (*eg,* noradrenergic, histaminic, muscarinic) also play a role in determining the adverse-effects profiles of different drugs [12].

PHARMACOKINETICS

The pharmacokinetics of antipsychotic drugs vary according to their chemistry. Antipsychotic drugs are generally well absorbed orally and undergo a marked first-pass hepatic effect. Volume of distribution and plasma binding are extensive. Small amounts are excreted unchanged in the kidney. Some antipsychotic drugs, such as chlorpromazine, have numerous metabolites (ie, more than 100). Although most metabolites are minor, some can be neuropharmacologically active. In the case of most antipsychotics, residual amounts can be found in humans weeks or even months after drug discontinuation. There is enormous interindividual variability in drug blood levels following oral administration of antipsychotic drugs. Although correlations have been reported between blood levels and clinical response for some drugs, the results are not entirely consistent, and routine blood levels do not seem justified at this time. Such measures may be useful if patients fail to respond to a seemingly adequate trial, develop severe or atypical adverse effects, if noncompliance is suspected, or if patients are receiving other drugs that may influence absorption or metabolism [13].

Antipsychotic drugs should be withdrawn slowly whenever possible because withdrawal reactions can occur. Parkinsonian side effects may persist for days or even weeks following drug discontinuation, and the continued use of antiparkinsonian drugs may occasionally be warranted.

PHARMACOECONOMICS

Atypical antipsychotic drugs are at least as effective as are conventional antipsychotics in treating psychotic symptoms, and they have a significantly lower propensity to cause extrapyramidal side effects. This extrapyramidal–side-effects advantage of the atypical antipsychotics translates into several "secondary" benefits (see Fig. 5-1). On the other hand, atypical antipsychotics tend to be about 10 to 20 times as expensive as are conventional antipsychotics. Most pharmacoeconomic studies suggest that the use of atypical antipsychotics is cost-effective, with most of the cost savings resulting from lower hospital costs suggesting greater effectiveness of these agents. At present, it is not known whether this greater effectiveness is due to better compliance, greater efficacy, fewer adverse effects, a combination of these factors, or some other factor.

REFERENCES

1. Janicak PG, Davis JM, Preskorn SH, Ayd FJ Jr: *Principles and Practice of Pharmacotherapy*, edn 2. Baltimore: William and Wilkins; 1997.

2. Kane JM, Honigfeld G, Singer J, Meltzer HY: Clozapine for the treatment-resistant schizophrenic: a double-blind comparison versus chlorpromazine/benztropine. *Arch Gen Psychiatry* 1988, 45:789–796.

3. Schulz SC : Schizophrenia: somatic treatment. In *Comprehensive Textbook of Psychiatry*, edn 6. Edited by Kaplan HI, Sadock BJ. Baltimore: William and Wilkins; 1995:987–998.

4. American Psychiatric Association: Practice guidelines for the treatment of patients with schizophrenia. *Am J Psychiatry* 1997, 154(suppl 4):1–63.

5. Jibson MD, Tandon R: Psychosis and schizophrenia. In *Primary Care Psychiatry*. Edited by Knesper DJ, Riba MB, Schwenk TL. Philadelphia: WB Saunders; 1997:163–183.

6. Kane JM, Marder SR: Psychopharmacologic treatment of schizophrenia. *Schizophr Bull* 1993, 19:287–302.

7. Casey DE: The relationship of pharmacology to side effects. *J Clin Psychiatry* 1997, 58(suppl 58):55–62.

8. Greden JF, Tandon R: Longterm treatment for lifelong disorders. *Arch Gen Psychiatry* 1995, 52:197–200.

9. Kane JM, Jeste DV, Barnes TRE, *et al.*: *American Task Force Report on Tardive Dyskinesia*. Washington DC: American Psychiatric Press; 1992.

10. Tandon R, Taylor SF, DeQuardo JR: Neurobiology of schizophrenia. In *Textbook of Psychopharmacology*. Edited by Ananth J. New Delhi: Jaypee Brothers; 1998.

11. Tandon R, Kane JM: Neuropharmacological basis of clozapine's unique clinical profile. *Arch Gen Psychiatry* 1992, 50:157–159.

12. Jibson MD, Tandon R: New atypical antipsychotic medications. *J Psychiatr Research* 1998, 32.

13. Goff DC, Baldessarini RJ: Drug interactions with antipsychotic agents. *J Clin Psychopharmacol* 1993, 13: 57–67.

RISPERIDONE

(Risperdal)

Risperidone is an antipsychotic agent that belongs to a new chemical class, the benzisoxazole derivatives. The mechanism of action is unknown; however, it has been proposed that the drug's antipsychotic activity is mediated through a combination of dopamine type 2 and serotonin type 2 antagonism. Risperidone also has α-adrenergic antagonist effects. It produces relatively few extrapyramidal effects at typical doses. There is a dose-related increase in the incidence of extrapyramidal side effects. It can produce sedation and orthostatic hypotension.

SPECIAL PRECAUTIONS

The neurologic syndromes that can occur with risperidone (parkinsonism, dystonia, akathisia, tardive dyskinesia, tardive dystonia) may be confused with other behavioral or neurologic syndromes.

Tardive dyskinesia, a syndrome of involuntary abnormal movements, may develop in patients treated with this drug. In some cases, these movements can be severe or persistent. The elderly are at highest risk, but it can occur at any age. The risk of developing tardive dyskinesia and the likelihood that it will become irreversible increase as the total duration and total cumulative dose of the antipsychotic administered to the patient increase. Tardive dystonia unassociated with tardive dyskinesia also has been reported with antipsychotic drug use. The condition is characterized by delayed onset of choreic or dystonic movements and may become irreversible.

A potentially fatal syndrome involving high fever, rigidity, autonomic instability, altered level of consciousness, and elevated creatine phosphokinase referred to as *neuroleptic malignant syndrome* can occur in patients receiving antipsychotic medications.

Risperidone apparently lengthens the Q-T interval in some patients, although there is no average increase in treated patients. Bradycardia, electrolyte imbalance, concomitant use with other drugs that prolong Q-T, or presence of congenital prolongation in Q-T can increase the risk for occurrence of torsades de pointes, a life-threatening arrhythmia.

Risperidone may induce orthostatic hypotension associated with dizziness, tachycardia, and syncope, especially during the initial dose titration period, probably reflecting the drug's α-adrenergic antagonistic properties. Dosage reduction should be considered if hypotension occurs. Risperidone should be used with particular caution in patients with known cardiovascular disease, cerebrovascular disease, and conditions that predispose patients to hypotension.

SPECIAL GROUPS

Race: Generally effective regardless of race; dosage requirements may vary.
Children: Safety and efficacy not established.
Elderly: Lower starting dose is recommended.
Renal impairment: Administer with caution. Use lower starting doses.
Hepatic impairment: Administer with caution. Use lower starting doses.
Pregnancy: Safety not established. Use only when potential benefit outweighs potential risk.
Breast-feeding: Antipsychotic drugs are excreted in low concentrations in breast milk. Women receiving risperidone should not breast-feed.

(Continued on next page)

In Brief

INDICATIONS

Manifestations of psychotic disorders, mania, severe behavioral disturbances associated with some organic mental syndromes or developmental disorders

CONTRAINDICATIONS

Known hypersensitivity to risperidone

INTERACTIONS

Other centrally active drugs, alcohol, antihypertensive agents, levodopa, dopamine agonists, carbamazepine, drugs that inhibit cytochrome $P_{450}IID_6$ (eg, quinidine) and other P_{450} isozymes as well as drugs metabolized by cytochrome $P_{450}IID_6$

ADVERSE EFFECTS

Extrapyramidal symptoms, dizziness, hyperkinesia, somnolence, nausea, anxiety, constipation, dyspepsia, rhinitis, rash, tachycardia, increased dream activity, increased duration of sleep, accommodation disturbances, increased or reduced salivation, micturition disturbances, diarrhea, weight gain, menorrhagia, diminished sexual desire, erectile dysfunction, ejaculatory dysfunction, orgasm dysfunction, aggressive reaction, headache, vomiting, abdominal pain, fever, torticollis, hypotonia, migraine, hyperreflexia, choreoathetosis, anorexia, flatulence, increased appetite, fatigue, increased pigmentation, photosensitivity, increased or decreased sweating, acne, alopecia, hyperkeratosis, pruritus, aggravated psoriasis, hypotension, AV block, ventricular tachycardia, hyponatremia, creatine phosphokinase increase, thirst, lactation, amenorrhea, increased AST, increased ALT, cholestatic hepatitis

PHARMACOKINETICS AND PHARMACODYNAMICS

Onset of action: variable
Peak plasma levels: mean of 1 h for risperidone; in extensive metabolizers, about 3 h for 9-hydroxyrisperidone; in poor metabolizers, about 17 h for 9-hydroxyrisperidone
Plasma half-life: about 3 h in extensive metabolizers and 20 h in poor metabolizers for risperidone; about 21 h in extensive metabolizers and 30 h in poor metabolizers for 9-hydroxyrisperidone; half-lives prolonged in the elderly; the overall mean elimination half-life is about 20 h
Bioavailability: relative bioavailability of 94%; absolute bioavailability of 70%
Metabolism: extensively metabolized in the liver by cytochrome $P_{450}IID_6$ to major active metabolite 9-hydroxyrisperidone, which is the predominant circulating metabolite and appears about equally effective with risperidone with respect to receptor-binding activity and some effects in animals. A second minor pathway is N-dealkylation. The enzyme-catalyzing hydroxylation is cytochrome $P_{450}IID_6$, also called debrisoquine hydroxylase, the enzyme responsible for metabolism of many neuroleptics, antidepressants, antiarrhythmics, and other drugs. Cytochrome $P_{450}IID_6$ is subject to genetic polymorphism (about 6%–8% of whites and a low percentage of Asians have little or no activity and are poor metabolizers) and to inhibition by various substrates and some nonsubstrates. Whereas extensive metabolizers convert risperidone rapidly into 9-hydroxyrisperidone, poor metabolizers convert it much more slowly. Extensive metabolizers therefore have lower risperidone and higher 9-hydroxyrisperidone concentrations than do poor metabolizers.

(Continued on next page)

RISPERIDONE (CONTINUED)

DOSAGE

Adults: *Usual initial dose*—Risperidone can be administered on either a twice-daily or a three-times-daily schedule. In early clinical trials, risperidone was generally administered at 1 mg twice a day initially, with increases in increments of 1 mg twice a day on the second and third day, as tolerated, to a target dose of 3 mg twice a day by the third day. Subsequent controlled trials have indicated that most patients tolerate equally well receiving these total daily doses in either twice a day or three times a day. However, regardless of which regimen if employed, a slower titration may be medically appropriate in some patients. Further dosage adjustments, if indicated, should generally occur at intervals of not less than 1 week. Maximal effect was generally seen in a range of 4 to 8 mg/d. Doses above 6 mg/d for twice-a-day dosing were not demonstrated to be more efficacious than were lower doses, were associated with more extrapyramidal symptoms and other adverse effects, and are not generally recommended. In a single study supporting dosing four times a day, the efficacy results were generally stronger for 8 mg than for 4 mg. Safety of doses above 16 mg/d has not been evaluated in clinical trials. For patients receiving maintenance treatment, attempts should be made to reduce dosage to the lower effective level after symptoms have been controlled for a reasonable period.

Elderly: Usually one third to one half the adult dose, and increase more gradually. The recommended initial dose is 0.5 mg twice a day. Dosage increases should be increments of no more than 0.5 mg twice a day. Increases to dosages above 1.5 mg twice a day should generally occur at intervals of at least 1 week. If a once-a-day dosing regimen in the elderly or debilitated patient is being considered, it is recommended that the patient be titrated on twice-a-day regimen for 2 to 3 days at the target dose. Subsequent switches to a once-a-day dosing regimen can be done thereafter.

PHARMACOKINETICS AND PHARMACODYNAMICS (CONTINUED)

Excretion: eliminated through the kidneys; 70% excreted in the urine and 15% in the feces (recovery at 1 wk); renal clearance prolonged in elderly

Effect of food: food does not affect either rate or extent of absorption; drug can be given with or without meals

Protein binding: plasma protein binding of about 90% for risperidone (increased with increasing concentrations of α_1-acid glycoprotein); plasma binding of 77% for 9-hydroxyrisperidone; parent drug and metabolite do not displace each other from plasma-binding sites

Renal impairment: clearance of the sum of risperidone and its active metabolite decreased by 60% in patients with moderate to severe renal disease

Hepatic impairment: pharmacokinetics of risperidone in patients with liver disease comparable to those in young healthy subjects; however, the mean free fraction of risperidone in plasma increases by about 35% because of the diminished concentration of both albumin and α-$_1$-acid glycoprotein

PROLONGED USE

Antipsychotic efficacy was established in short-term (6–8 wk) trials of schizophrenic inpatients; effectiveness in long-term use, *ie*, more than 6–8 wk, has not been systematically evaluated, and the physician who elects to use risperidone for extended periods should periodically reevaluate long-term usefulness of the drug for the individual patient

OVERDOSAGE

Experience with risperidone in acute overdosage is limited in the premarketing database (eight reports), with estimated doses ranging from 20–300 mg and no fatalities. Reported symptoms are those resulting from exaggeration of the drug's known pharmacologic effects (*ie*, drowsiness and sedation, tachycardia and hypotension, and extrapyramidal symptoms). One case involving an estimated overdosage of 240 mg was associated with hyponatremia, hypokalemia, prolonged Q-T, and widened QRS. Another case involving an estimated overdosage of 36 mg was associated with a seizure.

To manage a case of acute overdosage, establish and maintain an airway and ensure adequate oxygenation and ventilation. Gastric lavage (after intubation if patient is unconscious) and administration of activated charcoal together with a laxative should be considered. The possibility of obtundation, seizures, or dystonic reaction of the head and neck following overdosage may create a risk of aspiration with induced emesis. Cardiovascular monitoring should begin immediately and should include continuous ECG monitoring to detect possible arrhythmias. If antiarrhythmic therapy is administered, disopyramide, procainamide, and quinidine carry a theoretic hazard of Q-T–prolonging effects that might be additive to those of risperidone. Similarly, it is reasonable to expect that the α-blocking properties of bretylium might be additive to those of risperidone, resulting in problematic hypotension. There is no specific antidote to risperidone. Therefore, appropriate supportive measures should be instituted. The possibility of multiple-drug involvement should be considered. Hypotension and circulatory collapse should be treated with appropriate measures, such as IV fluids or sympathomimetic agents (epinephrine and dopamine should not be used because β stimulation may worsen hypotension in the setting of risperidone-induced α-blockade). In cases of severe extrapyramidal symptoms, anticholinergic medication should be administered. Close medical supervision and monitoring should continue until patient recovers.

(Continued on next page)

PATIENT INFORMATION

Patients should be given a list of common side effects and be instructed to report extrapyramidal symptoms. Patients should protect themselves from sun exposure. Caution should be used when performing activities requiring mental alertness. Patients should limit alcohol consumption. Given the likelihood that a proportion of patients exposed to antipsychotic drugs will develop tardive dyskinesia, all patients for whom long-term use is contemplated should be given information about this risk. The decision when to inform patients (or guardians) should take into account the clinical circumstances and the competency of the patient to understand the information provided. The risks of discontinuing treatment also must be described.

AVAILABILITY

Tablets—1, 2, 3, and 4 mg in 60s (bottles) and 100s (blister packs)
Concentrate—1 mg/mL in 100-mL bottles

HALOPERIDOL (Haldol), HALOPERIDOL DECANOATE

Haloperidol is an antipsychotic agent classified as a butyrophenone. It is one of the most widely used antipsychotic medications and is available in oral, injectable, and depot preparations. Haloperidol is considered a high-potency compound associated with a moderate to marked degree of extrapyramidal side effects. It has relatively little sedative effect or anticholinergic properties.

SPECIAL PRECAUTIONS

The neurologic syndromes that can occur with use of haloperidol (parkinsonism, dystonia, akathisia, tardive dyskinesia, tardive dystonia) may be confused with other behavioral or neurologic syndromes.

Tardive dyskinesia, a syndrome of involuntary abnormal movements, may develop in patients treated with this drug. In some cases, these movements can be severe or persistent. The elderly are at highest risk, but it can occur at any age. Tardive dystonia unassociated with tardive dyskinesia has also been reported with antipsychotic drug use. The condition is characterized by delayed onset of choreic or dystonic movements and may become irreversible.

A potentially fatal syndrome involving high fever, rigidity, autonomic instability, altered level of consciousness, and elevated creatine phosphokinase referred to as *neuroleptic malignant syndrome* can occur in patients receiving antipsychotic medications.

Avoid or use with caution in patients with a history of bone marrow depression or previous hypersensitivity reaction.

Administer with caution in patients with cardiovascular disease, chronic respiratory disorders, parkinsonism, epilepsy, myasthenia gravis, narrow-angle glaucoma, and those exposed to extreme heat or cold.

In Brief

INDICATIONS

Manifestations of psychotic disorders, mania, severe behavioral disturbances associated with some organic mental syndromes or developmental disorders, Tourette syndrome

CONTRAINDICATIONS

Known hypersensitivity, comatose states or depressed levels of consciousness of unknown cause, presence of large amounts of CNS depressants

INTERACTIONS

Lithium, anesthetics, opiates, alcohol, sedatives, antihistamines, antiparkinson agents

ADVERSE EFFECTS

Parkinson-like symptoms, akathisia, dystonia, tardive dyskinesia, tardive dystonia, insomnia, restlessness, anxiety, euphoria, agitation, vertigo, grand mal seizures, hallucinations, catatonic-like state, heatstroke, hyperpyrexia, muscle rigidity, altered mental status, tachycardia, diaphoresis, cardiac dysrhythmia, myoglobinuria, acute renal failure (occurs with neuroleptic malignant syndrome), hypotension, transient leukopenia and leukocytosis, agranulocytosis, impaired liver function and jaundice, maculopapular and acneiform skin reactions, loss of hair, photosensitivity, lactation, breast engorgement, mastalgia, menstrual irregularities, gynecomastia, impotence, increased libido, hyperglycemia, hypoglycemia, hyponatremia, anorexia, constipation, diarrhea, hypersalivation, dyspepsia, nausea and vomiting, dry mouth, blurred vision, urinary retention, diaphoresis, priapism, laryngospasm, bronchospasm, increased depth of respiration, cataracts, retinopathy, visual disturbances, sudden death

PHARMACOKINETICS AND PHARMACODYNAMICS

Onset of action: variable, depending on dose form
Peak plasma levels: *Oral*—3–5 h; *IM lactate*—20 min; *IM decanoate*—4–11 d
Plasma half-life: *Oral*—2 d; *IM lactate*—13 h–3 d; *IM decanoate*—3 wk
Bioavailability: *Oral*—60%; *IM lactate*—75%; *IM decanoate*—approaches 100%
Metabolism: metabolized in the liver; involves N-dealkylation, oxidation, and conjugation; although active hydroxy metabolite is formed, its role in action of drug unknown
Excretion: 40% in urine and 15% in bile
Effect of food: not known
Protein binding: 90%–92% protein bound

(Continued on next page)

(Continued on next page)

HALOPERIDAL, HALOPERIDOL DECANOATE (CONTINUED)

SPECIAL GROUPS
Race: Generally effective regardless of race; dosage requirements may vary.
Children: Use with caution. Do not use in children or adolescents whose symptoms suggest Reye syndrome. Tardive dyskinesia can occur in children.
Elderly: The prevalence of tardive dyskinesia is highest in the elderly. Use lower doses and increase more gradually; observe for hypotensive reactions.
Renal impairment: Administer with caution.
Hepatic impairment: Administer with caution—smaller doses may be required.
Pregnancy: Safety not established. Use only when potential benefit outweighs potential risk.
Breast-feeding: Antipsychotic drugs are excreted in low concentrations in breast milk. Use with caution.

DOSAGE
Adults: Oral route is appropriate for most patients during acute treatment; however, IM injections may be desirable for severely ill patients for the first 24 hours. Oral dosage initially 2.5 to 10 mg daily. (There appears to be little if any value in exceeding 20 mg/d for most patients.) IM (lactate) 2 to 5 mg every 2 to 8 hours until symptoms are controlled or oral medication can be substituted. *Depot preparation*—Adults initially should receive 10 to 15 times the daily oral dose or equivalent; however, dosage should also be influenced by clinical history, physical condition, and response to previous therapy. Initial dose should not exceed 100 mg. Maximum volume/injection site should not exceed 3 mL. The recommended interval between doses is 4 weeks. It may take 2 to 3 months for steady state to be achieved. Optimal dosage range for most patients is between 50 to 200 mg every 4 weeks. For Tourette syndrome, usual dose is 0.05 to 0.075 mg/kg/d. For patients receiving maintenance treatment, attempts should be made to reduce dosage to the lowest effective level after symptoms have been controlled for a reasonable time.
Elderly: 1 to 3 mg/d orally depending on condition, weight, and response. Depot drugs may be useful in some elderly individuals, but low doses should be administered with careful observation.
Children: Not recommended for use in children younger than 3 years or weighing less than 15 kg. Decanoate is not generally recommended for use in children under 12 years. For children aged 3 to 12 (or weight 15–40 kg), the initial dose is 0.5 mg/kg. Dosage in this age group has not been well established.

PHARMACOKINETICS AND PHARMACODYNAMICS (CONTINUED)
Renal impairment: effects not known; administer with caution
Hepatic impairment: impaired hepatic function may increase bioavailability and decrease elimination
Elderly: half-life may be extended

PROLONGED USE
Antipsychotic drugs may be indicated for maintenance and prophylactic treatment in some disorders (particularly schizophrenia). To lessen the likelihood of adverse reactions related to cumulative drug effects, patients on long-term therapy should be evaluated periodically to determine if dose can be lowered or drug therapy discontinued; short-acting IM preparations are not intended for long-term use. Patients should be examined periodically for the development of tardive dyskinesia or tardive dystonia.

OVERDOSAGE
Symptoms of overdosage are exaggeration of known pharmacologic effects and adverse reactions, the most prominent being severe extrapyramidal reactions, hypotension, or sedation. Patients appear comatose with respiratory depression and hypotension severe enough to produce shocklike state. Extrapyramidal reaction is manifested by muscular weakness or rigidity and generalized or localized tremor. The risk of ECG changes associated with torsades de pointes should be considered. Gastric lavage or induction of emesis should be done immediately and followed by administration of activated charcoal. Because there is no specific antidote, treatment is primarily supportive. Establish patent airway by use of oropharyngeal airway of endotracheal tube or, in prolonged cases of coma, tracheostomy. Counter respiratory depression by artificial respiration and mechanical respirators. Counter hypotension and circulatory collapse by IV fluids, plasma, or concentrated albumin; vasopressor agents, including metaraminol, phenylephrine, and norepinephrine, can be used; do *not* use epinephrine. In case of severe extrapyramidal reactions, administer antiparkinson medication. ECG and vital signs should be monitored, especially for signs of Q-T prolongation or dysrhythmia; monitoring should continue until ECG is normal. Severe arrhythmia should be treated with appropriate antiarrhythmic measures.

PATIENT INFORMATION
Given the likelihood that a proportion of patients exposed to antipsychotic drugs will develop tardive dyskinesia, all patients for whom long-term use is contemplated should be given information about this risk. The decision of when to inform patients (or guardian) should take into account the clinical circumstances and the competency of the patient to understand the information provided. The risks of discontinuing treatment must also be described.

AVAILABILITY
Tablets—0.5, 1, 2, and 5 mg in 100s, 500s, 1000s, and UD 100s; 10 and 20 mg in 100s, 500s, and UD 100s
Concentrate (lactate)—2 mg/mL in 15 and 120 mL and 5- and 10-mL UD 100s
Injection (lactate)—5 mg/mL in 1-mL amps, syringes, and vials with and without methyl and propyl parabens; in 2- and 2.5-mL vials without methyl and propyl parabens; and in 10-mL vials and 1-mL disposable syringes with methyl and propyl parabens
Injection (decanoate)—100 mg/mL in 1-mL amps and 5-mL vials in sesame oil with 1.2% benzyl alcohol

CLOZAPINE

(Clozaril)

Clozapine is an antipsychotic agent classified as a dibenzodiazepine that is relatively free of extrapyramidal side effects. The drug acts as an antagonist at dopamine, adrenergic, cholinergic, histaminergic, and serotoninergic receptors. Clozapine has a higher incidence of agranulocytosis than other antipsychotics and is therefore not considered a first-line medication. Clozapine is now frequently used to treat psychosis induced by dopamine agonists used in the treatment of Parkinson disease. Clozapine is the only drug thus far found to be superior to other antipsychotics in the treatment of poor or partial responders.

SPECIAL PRECAUTIONS

Because of the significant risk of agranulocytosis, clozapine should be reserved for treatment of severely ill schizophrenic patients who fail to show acceptable response to standard antipsychotic drug treatment. Before instituting treatment, it is strongly advised that a patient be given at least 2 trials with other medications.

Patients must have baseline WBC and differential counts before treatment with clozapine and counts every week throughout treatment as well as for 4 wk after discontinuation.

Caution should be used in administering clozapine to patients with a history of seizures or other predisposing factors. The incidence of seizures may be dose related.

Circulatory collapse, respiratory arrest, and cardiac arrest may represent a continuing risk in some patients. Some cases during initial treatment occurred in patients who were taking benzodiazepines.

A potentially fatal symptom complex sometimes referred to as *neuroleptic malignant syndrome* has been reported in association with clozapine.

Tardive dyskinesia, a syndrome consisting of potentially irreversible, involuntary, dyskinetic movements, may develop in patients treated with clozapine but appears to be significantly less of a risk than with other drugs. Both the risk of developing the syndrome and likelihood that it will become irreversible are believed to increase as duration of treatment and total cumulative doses administered to the patient increase.

Clozapine is available only through a patient management system that combines WBC testing, patient monitoring, and pharmacy and drug distribution services, all linked to compliance with required safety monitoring.

During therapy, patients may experience transient temperature elevations, with peak incidence within the first 3 weeks of treatment.

Administer with caution in patients with cardiovascular disease, chronic respiratory disorders, parkinsonism, epilepsy, myasthenia gravis, narrow-angle glaucoma, and those exposed to extreme heat or cold.

SPECIAL GROUPS

Race: Generally effective regardless of race; dosage requirements may vary.

Children: Dosage recommendations not available. Limited experience with adolescents suggest low end of adult dose. Risk of agranulocytosis may be higher in adolescents.

Elderly: Use lower doses and increase more gradually; observe for hypotensive reactions. Low doses, such as 12.5 to 50 mg, can be effective for the control of psychosis in patients with Parkinson disease.

Renal impairment: Administer with caution.

(Continued on next page)

In Brief

INDICATIONS

FDA-approved: Severely ill schizophrenic patients who fail to respond adequately to or cannot tolerate standard antipsychotic drug treatment

Off-label: Psychosis occurring in patients with Parkinson disease, refractory schizoaffective and bipolar disorders

CONTRAINDICATIONS

Myeloproliferative disorders, history of clozapine-induced agranulocytosis or severe granulocytopenia, simultaneous administration with agents having well-known potential to suppress bone marrow function, severe CNS depression, or comatose states from any cause

INTERACTIONS

Anticholinergics, antihypertensives, agents that suppress bone marrow function, highly protein-bound drugs, benzodiazepines, alcohol, antihistamines, sedatives, anesthetics, narcotics, antidepressants

ADVERSE EFFECTS

Drowsiness or sedation; dizziness or vertigo; tremor; syncope; disturbed sleep or nightmares; restlessness; hypokinesia; akinesia; agitation; seizures; rigidity; akathisia; confusion; fatigue; insomnia; hyperkinesia; weakness; lethargy; ataxia; slurred speech; depression; epileptiform movements; myoclonic jerks; anxiety; salivation; sweating; dry mouth; visual disturbances; pain in back, neck, and legs; muscle spasm; muscle weakness; tachycardia; hypotension; hypertension; chest pain or angina; cardiac abnormality; constipation; nausea; abdominal discomfort; vomiting; diarrhea; anorexia; urinary abnormalities; abnormal ejaculation; urinary incontinence; throat discomfort; dyspnea; nasal congestion; leukopenia; decreased WBC; neutropenia; agranulocytosis; eosinophilia; fever; weight gain; rash; sore or numb tongue

PHARMACOKINETICS AND PHARMACODYNAMICS

Onset of action: variable from days to weeks

Peak plasma levels: 2.5 h

Plasma half-life: about 12 h

Bioavailability: oral bioavailability averages 50%–60%

Metabolism: metabolized in the liver to inactive compounds; the desmethyl metabolite has limited activity, and the hydroxylated and N-oxide metabolites are inactive

Excretion: only trace amounts of unchanged drug detectable in urine and feces; 50% excreted in urine and 30% in feces as demethylated, hydroxylated, and N-oxide derivatives

Effect of food: food does not affect bioavailability

Protein binding: 95% bound to serum proteins; interaction between clozapine and other highly protein-bound drugs has not been fully evaluated but may be important

Renal impairment: effects not known

Hepatic impairment: impaired metabolism may increase bioavailability and decrease elimination

PROLONGED USE

For long-term therapy of severely ill schizophrenic patients who fail to respond to or are intolerant of standard antipsychotics. Antipsychotic drugs may be indicated for maintenance and prophylactic treatment in some disorders (particularly schizophrenia). To lessen the likelihood of adverse reactions related to cumulative drug effects, patients on long-term therapy should be evaluated periodically to determine if dose can be lowered or drug therapy discontinued. Patients should be examined periodically for the development of tardive dyskinesia or tardive dystonia.

CLOZAPINE (CONTINUED)

SPECIAL GROUPS (CONTINUED)

Hepatic impairment: Administer with caution—smaller doses may be required.

Pregnancy: Safety not established. Use only when potential benefit outweighs potential risk.

Breast-feeding: Antipsychotic drugs are excreted in low concentrations in breast milk. Use with caution.

DOSAGE

Adults: Use with caution in patients with cardiac, hepatic, and renal disease. Do not dispense more than a 1-week supply from the patient management system. *Initial*—12.5 to 25 mg once or twice daily and then continue with daily dose increments of 25 to 50 mg/d to target dose of 300 to 450 mg/d by the end of 2 weeks. Make subsequent dose increments no more than once or twice weekly in increments not to exceed 100 mg. *Dosage adjustment*—Continue daily dosing on divided basis to effective dosage level. Many patients respond adequately to dosages between 300 and 600 mg/d; it may be necessary to raise dosage to 600 to 900 mg/d. Do not exceed 900 mg/d. *Maintenance*—Continue at lowest level needed to maintain remission. Periodically reassess patients. *Discontinuation*—Gradual reduction over 1 and 2 weeks. *Reinitiation of treatment*—Follow original dose build-up guidelines. Reexposure might enhance risk of adverse reactions. Patients discontinued for WBC counts less than 2000/mm^3 or granulocyte counts less than 1000/mm^3 must *not* be restarted on clozapine.

Elderly: Use with caution. Risk of agranulocytosis higher in the elderly. Doses of 12.5 to 50 mg may be effective for the control of psychosis in patients with Parkinson disease.

Children: Not recommended for use in children younger than 16 years. In adolescents aged 16 to 18, follow adult dosages.

OVERDOSAGE

Symptoms include altered states of consciousness, tachycardia, hypotension, respiratory depression or failure, and hypersalivation. Seizures have occurred. Fatal overdoses have been reported. Establish and maintain patent airway; ensure adequate oxygen and ventilation. Activated charcoal may be more effective than emesis or lavage. Cardiac and vital signs should be monitored. Avoid epinephrine and derivatives when treating hypotension and quinidine and procainamide when treating cardiac arrhythmia. Forced diuresis, dialysis, hemoperfusion, and exchange transfusion are unlikely to be of benefit.

PATIENT INFORMATION

Patients should be warned about the significant risk of developing agranulocytosis. They should be informed that weekly blood tests are required and that clozapine tablets are available only through a special program designed to ensure the required blood monitoring. Patients should report immediately the appearance of lethargy, weakness, fever, sore throat, malaise, mucous membrane ulceration, or other possible signs of infection. Patients should be informed of the significant risk of seizures during treatment and to avoid driving and any other potentially hazardous activity. If patients stop taking clozapine for more than 2 d, they should not restart but contact their physician for dosing instructions. Patients should avoid alcohol and over-the-counter drugs.

AVAILABILITY

Tablets—25 and 100 mg in UD 100s and in total daily dose packages containing 1 wk of medication in various combinations of 150, 200, 250, 300, 400, 500, and 600 mg/d.

QUETIAPINE

(Seroquel)

Quetiapine is an antipsychotic agent classified as a dibenzothiazepine that is relatively free of extrapyramidal side effects. The drug acts as an antagonist at the dopaminergic, serotoninergic, adrenergic, and histaminergic receptors. Although its precise mechanism of action is unknown, it has been proposed that the drug's antipsychotic activity is mediated through a combination of dopamine type 2 and serotonin type 2A antagonism. It produces few extrapyramidal side effects at typical doses. It can produce sedation, orthostatic hypotension, and weight gain.

SPECIAL PRECAUTIONS

Quetiapine may induce orthostatic hypotension associated with dizziness, tachycardia, and syncope; dosage reduction should be considered if significant orthostatic hypotension develops. The risk of hypotension can be minimized by using a lower starting dose (25 mg twice a day). Quetiapine should be used with caution in patients with known cardiovascular disease, cerebrovascular disease, and conditions predisposing to hypotension.

(Continued on next page)

In Brief

INDICATIONS

Manifestations of psychotic disorders, mania, severe behavioral disturbances associated with some organic mental syndromes or developmental disorders

CONTRAINDICATIONS

Known hypersensitivity to quetiapine

INTERACTIONS

Other centrally active drugs; alcohol; antihypertensive agents; levodopa; dopamine agonists; drugs that inhibit cytochrome P$_{4503A}$ (eg, ketoconazole, erythromycin) or induce the enzyme (eg, phenytoin) may modify bioavailability of quetiapine; the risks of using quetiapine in combination with other drugs has not been extensively evaluated in clinical trials

ADVERSE EFFECTS

Drowsiness, dizziness, weight gain, headache, asthenia, nausea, anxiety, constipation, dyspepsia, rhinitis, rash, palpitations, dyspnea, tachycardia, increased duration of sleep, accommodation disturbances, increased or reduced salivation, micturition disturbances, extrapyramidal symptoms, hypertonia, tardive dyskinesia, aggressive reaction, nausea, vomiting, abdominal pain, fever, torticollis, hypotonia, migraine, hyperreflexia, choreoathetosis, anorexia, flatulence, increased appetite, fatigue, flu syndrome, increased or decreased sweating, peripheral edema, eczema, alopecia, seborrhea, increased AST and increased ALT

(Continued on next page)

SPECIAL PRECAUTIONS (CONTINUED)

The development of cataracts was observed in association with quetiapine treatment in chronic dog studies. Lens changes have also been observed in patients during long-term quetiapine treatment, but a causal relationship to quetiapine has not been established. Nevertheless, the possibility of lenticular changes can not be excluded at this time; therefore, examination of the lens by methods adequate to detect cataract formation, such as slit-lamp examination or other appropriately sensitive methods, is recommended at initiation of treatment or shortly thereafter and at 6-month intervals during chronic treatment.

Quetiapine should be used with caution in patients with a seizure disorder.

Transient elevations (up to threefold) in alanine aminotransferase (ALT) can occur in some patients, but levels generally return to normal within three weeks. About 0.4% of patients treated with quetiapine may experience elevations in thyroid-stimulating hormone, and about half of these may require thyroid replacement.

Esophageal dysmotility and aspiration have been associated with antipsychotic drug use. Like other antipsychotic drugs, quetiapine should be used with caution in patients at risk for aspiration pneumonia.

Tardive dyskinesia, a syndrome of involuntary abnormal movements, may develop in patients treated with this drug. In some cases, these movements can be severe or persistent. The elderly are at highest risk, but it can occur at any age. The risk of developing tardive dyskinesia and the likelihood that it will become irreversible increase as the total duration and total cumulative dose of the antipsychotic administered to the patient increase. Tardive dystonia unassociated with tardive dyskinesia also has been reported with antipsychotic drug use. The condition is characterized by delayed onset of choreic or dystonic movements and may become irreversible.

Neuroleptic malignant syndrome, a potentially fatal syndrome involving high fever, rigidity, autonomic instability, altered level of consciousness, and elevated creatine phosphokinase level can occur in patients receiving antipsychotic medications. Two possible cases (< 0.1%) among the over 2000 patients who have received quetiapine have been reported; however, the exact frequency with which this side effect occurs in patients treated with quetiapine is unknown.

SPECIAL GROUPS

Race: Generally effective regardless of race; there is no race effect on the pharmacokinetics of quetiapine.

Gender: There is no gender effect on the pharmacokinetics of quetiapine.

Children: Safety and efficacy not established.

Elderly: Oral clearance of quetiapine was reduced about 40% in elderly patients (> 65 years); lower starting and maintenance doses are recommended.

Renal impairment: Although severe renal dysfunction can reduce oral clearance by about 25%, quetiapine levels stay within the acceptable range. The need for dosage adjustments is unclear.

Hepatic impairment: Administer with caution. Use lower starting doses.

Pregnancy: Safety not established. Use only when potential benefit outweighs potential risk.

Breast-feeding: Antipsychotic drugs excreted in low concentrations in breast milk. Women receiving quetiapine should not breast-feed.

Smoking status: Smoking has no effect on the oral clearance of quetiapine.

PHARMACOKINETICS AND PHARMACODYNAMICS

Onset of action: variable

Peak plasma levels: about 1.5 h following oral dose

Plasma half-life: about 6 h

Bioavailability: about 100%; its bioavailability is marginally increased (15%–25%) by administration with food

Metabolism: extensively metabolized by the liver; the major metabolic pathways are sulfoxidation to the sulfoxide metabolite and oxidation to the parent acid metabolite; both metabolites are pharmacologically inactive; it appears that the P450 3A4 isoenzyme is involved in the metabolism of quetiapine to its major, but inactive, sulfoxide metabolite

Excretion: following a single oral dose of quetiapine, < 1% of the drug is excreted unchanged in the urine, indicating that the drug is highly metabolized; approximately 73% and 20% of the drug is excreted in the urine and feces, respectively

Effect of food: food does marginally affect the extent of absorption, increasing C_{max} and AUC values by 25% and 15%, respectively

Protein binding: plasma protein binding of about 83% for quetiapine at therapeutic concentrations

Renal impairment: patients with severe renal impairment exhibit a 25% lower mean oral clearance than do normal subjects; because quetiapine is highly metabolized before excretion and < 1% of the drug is excreted unchanged, however, renal dysfunction alone is unlikely to have a major impact on the pharmacokinetics of quetiapine

Hepatic impairment: since quetiapine is extensively metabolized by the liver, higher plasma levels are expected in the hepatically impaired population, and dosage adjustment may be necessary

PROLONGED USE

Antipsychotic efficacy was established in short-term (6- to 8-wk) trials of schizophrenic inpatients; effectiveness in long-term use (ie, more than 6 to 8 weeks) has not been systematically evaluated, and the physician who elects to use quetiapine for extended periods should periodically reevaluate long-term usefulness of the drug for the individual patient.

OVERDOSAGE

Experience with quetiapine in acute overdosage is limited in the premarketing database (six reports with doses ranging from 1200 to 9300 mg; no fatalities have been reported). Reported symptoms are those resulting from exaggeration of the drug's known pharmacologic effects (ie, drowsiness, sedation, tachycardia, and hypotension). To manage a case of acute overdosage, establish and maintain an airway and ensure adequate oxygenation and ventilation. Gastric lavage (after intubation if patient is unconscious) and administration of activated charcoal together with a laxative should be considered. The possibility of obtundation, seizures, or dystonic reaction of the head and neck following overdosage may create a risk of aspiration with induced emesis. Cardiovascular monitoring should begin immediately and should include continuous ECG monitoring to detect possible arrhythmias. If antiarrhythmic therapy is administered, disopyramide, procainamide, and quinidine carry a theoretic hazard of Q-T–prolonging effects that might be additive to those of quetiapine. There is no specific antidote to quetiapine overdosage; therefore, appropriate supportive measures should be instituted. The possibility of multiple-drug involvement should be considered. Hypotension and circulatory collapse should be treated with appropriate measures, such as IV fluids or sympathomimetic agents (epinephrine and dopamine should not be used because β stimulation may worsen hypotension in the setting of quetiapine-induced α blockade). Close medical supervision and monitoring should continue until patient recovers.

(Continued on next page)

QUETIAPINE (CONTINUED)

DOSAGE

Adults: *Usual dose*—Should generally be administered with an initial dose of 25 mg twice a day, with increases in increments of 25 to 50 mg twice a day on the second and third day, as tolerated, to a dosage of 300 mg/d by the fourth day, given twice or three times a day. Further dosage adjustments, if indicated, should generally occur at intervals of not less than 2 days. The safety of dosages above 800 mg/d has not been evaluated at this time. For patients receiving maintenance treatment, attempts should be made to reduce dosage to the lower effective level after symptoms have been controlled for a reasonable period.

Elderly: Slower rate of dose titration and a lower target dose should be employed.

PATIENT INFORMATION

Patients should be given a list of common side effects and be instructed to report all symptoms. Patients should protect themselves from sun exposure. Caution should be used when performing activities requiring mental alertness. Patients should limit alcohol consumption. Given the likelihood that a proportion of patients will develop tardive dyskinesia, all patients for whom long-term use is contemplated should be given information about this risk. The decision of when to inform patients (or guardians) should take into account the clinical circumstances and competency of the patient to understand the information provided. The risks of discontinuing treatment also must be described.

AVAILABILITY

Tablets—25-, 100-, and 200-mg tablets in bottles of 100 tablets, 1000 tablets, and hospital unit dose packages of 100 tablets

LOXAPINE

(Loxitane)

Loxapine is an antipsychotic agent classified as a dibenzoxazepine that belongs to a subclass of tricyclic antipsychotic agents. Loxapine is chemically distinct from the thioxanthenes, butyrophenones, and phenothiazines. It causes moderate extrapyramidal effects, moderate sedative effects, and minimal anticholinergic and hypotensive effects.

SPECIAL PRECAUTIONS

The neurologic syndromes that can occur with loxapine (parkinsonism, dystonia, akathisia, tardive dyskinesia, tardive dystonia) may be confused with other behavioral or neurologic syndromes.

Tardive dyskinesia, a syndrome of involuntary abnormal movements, may develop in patients treated with this drug. In some cases, these movements can be severe or persistent. The elderly are at highest risk, but it can occur at any age. Tardive dystonia unassociated with tardive dyskinesia has also been reported with antipsychotic drug use. The condition is characterized by delayed onset of choreic or dystonic movements and may become irreversible.

A potentially fatal syndrome involving high fever, rigidity, autonomic instability, altered level of consciousness, and elevated creatine phosphokinase referred to as *neuroleptic malignant syndrome* can occur in patients receiving antipsychotic medications,

Avoid or use with caution in patients with a history of bone marrow depression or previous hypersensitivity reaction.

Administer with caution in patients with cardiovascular disease, chronic respiratory disorders, parkinsonism, epilepsy, myasthenia gravis, or narrow-angle glaucoma, and those exposed to extreme heat or cold.

In Brief

INDICATIONS

Manifestations of psychotic disorders, mania, severe behavioral disturbances associated with some organic mental syndromes or developmental disorders

CONTRAINDICATIONS

Known hypersensitivity, comatose states or depressed levels of consciousness of unknown cause, presence of large amounts of CNS depressants

INTERACTIONS

Alcohol, barbiturates, sedatives, narcotics, antihistamines, anesthetics

ADVERSE EFFECTS

Tremor, rigidity, excessive salivation, tardive dyskinesia, masked facies, akathisia, tachycardia, hypotension, hypertension, orthostatic hypotension, lightheadedness, syncope, dermatitis, edema of face, pruritus, rash, alopecia, seborrhea, dry mouth, nasal congestion, constipation, blurred vision, urinary retention, paralytic ileus, nausea and vomiting, weight gain, weight loss, dyspnea, ptosis, hyperpyrexia, flushed facies, headache, paresthesia, polydipsia, agranulocytosis, thrombocytopenia, leukopenia, jaundice, hepatitis, galactorrhea, amenorrhea, gynecomastia, menstrual irregularity

PHARMACOKINETICS AND PHARMACODYNAMICS

Onset of action: variable
Peak plasma levels: 1.5–3 h
Plasma half-life: *Oral*—3–4 h; *IM*—12 h
Bioavailability: oral form incompletely absorbed, possibly because of first-pass metabolism; more complete and prolonged absorption by IM administration
Metabolism: metabolized extensively; partial metabolism in liver into five metabolites
Excretion: within 48 h of administration, 30%–40% excreted in urine as conjugates and in feces unconjugated
Hepatic impairment: impaired metabolism may increase bioavailability and decrease elimination
Elderly: half-life may be extended

SPECIAL GROUPS

Race: Generally effective regardless of race; dosage requirements may vary.

Children: Use with caution. Do not use in children or adolescents whose symptoms suggest Reye syndrome. Tardive dyskinesia can occur in children.

Elderly: Prevalence of tardive dyskinesia is highest in the elderly. Use lower doses and increase more gradually; observe for hypotensive reactions.

Renal impairment: Administer with caution.

Hepatic impairment: Administer with caution—smaller doses may be required.

Pregnancy: Safety not established. Use only when potential benefit outweighs potential risk.

Breast-feeding: Antipsychotic drugs are excreted in low concentrations in breast milk. Use with caution.

DOSAGE

Adults: Oral route is appropriate for most patients; however, IM injections may be desirable for severely ill patients during the first 24 hours. Oral doses can be initiated at 10 mg twice daily or up to a maximum of 50 mg/d for severely ill patients. Dosage can be increased over 7 to 10 days to usual range of 60 to 100 mg/d. Dosage should not exceed 250 mg/d. IM 12.5 to 50 mg every 4 to 6 hours. Substitute oral medication as soon as feasible.

Elderly: Use with caution; administer low end of adult dose.

Children: Not recommended in children younger than 16 years because inadequate dosing information is available. In adolescents 16 to 18, start low end of adult dose.

PROLONGED USE

Antipsychotic drugs may be indicated for maintenance and prophylactic treatment in some disorders (particularly schizophrenia). To lessen the likelihood of adverse reactions related to cumulative drug effects, patients on long-term therapy should be evaluated periodically to determine if dose can be lowered or drug therapy discontinued; short-acting IM preparations are not intended for long-term use. Patients should be examined periodically for the development of tardive dyskinesia or tardive dystonia.

OVERDOSAGE

Symptoms depend on amount ingested and individual patient tolerance. Clinical findings may range from mild depression of the CNS and cardiovascular system to profound hypotension, respiratory depression, and unconsciousness. Possibility of extrapyramidal symptoms and convulsive seizures should be kept in mind. Renal failure after overdose also has been reported. Treatment is essentially symptomatic and supportive. Early gastric lavage and extended dialysis might be beneficial. Centrally acting emetics have little effect. Emesis should be avoided because of possibility of aspiration of vomitus. Avoid analeptics, which may cause convulsions. Severe hypotension may respond to levarterenol or phenylephrine. *Epinephrine should not be used.* Severe extrapyramidal reactions should be treated with anticholinergic antiparkinson agents or diphenhydramine hydrochloride. Additional measures include oxygen and IV fluids.

PATIENT INFORMATION

Patients should be given a list of common side effects and be instructed to report extrapyramidal symptoms. Patients should protect themselves from sun exposure. Caution should be used when performing activities requiring mental alertness. Patients should limit alcohol consumption. Given the likelihood that a proportion of patients exposed to antipsychotic drugs will develop tardive dyskinesia, all patients for whom long-term use is contemplated should be given information about this risk. The decision when to inform patients (or guardian) should take into account the clinical circumstances and the competency of the patient to understand the information provided. The risks of discontinuing treatment must also be described.

AVAILABILITY

Capsules—5, 10, 25, and 50 mg in 100s
Capsules as succinate—5 mg in 100s and UD 100s; 10, 25, and 50 mg in 100s, 1000s, and UD 100s
Concentrate as HCl—25 mg/mL in 120 mL with dropper
Injection as HCl—50 mg/mL in 1-mL amps and 10-mL vials

MOLINDONE HYDROCHLORIDE

(Moban)

Molindone HCl is an antipsychotic agent classified as a dihydro-indolone with slight to no antiemetic, hypotensive, anticholinergic, or sedative effects. Molindone is structurally unrelated to the phenothiazines, butyrophenones, or thioxanthenes; the clinical actions of molindone are, however, similar to those of the piper-azine-type phenothiazines with somewhat fewer side effects, including a lower incidence of weight gain.

SPECIAL PRECAUTIONS

The neurologic syndromes that can occur with use of molindone (parkinsonism, dystonia, akathisia, tardive dyskinesia, tardive dystonia) may be confused with other behavioral or neurologic syndromes.

Tardive dyskinesia, a syndrome of involuntary abnormal move-ments, may develop in patients treated with this drug. In some cases, these movements can be severe or persistent. The elderly are at highest risk, but it can occur at any age. Tardive dystonia unassoci-ated with tardive dyskinesia has also been reported with antipsy-chotic drug use. The condition is characterized by delayed onset of choreic or dystonic movements and may become irreversible.

A potentially fatal syndrome involving high fever, rigidity, auto-nomic instability, altered level of consciousness, and elevated creati-nine phosphokinase referred to as *neuroleptic malignant syndrome* can occur in patients receiving antipsychotic medications.

Avoid or use with caution in patients with a history of bone marrow depression or previous hypersensitivity reaction.

Administer with caution in patients with cardiovascular disease, chronic respiratory disorders, parkinsonism, epilepsy, myasthenia gravis, narrow-angle glaucoma, and those exposed to extreme heat or cold.

SPECIAL GROUPS

Race: Generally effective regardless of race; dosage requirements may vary.

Children: Use with caution. Do not use in children or adolescents whose symptoms suggest Reye syndrome. Tardive dyskinesia can occur in children.

Elderly: The prevalence of tardive dyskinesia is highest in the elderly. Use lower doses and increase more gradually; observe for hypotensive reactions.

Renal impairment: Administer with caution.

Hepatic impairment: Administer with caution—smaller doses may be required.

Pregnancy: Safety not established. Use only when potential benefit outweighs potential risk.

Breast-feeding: Antipsychotic drugs are excreted in low concentra-tions in breast milk. Use with caution.

(Continued on next page)

In Brief

INDICATIONS

Manifestations of psychotic disorders, mania, severe behavioral distur-bances associated with some organic mental syndromes or develop-mental disorders

CONTRAINDICATIONS

Known hypersensitivity, comatose states or depressed levels of consciousness of unknown cause, presence of large amounts of CNS depressants

INTERACTIONS

None reported

ADVERSE EFFECTS

Drowsiness, depression, hyperactivity, euphoria, akinesia, motor restlessness, dystonic syndrome, tardive dyskinesia, blurred vision, tachycardia, nausea, dry mouth, salivation, urinary retention, consti-pation, leukopenia, leukocytosis, altered liver function, hypotension, lens opacities and pigmentary retinopathy, nonspecific skin rash, altered thyroid function, heavy menses, galactorrhea, gynecomastia

PHARMACOKINETICS AND PHARMACODYNAMICS

Onset of action: variable
Peak plasma levels: 1.5 h (unmetabolized drug)
Bioavailability: rapidly absorbed from the GI tract
Metabolism: rapidly metabolized with 36 recognized metabolites
Excretion: < 2% excreted unmetabolized in urine and < 1% excreted unmetabolized in feces
Hepatic impairment: impaired metabolism may increase bioavailability and decrease elimination

PROLONGED USE

Antipsychotic drugs may be indicated for maintenance and prophylac-tic treatment in some disorders (particularly schizophrenia). To lessen the likelihood of adverse reactions related to cumulative drug effects, patients on long-term therapy should be evaluated periodi-cally to determine if dose can be lowered or drug therapy discontin-ued; short-acting IM preparations are not intended for long-term use. Patients should be examined periodically for the development of tardive dyskinesia or tardive dystonia.

OVERDOSAGE

Symptomatic, supportive therapy should be the rule. Gastric lavage is indicated for reduction of absorption of molindone, which is freely soluble in water. Because the adsorption of molindone in activated charcoal has not been determined, use of this antidote must be considered of theoretic value. Emesis in a comatose patient is contraindicated. A significant increase in rate of removal of unmetab-olized molindone by forced diuresis, peritoneal dialysis, or renal dialysis would not be expected. Extrapyramidal symptoms have responded to diphenhydramine and synthetic anticholinergic antiparkinson agents.

PATIENT INFORMATION

Patients should be given a list of common side effects and instructed to report extrapyramidal symptoms. Patients should protect them-selves from sun exposure. Caution should be used when performing activities requiring mental alertness. Patients should limit alcohol consumption. Given the likelihood that a proportion of patients exposed to antipsychotic drugs will develop tardive dyskinesia, all patients for whom long-term use is contemplated should be given information about this risk. The decision of when to inform patients (or guardian) should take into account the clinical circumstances

(Continued on next page)

DOSAGE

Adults: Initial dosage is usually 50 to 75 mg/d increased to 100 mg/d in 3 to 4 days. Some patients may require up to 225 mg/d. For patients receiving maintenance treatment, attempts should be made to reduce dosage to the lowest effective level after symptoms have been controlled for a reasonable period.

Elderly: Use with caution, usually one third to half adult dose, and increase more frequently.

Children: Not recommended for children younger than 12 years; inadequate information available regarding dosage. Use lower end of adult dosage in children aged 12 to 18 years.

PATIENT INFORMATION (CONTINUED)

and the competency of the patient to understand the information provided. The risks of discontinuing treatment must also be described.

AVAILABILITY

Tablets—5, 10, 25, 50, and 100 mg in 100s
Concentrate—20 mg/mL with cherry flavor in 120 mL (with parabens and sodium metabisulfite)

CHLORPROMAZINE HYDROCHLORIDE

(Thorazine)

Chlorpromazine HCl is an antipsychotic agent classified as an aliphatic phenothiazine that was introduced into clinical practice more than 40 years ago and continues to be widely used. It has significant hypotensive properties and sedative effects as well as moderate anticholinergic and extrapyramidal effects.

SPECIAL PRECAUTIONS

The neurologic syndromes that can occur with use of chlorpromazine (parkinsonism, dystonia, akathisia, tardive dyskinesia, tardive dystonia) may be confused with other behavioral or neurologic syndromes.

Tardive dyskinesia, a syndrome of involuntary abnormal movements, may develop in patients treated with this drug. In some cases, these movements can be severe or persistent. The elderly are at highest risk, but it can occur at any age. Tardive dystonia unassociated with tardive dyskinesia has also been reported with antipsychotic drug use. The condition is characterized by delayed onset of choreic or dystonic movements and may become irreversible.

A potentially fatal syndrome involving high fever, rigidity, autonomic instability, altered level of consciousness, and elevated creatine phosphokinase referred to as neuroleptic malignant syndrome can occur in patients receiving antipsychotic medications.

Avoid or use with caution in patients with a history of bone marrow depression or previous hypersensitivity reaction.

Administer with caution in patients with cardiovascular disease, chronic respiratory disorders, parkinsonism, epilepsy, myasthenia gravis, narrow-angle glaucoma, and those exposed to extreme heat or cold.

In Brief

INDICATIONS

Manifestations of psychotic disorders; mania, severe behavioral disturbances associated with some organic mental syndromes or developmental disorders

CONTRAINDICATIONS

Hypersensitivity, comatose states or depressed levels of consciousness of unknown cause, presence of large amounts of CNS depressants

INTERACTIONS

Epinephrine, norepinephrine, valproic acid, oral anticoagulants, thiazide diuretics, propranolol, metrizamide, anesthetics, barbiturates, narcotics, organophosphorus insecticides, atropine, alcohol, antacids, anticholinergics, anticonvulsants, α-methyldopa, guanethidine, orphenadrine

ADVERSE EFFECTS

Cholestasis, drowsiness, jaundice, leukopenia, agranulocytosis, eosinophilia, hemolytic anemia, thrombocytopenic purpura, pancytopenia, aplastic anemia, postural hypotension, simple tachycardia, momentary fainting and dizziness, ECG changes, dystonia, akathisia and restlessness, pseudoparkinsonism, tardive dyskinesia, tardive dystonia, torticollis, extensor rigidity of back muscles, opisthotonos, trismus, oculogyric crisis, agitation, insomnia, cerebral edema, abnormal CSF proteins, skin rash, mild urticaria, exfoliative dermatitis, contact dermatitis, skin pigmentation, photosensitivity, corneal or lenticular deposits, gynecomastia, amenorrhea, hyperglycemia, hypoglycemia, dry mouth, nausea, constipation, urinary retention, miosis, atonic colon, mild fever (IM), increased appetite and weight gain, peripheral edema, sudden death, carpopedal spasm, difficulty swallowing, protrusion of tongue, catatonic-like states, convulsive seizures, hyperprolactinemia, breast engorgement, galactorrhea, nasal congestion, obstipation, adynamic ileus, priapism, mydriasis, ejaculatory disorders or impotence, hyperpyrexia, systemic lupus erythematosus–like syndrome

(Continued on next page)

CHLORPROMAZINE HYDROCHLORIDE (CONTINUED)

SPECIAL GROUPS

Race: Generally effective regardless of race; dosage requirements may vary.

Children: Use with caution. Do not use in children or adolescents whose symptoms suggest Reye syndrome. Tardive dyskinesia can occur in children.

Elderly: Prevalence of tardive dyskinesia is highest in the elderly. Use lower doses and increase more gradually; observe for hypotensive reactions.

Renal impairment: Administer with caution.

Hepatic impairment: Administer with caution—smaller doses may be required.

Pregnancy: Safety not established. Use only when potential benefit outweighs potential risk.

Breast-feeding: Antipsychotic drugs are excreted in low concentrations in breast milk. Use with caution.

DOSAGE

Adults: Oral route is appropriate for most patients; however, IM injections may be desirable in severely ill patients for the first 24 hours. Oral dosages can be initiated with 50 to 100 mg every 4 hours depending on age, weight, and severity of symptoms. Dosages between 300 to 800 mg are usually adequate, and higher doses rarely improve response. IM 25 to 50 mg every 4 to 6 hours. For patients receiving maintenance treatment, attempts should be made to reduce dosage to lowest effective level after symptoms have been controlled for a reasonable period.

Elderly: Usually one third to half usual adult dosage, and increase more gradually.

Children: 0.5 mg/kg every 4 to 6 hours as needed.

PHARMACOKINETICS AND PHARMACODYNAMICS

Onset of action: variable; 1–3 h following oral administration, 30–60 min following IM

Peak plasma levels: 2–3 h

Plasma half-life: 8–35 h

Bioavailability: 10%–40%

Metabolism: hepatic to numerous (100) metabolites

Excretion: 50% renal; 50% enterohepatic; 1% unchanged

Effect of food: variable

Protein binding: 90%–99%

Hepatic impairment: impaired metabolism may increase bioavailability and decrease elimination

Elderly: half-life may be extended

PROLONGED USE

Antipsychotic drugs may be indicated for maintenance and prophylactic treatment in some disorders (particularly schizophrenia). To lessen the likelihood of adverse reactions related to cumulative drug effects, patients on long-term therapy should be evaluated periodically to determine if dose can be lowered or drug therapy discontinued; short-acting IM preparations are not intended for long-term use. Patients should be examined periodically for the development of tardive dyskinesia or tardive dystonia.

OVERDOSAGE

Possible symptoms include dystonic reactions, hypothermia, tachycardia, tachypnea, cardiac arrhythmia, fever, autonomic reactions, hypotension, somnolence, and coma. There is no specific antidote. Early treatment should include gastric lavage. *Do not attempt to induce emesis.* If a vasoconstrictor is indicated, use norepinephrine (*not epinephrine*). Observe for bladder or intestinal distention. Hemodialysis is not effective. Use conservative symptomatic treatment for CNS depression. Extrapyramidal reactions can produce dysphagia and respiratory dysfunction.

PATIENT INFORMATION

Patients should be given a list of common side effects and instructed to report extrapyramidal symptoms. Patients should protect themselves from sun exposure. Caution should be used when performing activities requiring mental alertness. Patients should limit alcohol consumption. Given the likelihood that a proportion of patients exposed to antipsychotic drugs will develop tardive dyskinesia, all patients for whom long-term use is contemplated should be given information about this risk. The decision of when to inform patients (or guardian) should take into account the clinical circumstances and the competency of the patient to understand the information provided. The risks of discontinuing treatment must also be described.

AVAILABILITY

Tablets—10 mg in 100s, 1000s, and UD 100s; 25 mg in 100s, 1000s, and UD 100s; 50 mg in 100s, 1000s, and US 100s; 100 mg in 100s, 1000s, and UD 100s; 200 mg in 100s, 1000s, and UD 100s

Capsules (sustained release)—30, 75, 150, 200, and 300 mg in 50s, 500s, and UD 100s

Syrup—10 mg/5 mL wintergreen or orange-custard flavor in 120 mL

Concentrate—30mg/mL in 120 mL; 100 mg/mL in 60 and 240 mL with or without custard flavor

Suppositories (as base)—25 or 100 mg in 12s

Injection—25 mg/mL in 1- and 2-mL amps and 10-mL vials

TRIFLUPROMAZINE HYDROCHLORIDE

(Vesprin)

Triflupromazine HCl is an aliphatic-type phenothiazine antipsychotic agent. It has significant antiemetic and sedative effects and mild extrapyramidal effects. It has mild to moderate hypotensive properties. Triflupromazine has been shown to be equal in efficacy to chlorpromazine in a number of studies. This compound is not widely used at the present time, however, and is available only in an IM preparation.

SPECIAL PRECAUTIONS

The neurologic syndromes that occur with use of triflupromazine (parkinsonism, dystonia, akathisia, tardive dyskinesia, tardive dystonia) may be confused with other behavioral or neurologic syndromes.

Tardive dyskinesia, a syndrome of involuntary abnormal movements, may develop in patients treated with this drug. In some cases, these movements can be severe or persistent. The elderly are at highest risk, but it can occur at any age. Tardive dystonia unassociated with tardive dyskinesia has also been reported with antipsychotic drug use. The condition is characterized by delayed onset of choreic or dystonic movements and may become irreversible.

A potentially fatal syndrome involving high fever, rigidity, autonomic instability, altered level of consciousness, and elevated creatine phosphokinase referred to as neuroleptic malignant syndrome can occur in patients receiving antipsychotic medications.

Avoid or use with caution in patients with a history of bone marrow depression or previous hypersensitivity reaction.

Administer with caution in patients with cardiovascular disease, chronic respiratory disorders, parkinsonism, epilepsy, myasthenia gravis, narrow-angle glaucoma, and those exposed to extreme heat or cold.

SPECIAL GROUPS

Race: Generally effective regardless of race; dosage requirements may vary.
Children: Use with caution. Do not use in children or adolescents whose symptoms suggest Reye syndrome. Tardive dyskinesia can occur in children.
Elderly: Prevalence of tardive dyskinesia is highest in the elderly. Use lower doses and increase more gradually; observe for hypotensive reactions.
Renal impairment: Administer with caution.
Hepatic impairment: Administer with caution—smaller doses may be required.
Pregnancy: Safety not established. Use only when potential benefit outweighs potential risk.
Breast-feeding: Antipsychotic drugs are excreted in low concentrations in breast milk. Use with caution.

DOSAGE

Adults: 50 mg IM to a maximum of 150 mg/d.
Elderly: Use one third to half usual adult dose.
Children: Not generally indicated for use in children. Dose range 0.2 to 0.25 mg/kg to maximum of 10 mg/d.

In Brief

INDICATIONS
Short-term management of manifestations of psychotic disorders, mania, severe behavioral disturbances associated with some organic mental syndromes or developmental disorders

CONTRAINDICATIONS
Hypersensitivity; comatose states or depressed levels of consciousness of unknown cause; presence of large amounts of CNS depressants

INTERACTIONS
Epinephrine, valproic acid, oral anticoagulants, thiazide diuretics, propranolol, metrizamide, anesthetics, barbiturates, narcotics, atropine

ADVERSE EFFECTS
Dystonia, pseudoparkinsonism, tardive dyskinesia, drowsiness, agranulocytosis, eosinophilia, leukopenia, hemolytic anemia, postural hypotension, simple tachycardia, motor restlessness, agitation, akathisia, insomnia, abnormal CSF proteins, dry mouth, nasal congestion, urinary retention, miosis, mydriasis, hypotension, hyperprolactinemia, amenorrhea, weight gain

PHARMACOKINETICS AND PHARMACODYNAMICS
Onset of action: variable
Peak plasma levels: 1–3 h
Plasma half-life: 3–40 h
Bioavailability: unpredictable patterns of absorption; widely distributed in tissue
Metabolism: extensively metabolized in the liver
Excretion: half occurs in kidneys and half through enterohepatic circulation; < 1% excreted as unchanged drug
Effect of food: GI absorption modified unpredictably by food
Protein binding: 85%–95%
Renal impairment: effects not known
Hepatic impairment: metabolism may be delayed or modified
Elderly: half-life probably extended

PROLONGED USE
Because this is available only in a short-acting IM preparation, it is not appropriate for long-term use.

OVERDOSAGE
Possible symptoms include dystonic reactions, hypothermia, tachycardia, tachypnea, cardiac arrhythmia, fever, autonomic reactions, hypotension, somnolence, and coma. There is no specific antidote. Early treatment should include gastric lavage. *Do not attempt to induce emesis.* If a vasoconstrictor is indicated, use norepinephrine (*not epinephrine*). Observe for bladder or intestinal distention. Hemodialysis is not effective. Use conservative symptomatic treatment for CNS depression. Extrapyramidal reactions can produce dysphagia and respiratory dysfunction.

(Continued on next page)

TRIFLUPROMAZINE HYDROCHLORIDE *(CONTINUED)*

PATIENT INFORMATION

Patients should be given a list of common side effects and instructed to report extrapyramidal symptoms. Patients should protect themselves from sun exposure. Caution should be used when performing activities requiring mental alertness. Patients should limit alcohol consumption. Given the likelihood that a proportion of patients exposed to

antipsychotic drugs will develop tardive dyskinesia, all patients for whom long-term use is contemplated should be given information about this risk. The decision of when to inform patients (or guardian) should take into account the clinical circumstances and the competency of the patient to understand the information provided. The risks of discontinuing treatment must also be described.

AVAILABILITY

Injection—10 mg/mL in 10-mL multidose vials; 20 mg/mL in 1-multidose vials

ACETOPHENAZINE MALEATE

(Tindal)

Acetophenazine maleate is a member of the piperazine class of phenothiazine antipsychotics. It has not been widely studied in controlled trials; however, trials that have been conducted suggest it is as effective as chlorpromazine. Acetophenazine is not as sedative or as likely to produce hypotension as chlorpromazine. It has moderate extrapyramidal effects. This drug is not widely used at the present time.

SPECIAL PRECAUTIONS

The neurologic syndromes that can occur with use of acetophenazine (parkinsonism, dystonia, akathisia, tardive dyskinesia, tardive dystonia) may be confused with other behavioral or neurologic syndromes.

Tardive dyskinesia, a syndrome of involuntary abnormal movements, may develop in patients treated with this drug. In some cases, these movements can be severe or persistent. The elderly are at highest risk, but it can occur at any age. Tardive dystonia unassociated with tardive dyskinesia has also been reported with antipsychotic drug use. The condition is characterized by delayed onset of choreic or dystonic movements and may become irreversible.

A potentially fatal syndrome involving high fever, rigidity, autonomic instability, altered level of consciousness, and elevated creatine phosphokinase referred to as neuroleptic malignant syndrome can occur in patients receiving antipsychotic medications.

Avoid or use with caution in patients with a history of bone marrow depression or previous hypersensitivity reaction.

Administer with caution in patients with cardiovascular disease, chronic respiratory disorders, parkinsonism, epilepsy, myasthenia gravis, narrow-angle glaucoma, and those exposed to extreme heat or cold.

In Brief

INDICATIONS

Manifestations of psychotic disorders, mania, severe behavioral disturbances associated with some organic mental syndromes or developmental disorders

CONTRAINDICATIONS

Hypersensitivity, comatose states or depressed levels of consciousness of unknown cause, presence of large amounts of CNS depressants

INTERACTIONS

Sedatives, narcotics, anesthetics, tranquilizers, alcohol, oral anticoagulants, propranolol, guanethidine, thiazide diuretics, metrizamide
Drug/laboratory test interactions: False-positive PKU test results

ADVERSE EFFECTS

Pseudoparkinsonism, dystonia, tardive dyskinesia, tardive dystonia, akathisia, grand mal and petit mal convulsions, altered CSF proteins, cerebral edema, dry mouth, nasal congestion, headaches, nausea, constipation, obstipation, adynamic ileus, ejaculatory disorders or impotence, priapism, atonic colon, urinary retention, miosis, mydriasis, catatonic-like states, hypotension, sudden death, blood dyscrasias, liver damage, hyperprolactinemia, amenorrhea, skin disorders, peripheral edema, hyperpyrexia, increased appetite, increased weight, systemic lupus erythematosus–like syndrome, pigmentary retinopathy, skin pigmentation, epithelial keratopathy, neuroleptic malignant syndrome

PHARMACOKINETICS AND PHARMACODYNAMICS

Onset of action: erratic and variable
Peak plasma levels: 2–3 h
Plasma half-life: 10–30 h
Bioavailability: variable
Metabolism: hepatic, no active metabolites known
Excretion: primary route is hepatic clearance; little unchanged drug excreted in urine
Protein binding: bound significantly to plasma proteins
Renal impairment: administer cautiously; effects not known
Hepatic impairment: impaired hepatic function may increase bioavailability and extend half-life; administer with caution

(Continued on next page)

SPECIAL GROUPS

Race: Generally effective regardless of race; dosage requirements may vary.

Children: Use with caution. Do not use in children or adolescents whose symptoms suggest Reye syndrome. Tardive dyskinesia can occur in children.

Elderly: Prevalence of tardive dyskinesia is highest in the elderly. Use lower doses, and increase more gradually; observe for hypotensive reactions.

Renal impairment: Administer with caution.

Hepatic impairment: Administer with caution—smaller doses may be required.

Pregnancy: Safety for use during pregnancy has not been established. Use only when potential benefit outweighs potential risk.

Breast-feeding: Antipsychotic drugs are excreted in low concentrations in breast milk. Use with caution.

DOSAGE

Adults: Initially 60 mg/d in divided doses. Optimum dosage usually 80 to 120 mg/d for acute treatment. For patients receiving maintenance treatment, attempts should be made to reduce dosage to the lowest effective level after symptoms have been controlled for a reasonable time period.

Elderly: Use lower doses and monitor closely.

Children: Dosage guidelines not established.

PROLONGED USE

Antipsychotic drugs may be indicated for maintenance and prophylactic treatment in some disorders (particularly schizophrenia). To lessen the likelihood of adverse reactions related to cumulative drug effects, patients on long-term therapy should be evaluated periodically to determine if dose can be lowered or drug therapy discontinued; short-acting IM preparations are not intended for long-term use. Patients should be examined periodically for the development of tardive dyskinesia or tardive dystonia.

OVERDOSAGE

Possible symptoms include dystonic reactions, hypothermia, tachycardia, tachypnea, cardiac arrhythmia, fever, autonomic reactions, hypotension, somnolence, and coma. There is no specific antidote. Early treatment should include gastric lavage. *Do not attempt to induce emesis.* If a vasoconstrictor is indicated, use norepinephrine (*not epinephrine*). Observe for bladder or intestinal distention. Hemodialysis is not effective. Use conservative symptomatic treatment for CNS depression. Extrapyramidal reactions can produce dysphagia and respiratory dysfunction.

PATIENT INFORMATION

Patients should be given a list of common side effects and instructed to report extrapyramidal symptoms. Patients should protect themselves from sun exposure. Caution should be used when performing activities requiring mental alertness. Patients should limit alcohol consumption. Given the likelihood that a proportion of patients exposed to antipsychotic drugs will develop tardive dyskinesia, all patients for whom long-term use is contemplated should be given information about this risk. The decision of when to inform patients (or guardian) should take into account the clinical circumstances and the competency of the patient to understand the information provided. The risks of discontinuing treatment must also be described.

AVAILABILITY

Tablets—20 mg sugar-coated in 100s

FLUPHENAZINE HYDROCHLORIDE

(Prolixin),

FLUPHENAZINE ENANTHATE

(Prolixin Enanthate),

FLUPHENAZINE DECANOATE

(Prolixin Decanoate)

Fluphenazine is a member of the piperazine subclass of the pheno-thiazine antipsychotic drug class. It is a widely used and extensively studied compound that has the advantage of also being available in a depot, injectable, long-acting preparation. Fluphenazine is considered a high-potency compound with substantial extrapyramidal effects but relatively little sedative, anticholinergic, and hypotensive effects. Fluphenazine decanoate and enanthate are both depot preparations of fluphenazine. The decanoate may be somewhat longer acting and may have fewer adverse effects. Fluphenazine is one of the highest potency antipsychotic drugs, being approximately 50 times more potent than is chlorpromazine on a milligram-for-milligram basis.

SPECIAL PRECAUTIONS

The neurologic syndromes that can occur with fluphenazine (parkinsonism, dystonia, akathisia, tardive dyskinesia, tardive dystonia) may be confused with other behavioral or neurologic syndromes.

Tardive dyskinesia, a syndrome of involuntary abnormal movements, may develop in patients treated with this drug. In some cases, these movements can be severe or persistent. The elderly are at highest risk, but it can occur at any age. Tardive dystonia unassociated with tardive dyskinesia has also been reported with antipsychotic drug use. The condition is characterized by delayed onset of choreic or dystonic movements and may become irreversible. There is no clear evidence that depot preparations of antipsychotic drugs have a greater liability for tardive dyskinesia or tardive dystonia when equivalent dosages are contrasted.

A potentially fatal syndrome involving high fever, rigidity, autonomic instability, altered level of consciousness, and elevated creatine phosphokinase referred to as *neuroleptic malignant syndrome* can occur in patients receiving antipsychotic medications. Some reports have suggested a higher incidence of neuroleptic malignant syndrome with depot drugs; however, it is difficult to draw definitive conclusions, and there is no substantial evidence that mortality is higher when a depot drug has been used (assuming prompt diagnosis and treatment).

Avoid or use with caution in patients with a history of bone marrow depression or previous hypersensitivity reaction.

Administer with caution in patients with cardiovascular disease, chronic respiratory disorders, parkinsonism, epilepsy, myasthenia gravis, narrow-angle glaucoma, and those exposed to extreme heat or cold.

(Continued on next page)

In Brief

INDICATIONS
Manifestations of psychotic disorders, mania, severe behavioral disturbances associated with some organic mental syndromes or developmental disorders; *fluphenazine decanoate or enanthate*—management of patients requiring prolonged antipsychotic treatment

CONTRAINDICATIONS
Hypersensitivity, comatose states or depressed levels of consciousness of unknown cause, presence of large amounts of CNS depressants

INTERACTIONS
Epinephrine, norepinephrine, valproic acid, oral anticoagulants, thiazide diuretics, propranolol, metrizamide, anesthetics, barbiturates, narcotics, organophosphorous insecticides, atropine, alcohol, antacids, anticonvulsants, α-methyldopa, guanethidine, orphenadrine

ADVERSE EFFECTS
Pseudoparkinsonism, dystonia, tardive dyskinesia, tardive dystonia, leukocytosis, elevated creatine kinase, liver function abnormalities, acute renal failure, drowsiness, lethargy, catatonic-like state, restlessness and akathisia, excitement, bizarre dreams, hypertension, nausea, salivation, perspiration, headaches, blurred vision, bladder paralysis, paralytic ileus, nasal congestion, weight change, abnormal lactation, menstrual irregularities, impotency, leukopenia, skin disorders, agranulocytosis, thrombocytopenia, eosinophilia, cholestatic jaundice, systemic lupus erythematosus–like syndrome, cardiac arrest, altered CSF proteins, asthma, laryngeal edema, angioneurotic edema, skin pigmentation, lenticular and corneal opacities, local tissue reactions (IM or SC), sudden death, hyperprolactinemia, hypotension, loss of appetite, polyuria, dry mouth, constipation, glaucoma, fecal impaction, tachycardia, peripheral edema, gynecomastia, purpura, pancytopenia

PHARMACOKINETICS AND PHARMACODYNAMICS
Onset of action: *Oral*—variable 1–3 h; *IM*—30–60 min; *Depot*—24–72 h
Peak plasma levels: *HCl*—2–4 h; *Decanoate*—1–3 d; *Enanthate*—2–4 d
Plasma half-life: *HCl*—12–20 h; *Decanoate*—variable 4–12 d; *Enanthate*—variable 4–6 d
Bioavailability: readily but incompletely absorbed; higher with IM preparations
Metabolism: metabolized extensively in the liver; the 7-hydroxy-metabolite may be active
Excretion: primary route is hepatic clearance; little unchanged drug excreted
Effect of food: does not affect bioavailability; substances containing caffeine, tannics, or pectinates may interfere
Protein binding: > 90%
Renal impairment: administer with caution
Hepatic impairment: impaired hepatic function extends half-life and drug's kinetic effects

PROLONGED USE
Antipsychotic drugs may be indicated for maintenance and prophylactic treatment in some disorders (particularly schizophrenia). To lessen the likelihood of adverse reactions related to cumulative drug effects, patients on long-term therapy should be evaluated periodically to determine if dose can be lowered or drug therapy discontinued; short-acting IM preparations are not intended for long-term use. Patients should be examined periodically for the development of tardive dyskinesia or tardive dystonia.

SPECIAL PRECAUTIONS (CONTINUED)

Although some situations might warrant the use of depot drugs for acute treatment, routine clinical practice should involve the use of short-acting IM or oral forms before the introduction of depot injections. Careful supervision should occur when switching from oral to depot.

SPECIAL GROUPS

Race: Generally effective regardless of race; dosage requirements may vary.

Children: Use with caution. Do not use in children or adolescents whose symptoms suggest Reye syndrome. Tardive dyskinesia can occur in children.

Elderly: Prevalence of tardive dyskinesia is highest in the elderly. Use lower doses, and increase more gradually; observe for hypotensive reactions.

Renal impairment: Administer with caution.

Hepatic impairment: Administer with caution—smaller doses may be required.

Pregnancy: Safety for use during pregnancy has not been established. Use only when potential benefit outweighs potential risk.

Breast-feeding: Antipsychotic drugs are excreted in low concentrations in breast milk. Use with caution.

DOSAGE

Adults: *Oral*—initially 2.5 to 10 mg daily. (There appears to be little if any value in exceeding 20 mg/d.) *IM, short-acting preparation*—1.25 to 5.0 mg every 2 to 8 hours until symptoms are controlled or oral medication can be substituted. *Depot preparations*—Adults initially 12.5 mg, but dosage must be individualized. There is no precise conversion formula; however, 10 mg/d of oral medication might be roughly equivalent to 12.5 mg of depot given every 2 to 3 weeks. It may take 2 to 3 months for steady-state to be achieved. Dosage should rarely exceed 50 mg every 2 weeks. For patients receiving maintenance treatment, attempts should be made to reduce dosage to lowest effective level after symptoms have been controlled for a reasonable period.

Elderly: 1 to 3 mg/d orally depending on condition, weight, and response. Depot drugs may be useful in some elderly individuals, but low doses should be administered with careful observation.

Children: There is inadequate information to make firm recommendations; however, dosages ranging from 0.5 to 10 mg have been used in children between the ages of 6 and 12 years. Fluphenazine depot preparations are not recommended for use in children younger than 12 years.

OVERDOSAGE

Possible symptoms include dystonic reactions, hypothermia, tachycardia, tachypnea, cardiac arrhythmia, fever, autonomic reactions, hypotension, somnolence, and coma. There is no specific antidote. Early treatment should include gastric lavage. *Do not attempt to induce emesis.* If a vasoconstrictor is indicated, use norepinephrine (*not epinephrine*). Observe for bladder or intestinal distention. Hemodialysis is not effective. Use conservative symptomatic treatment for CNS depression. Extrapyramidal reactions can produce dysphagia and respiratory dysfunction.

PATIENT INFORMATION

Patients should be given a list of common side effects and instructed to report extrapyramidal symptoms. Patients should protect themselves from sun exposure. Caution should be used when performing activities requiring mental alertness. Patients should limit alcohol consumption. Given the likelihood that a proportion of patients exposed to antipsychotic drugs will develop tardive dyskinesia, all patients for whom long-term use is contemplated should be given information about this risk. The decision of when to inform patients (or guardian) should take into account the clinical circumstances and the competency of the patient to understand the information provided. The risks of discontinuing treatment must also be described.

AVAILABILITY

HCl

Tablets—1 and 10 mg in 50s, 100s, 500s, 10,000s, and UD 100s; 2.5 and 5 mg in 50s, 100s, 500s, and UD 100s
Elixir—2.5 mg/mL in 60 mL with dropper and 473 mL
Concentrate—5 mg/mL in 188 and 120 mL with dropper
Injection—2.5 mg/mL in 10-mL vials

Enanthate

Injection—25 mg/mL in 5-mL vials

Decanoate

Injection—25 mg/mL in 5-mL vials and 1-mL Unimatic syringes

PERPHENAZINE
(Trilafon)

Perphenazine is a member of the piperazine class of phenothiazines. It has proven to be an effective antipsychotic drug in several placebo-controlled trials. It has modest anticholinergic effects and minimal hypotensive and sedative effects. Extrapyramidal reactions, however, are common. Piperazine compounds in general appear to have a low incidence of blood dyscrasias, jaundice, or ocular changes.

SPECIAL PRECAUTIONS

The neurologic syndromes that can occur with use of perphenazine (parkinsonism, dystonia, akathisia, tardive dyskinesia, tardive dystonia) may be confused with other behavioral or neurologic syndromes.

Tardive dyskinesia, a syndrome of involuntary abnormal movements, may develop in patients treated with this drug. In some cases, these movements can be severe or persistent. The elderly are at highest risk, but it can occur at any age. Tardive dystonia unassociated with tardive dyskinesia has also been reported with antipsychotic drug use. The condition is characterized by delayed onset of choreic or dystonic movements and may become irreversible.

A potentially fatal syndrome involving fever, rigidity, autonomic instability, altered level of consciousness, and elevated creatine phosphokinase referred to as neuroleptic malignant syndrome can occur in patients receiving phenothiazines.

Avoid or use with caution in patients with a history of bone marrow depression or previous hypersensitivity reaction.

Administer with caution in patients with cardiovascular disease, chronic respiratory disorders, parkinsonism, epilepsy, myasthenia gravis, narrow-angle glaucoma, and those exposed to extreme heat or cold.

SPECIAL GROUPS

Race: Generally effective regardless of race; dosage requirements may vary.
Children: Use with caution. Do not use in children or adolescents whose symptoms suggest Reye syndrome. Tardive dyskinesia can occur in children.
Elderly: Prevalence of tardive dyskinesia is highest in the elderly. Use lower doses, and increase more gradually; observe for hypotensive reactions.
Renal impairment: Administer with caution.
Hepatic impairment: Administer with caution—smaller doses may be required.
Pregnancy: Safety not established. Use only when potential benefit outweighs potential risk.
Breast-feeding: Antipsychotic drugs are excreted in low concentrations in breast milk. Use with caution.

DOSAGE

Adults: *Oral*—initially 8 to 16 mg in divided dose. Dosage in excess of 50 to 60 mg are not indicated. *IM*—5 mg every 6 hours; not to exceed 20 to 30 mg/d.
Elderly: One third to half usual adult dosage.
Children: Not usually recommended in children younger than 12 years. If indicated, 4 to 6 mg/d oral dosage.

In Brief

INDICATIONS
Short-term management of manifestations of psychotic disorders, mania, severe behavioral disturbances associated with some organic mental syndromes or developmental disorders

CONTRAINDICATIONS
Known hypersensitivity, comatose states or depressed levels of consciousness of unknown cause, presence of large amounts of CNS depressants

INTERACTIONS
Alcohol, antacids, amphetamines, general anesthetics, antianxiety drugs, anticholinergic drugs, antidepressants, antidiabetic agents, bacitracin, barbiturates, bromocriptine, capreomycin, charcoal, CNS depressants, colistimethate, diazoxide, guanethidine, hydantoins, lithium carbonate, meperidine, metoprolol, narcotics, phenytoin, polymycin B, propranolol, quinidine, succinylcholine, tricyclic antidepressants

ADVERSE EFFECTS
Opisthotonos, trismus, torticollis, retrocollis, aching and numbness of limbs, motor restlessness, oculogyric crisis, hyperreflexia, dystonia, tonic spasm of masticatory muscles, tight feeling in throat, slurred in speech, dysphagia, akathisia, parkinsonism, tardive dyskinesia, tardive dystonia, ataxia, cerebral edema, abnormality of CSF proteins, convulsive seizures, drowsiness, catatonic-like states, paranoid reactions, lethargy, paradoxic excitement, hyperactivity, nocturnal confusion, bizarre dreams, dry mouth, salivation, nausea, diarrhea, anorexia, constipation, obstipation, fecal impaction, urinary retention, urinary frequency or incontinence, bladder paralysis, polyuria, nasal congestion, pallor, myosis, mydriasis, blurred vision, glaucoma, perspiration, hypertension, change in pulse rate, adynamic ileus, hyperprolactinemia, galactorrhea, breast enlargement, gynecomastia, disturbances in menstrual cycle, amenorrhea, changes in libido, inhibition of ejaculation, hyperglycemia, hypoglycemia, glycosuria, tachycardia, bradycardia, cardiac arrest, sudden death, agranulocytosis, eosinophilia, leukopenia, hemolytic anemia, thrombocytopenic purpura, pancytopenia, liver damage, jaundice

PHARMACOKINETICS AND PHARMACODYNAMICS
Onset of action: variable 30 min–1 h IM; oral 1–3 h
Peak plasma levels: 2–3 h oral; 1–2 h IM
Plasma half-life: 10–15 h
Bioavailability: variable; large first-pass hepatic effect when given orally
Metabolism: hepatic; several metabolites; no major metabolites are known to be active
Excretion: 50% kidney; 50% enterohepatic < 1% unchanged
Effect of food: variable—do not administer concentrate with substances containing caffeine, tannins, or pectinates
Protein binding: > 90%
Renal impairment: effects not known
Hepatic impairment: half-life may be extended

PROLONGED USE
Antipsychotic drugs may be indicated for maintenance and prophylactic treatment in some disorders (particularly schizophrenia). To lessen the likelihood of adverse reactions related to cumulative drug effects, patients on long-term therapy should be evaluated periodically to determine if dose can be lowered or drug therapy discontinued; short-acting IM preparations are not intended for long-term use. Patients should be examined periodically for the development of tardive dyskinesia or tardive dystonia.

(Continued on next page)

142

OVERDOSAGE

Possible symptoms include dystonic reactions, hypothermia, tachycardia, tachypnea, cardiac arrhythmia, fever, autonomic reactions, hypotension, somnolence, and coma. There is no specific antidote. Early treatment should include gastric lavage. *Do not attempt to induce emesis.* If a vasoconstrictor is indicated, use norepinephrine (*not epinephrine*). Observe for bladder or intestinal distention. Hemodialysis is not effective. Use conservative symptomatic treatment for CNS depression. Extrapyramidal reactions can produce dysphagia and respiratory dysfunction.

PATIENT INFORMATION

Patients should be given a list of common side effects and instructed to report extrapyramidal symptoms. Patients should protect themselves from sun exposure. Caution should be used when performing activities requiring mental alertness. Patients should limit alcohol consumption. Given the likelihood that a proportion of patients exposed to antipsychotic drugs will develop tardive dyskinesia, all patients for whom long-term use is contemplated should be given information about this risk. The decision when to inform patients (or guardian) should take into account the clinical circumstances and the competency of the patient to understand the information provided. The risks of discontinuing treatment must also be described.

AVAILABILITY

Tablets—2, 4, and 16 mg in 100s and 500s; 8 mg in 100s, 250s, and 500s
Concentrate—16 mg/5 mL in 118 mL with dropper
Injection—5 mg/mL in 1-mL amps

PROCHLORPERAZINE

(Compazine)

Prochlorperazine is an antipsychotic agent classified as a piperazine-type phenothiazine with moderate extrapyramidal and antiemetic effects, moderate sedative effects, and minimal anticholinergic and hypotensive effects.

SPECIAL PRECAUTIONS

The neurologic syndromes that can occur with use of prochlorperazine (parkinsonism, dystonia, akathisia, tardive dyskinesia, tardive dystonia) may be confused with other behavioral or neurologic syndromes.

Tardive dyskinesia, a syndrome of involuntary abnormal movements, may develop in patients treated with this drug. In some cases, these movements can be severe or persistent. The elderly are at highest risk, but it can occur at any age. Tardive dystonia unassociated with tardive dyskinesia has also been reported with antipsychotic drug use. The condition is characterized by delayed onset of choreic or dystonic movements and may become irreversible.

A potentially fatal syndrome involving high fever, rigidity, autonomic instability, altered level of consciousness, and elevated creatine phosphokinase referred to as *neuroleptic malignant syndrome* can occur in patients receiving antipsychotic medications.

Avoid or use with caution in patients with a history of bone marrow depression or previous hypersensitivity reaction.

Administer with caution in patients with cardiovascular disease, chronic respiratory disorders, parkinsonism, epilepsy, myasthenia gravis, narrow-angle glaucoma, and those exposed to extreme heat or cold.

In Brief

INDICATIONS
Manifestations of psychotic disorders, mania, severe behavioral disturbances associated with some organic mental syndromes or developmental disorders

CONTRAINDICATIONS
Known hypersensitivity, comatose states, depressed level of consciousness or in presence of large amounts of CNS depressants

INTERACTIONS
Alcohol, anesthetics, narcotics, guanethidine, propranolol, phenytoin, metrizamide, oral anticoagulants, levodopa, thiazide diuretics
Drug/laboratory test interactions: False-positive PKU test results

ADVERSE EFFECTS
Drowsiness; dizziness; amenorrhea; blurred vision; hypotension; cholestatic jaundice; leukopenia; agranulocytosis; agitation; insomnia; neck muscle spasm; torticollis; extensor rigidity of back muscles; opisthotonos; carpopedal spasm; trismus; difficulty swallowing; oculogyric crisis; protrusion of tongue; masklike facies; drooling; tremors; pill-rolling motion; cogwheel rigidity; shuffling gait; involuntary movements of tongue, face, mouth, or jaw; contact dermatitis; extrapyramidal symptoms; grand mal and petit mal convulsions; altered CSF proteins; cerebral edema; dry mouth; nasal congestion; headache; nausea; constipation; obstipation; adynamic ileus; ejaculatory disorders; priapism, atonic colon; urinary retention; miosis; mydriasis; hypotension (sometimes fatal); cardiac arrest; catatonic-like states; blood dyscrasias; jaundice; biliary stasis; endocrine disturbances; skin disorders; asthma; laryngeal edema; angioneurotic edema; anaphylactoid reactions; hyperpyrexia; systemic lupus erythematosus–like syndrome; pigmentary retinopathy; ECG changes; sudden death

(Continued on next page)

PROCHLORPERAZINE
(CONTINUED)

SPECIAL GROUPS

Race: Generally effective regardless of race; dosage requirements may vary.

Children: Use with caution. Do not use in children or adolescents whose symptoms suggest Reye syndrome. Tardive dyskinesia can occur in children.

Elderly: Prevalence of tardive dyskinesia is highest in the elderly. Use lower doses, and increase more gradually; observe for hypotensive reactions.

Renal impairment: Administer with caution.

Hepatic impairment: Administer with caution—smaller doses may be required.

Pregnancy: Safety not established. Use only when potential benefit outweighs potential risk.

Breast-feeding: Antipsychotic drugs are excreted in low concentrations in breast milk. Use with caution.

DOSAGE

Adults: Oral route is appropriate for most patients; however, IM injections may be desirable in severely ill patients for the first 24 hours. *Oral*—Dosages can be initiated at 5 to 10 mg three or four times daily. In moderate to severe conditions for hospitalized or adequately supervised patients, give 10 mg three or four times daily. Increase dosage gradually until symptoms are controlled or side effects become bothersome. When dosage is increased by small increments every two or three days, side effects either do not occur or are easily controlled. Some patients respond to 50 to 75 mg/d. In some cases, optimum dose is 100 to 150 mg/d. *IM*—10 to 20 mg. If necessary, repeat every two to four hours. More than three or four doses seldom necessary. After control is achieved, switch patient to oral drug at same dosage level or higher.

Elderly: Same as adult except use lowest possible dose; monitor patients carefully.

Children: Follow general instructions under adult dosage. Do not use in children younger than 2 years or weighing less than 20 lb. Use lowest effective doses. Tell parents not to exceed prescribed doses. Take particular precaution in administering to children with acute illnesses or dehydration. When writing a prescription for the 2 1/2-mg size suppository, write 2 1/2, not 2.5 to avoid confusion with 25-mg adult size. Occasionally, patients may react to drug with signs of restlessness and excitement; if this occurs, do not administer additional doses. *Oral or rectal*—In children 2 to 12 years, 2.5 mg two or three times daily. Do not give more than 10 mg on first day. Increase dosage according to patient response. In children 2 to 5 years, do not exceed 20 mg total daily dose. In children 6 to 12 years, do not exceed 25 mg total daily dose. In children 12 to 18 years, use adult dosage. *IM*—In children 2 to 12 years, 0.03 mg/kg (0.06 mg/lb) by deep IM injection. After control is achieved (usually after 1 dose), switch to oral form at same dosage level or higher. In children 12 to 18 years, use adult dosage.

PHARMACOKINETICS AND PHARMACODYNAMICS

Onset of action: erratic and variable

Peak plasma levels: 2–3 h

Plasma half-life: initial (distribution phase) 4–5 h; final (elimination phase) 3–40 h; may be prolonged in the elderly

Bioavailability: unpredictable patterns of absorption, particularly after oral administration; parenteral administration can increase bioavailability of active drug by 4–10 times; widely distributed in tissue and CNS, and drug accumulates in brain, lung, and other tissue with high blood supply; also enters fetal circulation easily

Metabolism: extensively metabolized in intestinal wall and liver. Main routes of metabolism by oxidative processes mediated largely by hepatic microsomal and other drug-metabolizing enzymes. Conjugation with glucuronic acid is prominent route of metabolism

Excretion: half occurs in kidneys and half through enterohepatic circulation; < 1% excreted as unchanged drug

Effect of food: GI absorption modified unpredictably by food and probably decreased by antacids

Protein binding: bound significantly to plasma proteins; > 85% bound to albumin

Hepatic impairment: metabolism may increase bioavailability and decrease elimination

Elderly: half-life may be extended

PROLONGED USE

Antipsychotic drugs may be indicated for maintenance and prophylactic treatment in some disorders (particularly schizophrenia). To lessen the likelihood of adverse reactions related to cumulative drug effects, patients on long-term therapy should be evaluated periodically to determine if dosage can be lowered or drug therapy discontinued; short-acting IM preparations are not intended for long-term use. Patients should be examined periodically for the development of tardive dyskinesia or tardive dystonia.

OVERDOSAGE

Primary symptoms are those of CNS depression to the point of somnolence or coma. Hypotension and extrapyramidal symptoms also occur. Others include agitation and restlessness, convulsions, fever, autonomic reactions, ECG changes, and cardiac arrhythmia. Before treating, it is important to determine other medications being taken by the patient. Treatment is essentially symptomatic and supportive. Early gastric lavage is helpful. Keep patient under observation, and maintain open airway because involvement of the extrapyramidal mechanism may produce dysphagia and respiratory difficulty in severe overdose. *Do not attempt to induce emesis because a dystonic reaction of the head or neck may develop and result in aspiration of vomitus.* Extrapyramidal symptoms can be treated with antiparkinsonism drugs or barbiturates. Care should be taken to avoid increasing respiratory depression. If administration of a stimulant is desirable, amphetamine, dextroamphetamine, or caffeine with sodium benzoate is recommended. Stimulants that can cause convulsions should be avoided. If hypotension occurs, the standard measures for managing circulatory shock should be initiated. If a vasoconstrictor is administered, use norepinephrine or phenylephrine; other pressor agents, including epinephrine, are not recommended. Limited experience indicates that prochlorperazine is not dialyzable. If patient was given sustained-release capsules, therapy directed at reversing the effects of ingested drug and at supporting the patient should be continued for as long as overdose symptoms remain. Saline cathartics are useful for hastening evacuation of pellets that have not already released medication.

(Continued on next page)

PATIENT INFORMATION

Patients should be given a list of common side effects and instructed to report extrapyramidal symptoms. Patients should protect themselves from sun exposure. Caution should be used when performing activities requiring mental alertness. Patients should limit alcohol consumption. Given the likelihood that a proportion of patients exposed to antipsychotic drugs will develop tardive dyskinesia, all patients for whom long-term use is contemplated should be given information about this risk. The decision when to inform patients (or guardian) should take into account the clinical circumstances and the competency of the patient to understand the information provided. The risks of discontinuing treatment must also be described.

AVAILABILITY

Tablets—5 and 10 mg in 30s, 100s, 1000s, and 100 UDs (100 UDs for institutional use only); 25 mg in 100s, 1000s, and UD 100s (UD 100s for institutional use only)

Spansule capsules (sustained release)—10, 15, and 30 mg in 50s, 500s, and UD 100s

Injection—5 mg/mL in 10 mL vials; 5 mg/mL (as edisylate) in 2-mL amps with and without sodium sulfite and sodium bisulfite, 2- and 10-mL vials with and without sodium saccharin and benzyl alcohol, and 2-mL disposable syringes with sodium saccharin and benzyl alcohol

Syrup—5 mg/5 mL with fruit flavor in 120 mL

Suppositories—2 1/2 mg in 12s for young children; 5 mg in 12s for older children; 25 mg in 12s for adults

TRIFLUOPERAZINE HYDROCHLORIDE

(Stelazine)

Trifluoperazine HCl is an antipsychotic agent classified as a piperazine-type phenothiazine. Trifluoperazine is considered a high potency compound, generally considered to be 20 times more potent than chlorpromazine on a milligram-for-milligram basis. It has relatively weak hypotensive, antichlolinergic, and sedative effects but marked extrapyramidal effects and potent antiemetic properties. Piperazine compounds in general appear to have relatively low risk of jaundice or blood dyscrasias.

SPECIAL PRECAUTIONS

The neurologic syndromes that can occur with use of trifluoperazine (parkinsonism, dystonia, akathisia, tardive dyskinesia, tardive dystonia) may be confused with other behavioral or neurologic syndromes.

Tardive dyskinesia, a syndrome of involuntary abnormal movements, may develop in patients treated with this drug. In some cases, these movements can be severe or persistent. The elderly are at highest risk, but it can occur at any age. Tardive dystonia unassociated with tardive dyskinesia has also been reported with antipsychotic drug use. The condition is characterized by delayed onset of choreic or dystonic movements and may become irreversible.

A potentially fatal syndrome involving high fever, rigidity, autonomic instability, altered level of consciousness, and elevated creatine phosphokinase referred to as *neuroleptic malignant syndrome* can occur in patients receiving antipsychotic medications.

Avoid or use with caution in patients with a history of bone marrow depression or previous hypersensitivity reaction.

Administer with caution in patients with cardiovascular disease, chronic respiratory disorders, parkinsonism, epilepsy, myasthenia gravis, narrow-angle glaucoma, and those exposed to extreme heat or cold.

Trifluoperazine can rarely produce retinopathy.

In Brief

INDICATIONS

Manifestations of psychotic disorders, mania, severe behavioral disturbances associated with some organic mental syndromes or developmental disorders

CONTRAINDICATIONS

Known hypersensitivity, comatose states or depressed levels of consciousness of unknown cause, presence of large amounts of CNS depressants

INTERACTIONS

Alcohol, sedatives, narcotics, anesthetics, tranquilizers, epinephrine, oral anticoagulants, propranolol, guanethidine, metrizamide, organophosphorus insecticides, atropine, antihistamines, opiates

ADVERSE EFFECTS

Pseudoparkinsonism, dystonia, akathisia, tardive dyskinesia, tardive dystonia, grand mal and petit mal convulsions, altered CSF proteins, cerebral edema, dry mouth, nasal congestion, headaches, nausea, constipation, obstipation, adynamic ileus, ejaculatory disorders or impotence, priapism, atonic colon, urinary retention, miosis, mydriasis, changes in cardiac rate or rhythm, hypotension, cardiac arrest, blood dyscrasias, jaundice, endocrine disturbances, hyperprolactinemia, oligomenorrhea, amenorrhea, galactorrhea, skin disorders, peripheral edema, hyperpyrexia, mild fever (large IM doses), increased weight, increased appetite, pigmentary retinopathy, epithelial keratopathy (prolonged administration), lenticular and corneal deposits (prolonged administration), sudden death, neuroleptic malignant syndrome

PHARMACOKINETICS AND PHARMACODYNAMICS

Onset of action: variable 1–3 h following oral administration; 30–60 min following IM

Peak plasma level: 1–6 h

Plasma half-life: 6–18 h

Bioavailability: variable

Metabolism: hepatic, large number of metabolites; none known to be active

Excretion: enterohepatic and renal; < 100% unchanged

Protein binding: > 95%

Hepatic impairment: impaired metabolism may increase bioavailability and decrease elimination

Elderly: half-life may be extended

(Continued on next page)

145

TRIFLUOPERAZINE HYDROCHLORIDE (CONTINUED)

SPECIAL GROUPS

Race: Generally effective regardless of race; dosage requirements may vary.

Children: Use with caution. Do not use in children or adolescents whose symptoms suggest Reye syndrome. Tardive dyskinesia can occur in children.

Elderly: Prevalence of tardive dyskinesia is highest in the elderly. Use lower doses, and increase more gradually; observe for hypotensive reactions.

Renal impairment: Administer with caution.

Hepatic impairment: Administer with caution—smaller doses may be required.

Pregnancy: Safety not established. Use only when potential benefit outweighs potential risk.

Breast-feeding: Antipyschotic drugs are excreted in low concentrations in breast milk. Use with caution.

DOSAGE

Adult: Oral route is appropriate for most patients; however, IM injections may be desirable in severely ill patients for the first 24 hours. Oral dosages can be initiated with 4 to 20 mg/d in divided doses depending on age, weight, and severity of symptoms. Dosages between 10 and 40 mg/d are usually adequate, and higher doses rarely improve response. IM 1 to 2 mg every 4 to 6 hours. For patients receiving maintenance treatment, attempts should be made to reduce dosage to the lowest effective level after symptoms have been controlled for a reasonable period.

Elderly: Usually one third to half the usual adult dose, and increase more gradually.

Children: Not recommended in children younger than 6 years. Ages 6 to 12 years, 1 to 2 mg initial daily dose. It should not be necessary to exceed 15 mg/d. IM 1 to 2 mg/d.

PROLONGED USE

Antipsychotic drugs may be indicated for maintenance and prophylactic treatment in some disorders (particularly schizophrenia). To lessen the likelihood of adverse reactions related to cumulative drug effects, patients on long-term therapy should be evaluated periodically to determine if dosage can be lowered or drug therapy discontinued; short-acting IM preparations are not intended for long-term use. Patients should be examined periodically for the development of tardive dyskinesia or tardive dystonia.

OVERDOSAGE

Possible symptoms include dystonic reactions, hypothermia, tachycardia, tachypnea, cardiac arrhythmia, fever, autonomic reactions, hypotension, somnolence, and coma. There is no specific antidote. Early treatment should include gastric lavage. *Do not attempt to induce emesis.* If a vasoconstrictor is indicated, use norepinephrine (*not epinephrine*). Observe for bladder or intestinal distention. Hemodialysis is not effective. Use conservative symptomatic treatment for CNS depression. Extrapyramidal reactions can produce dysphagia and respiratory dysfunction.

PATIENT INFORMATION

Patients should be given a list of common side effects and instructed to report extrapyramidal symptoms. Patients should protect themselves from sun exposure. Caution should be used when performing activities requiring mental alertness. Patients should limit alcohol consumption. Given the likelihood that a proportion of patients exposed to antipsychotic drugs will develop tardive dyskinesia, all patients for whom long-term use is contemplated should be given information about this risk. The decision of when to inform patients (or guardian) should take into account the clinical circumstances and the competency of the patient to understand the information provided. The risks of discontinuing treatment must also be described.

AVAILABILITY

Tablets—1, 5, and 10 mg in 100s, 500s, 1000s, and UD 100s; 2 mg in 100s, 500s, 1000s, UD 100s and UD 1000s

Concentrate—10 mg/mL in 60 mL without dropper and banana-vanilla flavor with dropper

Injection—2 mg/mL in 10-mL vials with and without sodium saccharin and 0.75% benzyl alcohol

MESORIDAZINE BESYLATE

(Serentil)

Mesoridazine besylate is a piperidine-type phenothiazine. It is the major active metabolite of thioridazine. This compound has pronounced anticholinergic, sedative, and hypotensive effects. It is a potent antiemetic. It produces relatively few extrapyramidal effects. Mesoridazine is considered a low potency antipsychotic. It is considered to be twice as potent as thioridazine and chlorpromazine on a milligram-for-milligram basis. In general, mesoridazine shares the characteristics of thioridazine, and the latter's clinical effects may be largely due to mesoridazine.

SPECIAL PRECAUTIONS

The neurologic syndromes that can occur with use of mesoridazine (parkinsonism, dystonia, akathisia, tardive dyskinesia, tardive dystonia) may be confused with other behavioral or neurologic syndromes.

Tardive dyskinesia, a syndrome of involuntary abnormal movements, may develop in patients treated with this drug. In some cases, these movements can be severe or persistent. The elderly are at highest risk, but it can occur at any age. Tardive dystonia unassociated with tardive dyskinesia has also been reported with antipsychotic drug use. The condition is characterized by delayed onset of choreic or dystonic movements and may become irreversible.

A potentially fatal syndrome involving high fever, rigidity, autonomic instability, altered level of consciousness, and elevated creatine phosphokinase referred to as *neuroleptic malignant syndrome* can occur in patients receiving antipsychotic medications.

Avoid or use with caution in patients with a history of bone marrow depression or previous hypersensitivity reaction.

Administer with caution in patients with cardiovascular disease, chronic respiratory disorders, parkinsonism, epilepsy, myasthenia gravis, narrow-angle glaucoma, and those exposed to extreme heat or cold.

Given the risk of pigmentary retinopathy, doses in excess of 400 mg should not be used.

Sexual dysfunction, particularly retrograde ejaculation, is seen with some frequency.

SPECIAL GROUPS

Race: Generally effective regardless of race; dosage requirements may vary.
Children: Use with caution. Do not use in children or adolescents whose symptoms suggest Reye syndrome. Tardive dyskinesia can occur in children.
Elderly: Prevalence of tardive dyskinesia is highest in the elderly. Use lower doses, and increase more gradually; observe for hypotensive reactions.
Renal impairment: Administer with caution.
Hepatic impairment: Administer with caution—smaller doses may be required.
Pregnancy: Safety not established. Use only when potential benefit outweighs potential risk.
Breast-feeding: Antipsychotic drugs are excreted in low concentrations in breast milk. Use with caution.

In Brief

INDICATIONS
Manifestations of psychotic disorders, mania, severe behavioral disturbances associated with some organic mental syndromes or developmental disorders

CONTRAINDICATIONS
Known hypersensitivity, comatose states or depressed levels of consciousness of unknown cause, presence of large amounts of CNS depressants

INTERACTIONS
Alcohol, anesthetics, opiates, sedatives, barbiturates, phosphorus insecticides, atropine, epinephrine, guanethidine, antacids, anticonvulsants, anticholinergic agents

ADVERSE EFFECTS
Drowsiness, pseudoparkinsonism, dizziness, weakness, tremor, restlessness, ataxia, dystonia, slurring, akathisia, opisthotonos, tardive dyskinesia, tardive dystonia, dry mouth, nausea and vomiting, fainting, stuffy nose, photophobia, constipation, blurred vision, inhibition of ejaculation, impotence, retrograde ejaculation, enuresis, incontinence, itching, rash, hypertrophic papillae of tongue, angioneurotic edema, hypotension, tachycardia, miosis, obstipation, anorexia, paralytic ileus, erythema, exfoliative dermatitis, contact dermatitis, contact dermatitis, leukopenia, thrombocytopenia, agranulocytosis, eosinophilia, anemia, corneal and lenticular opacities, pigmentary retinopathy, neuroleptic malignant syndrome, aplastic anemia, pancytopenia, fever, laryngeal edema, angioneurotic edema, asthma, jaundice, hyperprolactinemia, biliary stasis, menstrual irregularities, altered libido, gynecomastia, lactation, weight gain, edema, urinary retention, hyperpyrexia, systemic lupus erythematosus–like syndrome

PHARMACOKINETICS AND PHARMACODYNAMICS
Peak plasma levels: 1–4 h
Plasma half-life: 20–36 h
Bioavailability: 50%–60%
Metabolism: hepatic, little information about metabolites
Excretion: urinary and enterohepatic
Protein binding: > 95%
Hepatic impairment: impaired metabolism may increase bioavailability and decrease elimination
Elderly: half-life may be extended

PROLONGED USE
Antipsychotic drugs may be indicated for maintenance and prophylactic treatment in some disorders (particularly schizophrenia). To lessen the likelihood of adverse reactions related to cumulative drug effects, patients on long-term therapy should be evaluated periodically to determine if dose can be lowered or drug therapy discontinued; short-acting IM preparations are not intended for long-term use. Patients should be examined periodically for the development of tardive dyskinesia or tardive dystonia.

OVERDOSAGE
Possible symptoms include dystonic reactions, hypothermia, tachycardia, tachypnea, cardiac arrhythmia, fever, autonomic reactions, hypotension, somnolence, and coma. There is no specific antidote. Early treatment should include gastric lavage. *Do not attempt to induce emesis.* If a vasoconstrictor is indicated, use norepinephrine (*not epinephrine*). Observe for bladder or intestinal distention. Hemodialysis is not effective. Use conservative symptomatic treatment of CNS depression. Extrapyramidal reactions can produce dysphagia and respiratory dysfunction.

(Continued on next page)

MESORIDAZINE BESYLATE
(CONTINUED)

DOSAGE

Adult: Oral route appropriate for most patients; however, IM injections may be desirable in severely ill patients for the first 24 hours. Oral dosage can be initiated with 50 mg twice or three times daily, increasing to 200 to 400 mg/d. IM 25 mg initially, repeat as indicated to maximum of 100 to 200 mg/d. For patients receiving maintenance treatment, attempts should be made to reduce dosage to the lowest effective level after symptoms have been controlled for a reasonable period.

Elderly: Usually one third to half the usual adult dose, and increase more gradually.

Children: Dosage guidelines not established for children younger than 12 years. Ages 12 to 18 use low end of adult dosage.

PATIENT INFORMATION

Patients should be given a list of common side effects and instructed to report extrapyramidal symptoms. Patients should protect themselves from sun exposure. Caution should be used when performing activities requiring mental alertness. Patients should limit alcohol consumption. Given the likelihood that a proportion of patients exposed to antipsychotic drugs will develop tardive dyskinesia, all patients for whom long-term use is contemplated should be given information about this risk. The decision of when to inform patients (or guardian) should take into account the clinical circumstances and the competency of the patient to understand the information provided. The risks of discontinuing treatment must also be described.

AVAILABILITY

Tablets—10, 25, 50, and 100 mg in 100s
Concentrate—25 mg/mL in 118 mL with dropper
Injection—25 mg/mL in 1-mL amps

THIORIDAZINE HYDROCHLORIDE

(Mellaril)

Thioridazine HCl is an antipsychotic agent classified as a piperidine-type phenothiazine. It has strong sedative, hypotensive, and anticholinergic effects and weak extrapyramidal and antiemetic properties. Thioridazine is a low potency compound considered equivalent to chlorpromazine on a milligram-for-milligram basis. Thioridazine's clinical effects may be due in large part to its active metabolite, mesoridazine, which is also available commercially. Although thioridazine has weak extrapyramidal effects, it is capable of producing pseudoparkinsonism and tardive dyskinesia.

SPECIAL PRECAUTIONS

The neurologic syndromes that can occur with use of thioridazine (parkinsonism, dystonia, akathisia, tardive dyskinesia, tardive dystonia) may be confused with other behavioral or neurologic syndromes.

Tardive dyskinesia, a syndrome of involuntary abnormal movements, may develop in patients treated with this drug. In some cases, these movements can be severe or persistent. The elderly are at highest risk, but it can occur at any age. Tardive dystonia unassociated with tardive dyskinesia has also been reported with antipsychotic drug use. The condition is characterized by delayed onset of choreic or dystonic movements and may become irreversible.

A potentially fatal syndrome involving high fever, rigidity, autonomic instability, altered level of consciousness, and elevated creatine phosphokinase referred to as *neuroleptic malignant syndrome* can occur in patients receiving antipsychotic medications.

Avoid or use with caution in patients with a history of bone marrow depression or previous hypersensitivity reaction.

Administer with caution in patients with cardiovascular disease, chronic respiratory disorders, parkinsonism, epilepsy, myasthenia gravis, narrow-angle glaucoma, and those exposed heat or cold.

Given the risk of pigmentary retinopathy, doses in excess of 800 mg should not be used.

Sexual dysfunction, particularly retrograde ejaculation, is seen with some frequency.

In Brief

INDICATIONS

Manifestations of psychotic disorders, mania, severe behavioral disturbances associated with some organic mental syndromes or developmental disorders

CONTRAINDICATIONS

Known hypersensitivity, comatose states or depressed levels of consciousness of unknown causes, presence of large amounts of CNS depressants

INTERACTIONS

Alcohol, barbiturates, sedatives, anesthetics, opiates, propranolol, pindolol, epinephrine, atropine, phosphorus insecticides, antacids, guanethidine, antihypertensives, anticholinergics

ADVERSE EFFECTS

Miosis, obstipation, anorexia, paralytic ileus, erythema, exfoliative dermatitis, contact dermatitis, agranulocytosis, leukopenia, eosinophilia, thrombocytopenia, anemia, aplastic anemia, pancytopenia, fever, laryngeal edema, angioneurotic edema, asthma, jaundice, biliary stasis, hypotension, tachycardia, cardiac arrhythmia, akathisia, agitation, motor restlessness, oculogyric crisis, pseudoparkinsonism, neuroleptic malignant syndrome, tardive dyskinesia, tardive dystonia, hyperpyrexia, diaphoresis, cardiac dysrhythmia, menstrual irregularities, hyperprolactinemia, retrograde ejaculation, impotence, priapism, altered libido, gynecomastia, lactation, weight gain, edema, urinary retention, incontinence, opacities of anterior lens and cornea, pigmentary retinopathy, systemic lupus erythematosus–like syndrome, sudden death

(Continued on next page)

148

SPECIAL GROUPS

Race: Generally effective regardless of race; dosage requirements may vary.

Children: Use with caution. Do not use in children or adolescents whose symptoms suggest Reye syndrome. Tardive dyskinesia can occur in children.

Elderly: The prevalence of tardive dyskinesia is highest in the elderly. Use lower doses, and increase more gradually; observe for hypotensive reactions.

Renal impairment: Administer with caution.

Hepatic impairment: Administer with caution—smaller doses may be required.

Pregnancy: Safety not established. Use only when potential benefit outweighs potential risk.

Breast-feeding: Antipsychotic drugs are excreted in low concentrations in breast milk. Use with caution.

DOSAGE

Adults: Initially 150 to 300 mg/d in divided doses, increasing gradually to 400 to 600 mg with a maximum of 800 mg. For patients receiving maintenance treatment, attempts should be made to reduce dosage to the lowest effective level after symptoms have been controlled for a reasonable period.

Elderly: One third to half usual adult dose.

Children: 1 mg/kg daily in divided doses. Safety, efficacy, and dosage not established for children younger than 2 years.

PHARMACOKINETICS AND PHARMACODYNAMICS

Onset of action: variable
Peak plasma levels: 1–4 h
Plasma half-life: 16–36 h
Bioavailability: 50%–60%
Metabolism: hepatic; numerous metabolites; mesoridazine (the 2-sulfoxide) is active
Excretion: largely in bile and feces; < 1% unchanged
Protein binding: > 95%
Hepatic impairment: impaired metabolism may increase bioavailability and decrease elimination

PROLONGED USE

Antipsychotic drugs may be indicated for maintenance and prophylactic treatment in some disorders (particularly schizophrenia). To lessen the likelihood of adverse reactions related to cumulative drug effects, patients on long-term therapy should be evaluated periodically to determine if dose can be lowered or drug therapy discontinued; short-acting IM preparations are not intended for long-term use. Patients should be examined periodically for the development of tardive dyskinesia or tardive dystonia.

OVERDOSAGE

Possible symptoms include dystonic reactions, hypothermia, tachycardia, tachypnea, cardiac arrhythmia, fever, autonomic reactions, hypotension, somnolence, and coma. There is no specific antidote. Early treatment should include gastric lavage. *Do not attempt to induce emesis.* If a vasoconstrictor is indicated, use norepinephrine (*not epinephrine*). Observe for bladder or intestinal distention. Hemodialysis is not effective. Use conservative symptomatic treatment for CNS depression. Extrapyramidal reactions can produce dysphagia and respiratory dysfunction.

PATIENT INFORMATION

Patients should be given a list of common side effects and instructed to report extrapyramidal symptoms. Patients should protect themselves from sun exposure. Caution should be used when performing activities requiring mental alertness. Patients should limit alcohol consumption. Given the likelihood that a proportion of patients exposed to antipsychotic drugs will develop tardive dyskinesia, all patients for whom long-term use is contemplated should be given information about this risk. The decision of when to inform patients (or guardian) should take into account the clinical circumstances and the competency of the patient to understand the information provided. The risks of discontinuing treatment must also be described.

AVAILABILITY

Tablets—10, 15, 25, 50, 100, 150, and 200 mg in 100s, 500s, 1000s, and UD 100s
Concentrate—30 mg/mL in 118 mL with dropper and 120 mL with or without dropper; 100 mg/mL in 118 mL with dropper, 120 mL with or without dropper, and 3.4 mL (UD 100s)
Suspension—25 and 100 mg/5 mL with buttermint flavor in pint bottles

OLANZAPINE
(Zyprexa)

Olanzapine is an antipsychotic agent, classified as a thienobenzodiazepine, that is relatively free of extrapyramidal side effects. The drug acts as an antagonist at the dopaminergic, serotoninergic, muscarinic, adrenergic, and histaminergic receptors. Although its precise mechanism of action is unknown, it has been proposed that the drug's antipsychotic activity is mediated through a combination of dopamine type 2 and serotonin type 2A antagonism. It produces few extrapyramidal side effects at typical doses. It can produce sedation, orthostatic hypotension, and weight gain.

SPECIAL PRECAUTIONS

Olanzapine may induce orthostatic hypotension associated with dizziness, tachycardia, and syncope; dosage reduction should be considered if significant orthostatic hypotension develops. The risk of hypotension can be minimized by using a lower starting dosage (2.5 or 5 mg/d). Olanzapine should be used with caution in patients with known cardiovascular disease, cerebrovascular disease, and conditions predisposing to hypotension.

Olanzapine should be used with caution in patients with a seizure disorder.

Significant elevations in ALT (up to threefold) can occur in some patients. Caution should be exercised in patients with signs and symptoms of hepatic impairment.

Esophageal dysmotility and aspiration have been associated with antipsychotic drug use. Like other antipsychotic drugs, olanzapine should be used with caution in patients at risk for aspiration pneumonia.

Olanzapine exhibits moderate anticholinergic activity *in vivo*, and patients being treated with olanzapine exhibit an increased frequency of anticholinergic side effects such as constipation, dry mouth, and tachycardia. Consequently, olanzapine should be used with caution in patients with clinically significant prostatic hypertrophy, narrow-angle glaucoma, and paralytic ileus.

Tardive dyskinesia, a syndrome of involuntary abnormal movements, may develop in patients treated with this drug. In some cases, these movements can be severe or persistent. The elderly are at highest risk, but it can occur at any age. The risk of developing tardive dyskinesia and the likelihood that it will become irreversible increase as the total duration and total cumulative dose of the antipsychotic administered to the patient increase. The risk of this side effect may be lower in patients treated with olanzapine than in those treated with typical antipsychotics; however, additional data are necessary to make this assertion confidently. Tardive dystonia unassociated with tardive dyskinesia also has been reported with antipsychotic drug use. The condition is characterized by delayed onset of choreic or dystonic movements and may become irreversible.

Neuroleptic malignant syndrome, a potentially fatal syndrome involving high fever, rigidity, autonomic instability, altered level of consciousness, and elevated creatine phosphokinase, can occur in patients receiving antipsychotic medications. The frequency with which this side effect occurs in patients treated with olanzapine is unknown.

(Continued on next page)

In Brief

INDICATIONS
Manifestations of psychotic disorders, mania, severe behavioral disturbances associated with some organic mental syndromes or developmental disorders

CONTRAINDICATIONS
Known hypersensitivity to olanzapine

INTERACTIONS
Other centrally active drugs, alcohol, antihypertensive agents, levodopa, dopamine agonists, carbamazepine; drugs (eg, fluvoxamine) that inhibit cytochrome $P_{450}1A_2$ or induce $P_{450}1A_2$ (eg, omeprazole and rifampin) isozymes may modify bioavailability of olanzapine. The risks of using olanzapine in combination with other drugs has not been extensively evaluated in clinical trials.

ADVERSE EFFECTS
Drowsiness, dizziness, weight gain, extrapyramidal symptoms, hyperkinesia, tardive dyskinesia, nausea, anxiety, constipation, dyspepsia, rhinitis, rash, dyspnea, tachycardia, increased duration of sleep, accommodation disturbances, increased or reduced salivation, micturition disturbances, menorrhagia and metrorrhagia, diminished sexual desire, erectile dysfunction, ejaculatory dysfunction, orgasm dysfunction, aggressive reaction, headache, nausea, vomiting, abdominal pain, fever, torticollis, hypotonia, migraine, hyperreflexia, choreoathetosis, anorexia, flatulence, increased appetite, fatigue, increased or decreased sweating, eczema, alopecia, seborrhea, flu-like syndrome, diabetes mellitus, increased creatine phosphokinase, thirst, lactation, amenorrhea, increased AST, increased ALT, hepatitis, agitation

PHARMACOKINETICS AND PHARMACODYNAMICS
Onset of action: variable
Peak plasma levels: about 6 hours following oral dose
Plasma half-life: ranges from 20–55 h, with a mean half-life of about 30 h
Bioavailability: well absorbed; it is eliminated extensively by first-pass metabolism, with approximately 40% of the dose being metabolized before reaching systemic circulation
Metabolism: direct glucuronidation and cytochrome P450 (CYP)-mediated oxidation are the primary metabolic pathways for olanzapine; *in vitro* studies suggest that CYPs 1A2 and 2D6, and the flavin-containing monooxygenase systems are involved in olanzapine oxidation; CYP2D6-mediated oxidation appears to be a minor metabolic pathway *in vivo*, because the clearance of olanzapine is not reduced in subjects who are deficient in this enzyme
Excretion: following a single oral dose of olanzapine, about 7% of the drug is excreted unchanged in the urine, indicating that the drug is highly metabolized; approximately 57% and 30% of the drug are excreted in the urine and feces, respectively; after multiple dosing, the major circulating metabolites are 10-N-glucuronide at 44 % and 4-N-desmethyl olanzapine at 31% of the concentration of olanzapine; both metabolites lack pharmacologic activity at these concentrations
Effect of food: food does not affect either rate or extent of absorption; drug can be given with or without meals
Protein binding: plasma protein binding of about 93% for olanzapine; it binds principally to albumin and α_1-acid glycoprotein
Renal impairment: because olanzapine is highly metabolized before excretion and only 7% of the drug is excreted unchanged, renal dysfunction alone is unlikely to have a major impact on the pharmacokinetics of olanzapine
Hepatic impairment: although the presence of hepatic dysfunction may be expected to reduce the clearance of olanzapine, there is as yet no definite evidence that it does

SPECIAL GROUPS

Race: Generally effective regardless of race; dosage requirements may vary but no specific modifications for race are recommended at this time.

Gender: Clearance of olanzapine is approximately 30% lower in women than in men; however, no dosage modifications based on gender are recommended at this time.

Children: Safety and efficacy not established.

Elderly: Lower starting dose is recommended.

Renal impairment: Administer with caution even though only 7% of the drug is excreted unchanged and renal dysfunction by itself appears to have little impact on its pharmacokinetics.

Hepatic impairment: Administer with caution. Use lower starting doses.

Pregnancy: Safety not established. Use only when potential benefit outweighs potential risk.

Breast-feeding: Antipsychotic drugs excreted in low concentrations in breast milk. Women receiving olanzapine should not breast-feed.

Smoking: Olanzapine clearance is about 40% higher in smokers than in nonsmokers, although dosage modifications are not routinely recommended.

Combined effects: The combined effects of age, smoking, and gender could lead to substantial pharmacokinetic differences that might necessitate dosage adjustments.

DOSAGE

Adults: *Usual dose*—Olanzapine can be administered on an every-day schedule. The initial dosage should be 5 to 10 mg/d, with a target dosage of 10 to 20 mg/d. Olanzapine can be administered without regard to meals and is best administered at bedtime. The safety of dosages above 20 mg/d has not been evaluated at this time. For patients receiving maintenance treatment, attempts should be made to reduce dosage to the lower effective level after symptoms have been controlled for a reasonable period.

Elderly: One half the adult dose, and increase more gradually. The recommended initial dose is 2.5 mg/d. Dosage increases should be increments of no more than 2.5 mg/d. If a once-a-day dosing regimen in the elderly or debilitated patient is being considered, it is recommended that the patient be titrated on twice-a-day regimen for 2 to 3 days at the target dose. Subsequent switches to a once-a-day dosing regimen can be done thereafter.

PROLONGED USE

Antipsychotic efficacy was established in short-term (6- to 8-wk) trials of schizophrenic inpatients; effectiveness in long-term use (*ie*, more than 6 to 8 weeks) has not been systematically evaluated, and the physician who elects to use olanzapine for extended periods should periodically reevaluate long-term usefulness of the drug for the individual patient

OVERDOSAGE

Experience with olanzapine in acute overdosage is limited in the premarketing database; (67 reports), with a maximum dose of 300 mg. No fatalities have been reported. Reported symptoms are those resulting from exaggeration of the drug's known pharmacologic effects (*ie*, drowsiness, sedation, and slurred speech).

To manage a case of acute overdosage, establish and maintain an airway and ensure adequate oxygenation and ventilation. Gastric lavage (after intubation if patient is unconscious) and administration of activated charcoal, together with a laxative, should be considered. The possibility of obtundation, seizures, or dystonic reaction of the head and neck following overdosage may create a risk of aspiration with induced emesis. Cardiovascular monitoring should begin immediately and should include continuous ECG monitoring to detect possible arrhythmias. There is no specific antidote to olanzapine overdosage. Therefore, appropriate supportive measures should be instituted. The possibility of multiple-drug involvement should be considered. Hypotension and circulatory collapse should be treated with appropriate measures, such as IV fluids or sympathomimetic agents (epinephrine and dopamine should not be used because β stimulation may worsen hypotension in the setting of olanzapine-induced α blockade). Close medical supervision and monitoring should continue until patient recovers.

PATIENT INFORMATION

Patients should be given a list of common side effects and be instructed to report all symptoms. Patients should protect themselves from sun exposure. Caution should be used when performing activities requiring mental alertness. Patients should limit alcohol consumption. Given the likelihood that a proportion of patients will develop tardive dyskinesia, all patients for whom long-term use is contemplated should be given information about this risk. The decision of when to inform patients (or guardians) should take into account the clinical circumstances and competency of the patient to understand the information provided. The risks of discontinuing treatment also must be described.

AVAILABILITY

Tablets—2.5, 5, 7.5, and 10 mg in 60s (bottles) and 100s (blister packs)

CHLORPROTHIXENE
(Taractan)

Chlorprothixene is an antipsychotic agent classified as a thioxanthene derivative. This compound has significant sedative, hypotensive, and antiemetic effects. It is moderately anticholinergic and produces a moderate degree of extrapyramidal side effects. Chlorprothixene is structurally similar to the phenothiazine class of antipsychotics and has clinical potency and an adverse effects profile similar in many respects to chlorpromazine.

SPECIAL PRECAUTIONS

The neurologic syndromes that can occur with use of chlorprothixene (parkinsonism, dystonia, akathisia, tardive dyskinesia, tardive dystonia) may be confused with other behavioral or neurologic syndromes.

Tardive dyskinesia, a syndrome of involuntary abnormal movements, may develop in patients treated with this drug. In some cases, these movements can be severe or persistent. The elderly are at highest risk, but it can occur at any age. Tardive dystonia unassociated with tardive dyskinesia has also been reported with antipsychotic drug use. The condition is characterized by delayed onset of choreic or dystonic movement and may become irreversible.

A potentially fatal syndrome involving high fever, rigidity, autonomic instability, altered level of consciousness, and elevated creatine phosphokinase referred to as *neuroleptic malignant syndrome* can occur in patients receiving antipsychotic medications.

Avoid or use with caution in patients with a history of bone marrow depression or previous hypersensitivity reaction.

Administer with caution in patients with cardiovascular disease, chronic respiratory disorders, parkinsonism, epilepsy, myasthenia gravis, narrow-angle glaucoma, and those exposed to extreme heat or cold.

SPECIAL GROUPS

Race: Generally effective regardless of race; dosage requirements may vary.

Children: Use with caution. Do not use in children or adolescents whose symptoms suggest Reye syndrome. Tardive dyskinesia can occur in children.

Elderly: Prevalence of tardive dyskinesia is highest in the elderly. Use lower doses, and increase more gradually; observe for hypotensive reactions.

Renal impairment: Administer with caution.

Hepatic impairment: Administer with caution—smaller doses may be required.

Pregnancy: Safety not established. Use only when potential benefit outweighs potential risk.

Breast-feeding: Antipsychotic drugs are excreted in low concentrations in breast milk. Use with caution.

In Brief

INDICATIONS

Manifestations of psychotic disorders, mania, severe behavioral disturbances associated with some organic syndromes or developmental disorders

CONTRAINDICATIONS

Known hypersensitivity, comatose states or depressed levels of consciousness of unknown cause, presence of large amounts of CNS depressants

INTERACTIONS

Alcohol, barbiturates, sedatives, narcotics, atropine and related drugs, phosphorus insecticides, antihistamines, norepinephrine

ADVERSE EFFECTS

Tardive dyskinesia, tardive dystonia, dystonia, akathisia, pseudoparkinsonism, sudden death, hypotension, cardiac arrest, asphyxia (failure of cough reflex), hyperactivity, convulsions, ataxia, dry mouth, nasal stuffiness, visual changes, constipation, headaches, gastric upset, postural hypotension, tachycardia, dizziness, dermatitis, urticarial-type skin reactions, photosensitivity, jaundice, agranulocytosis, eosinophilia, leukopenia, hemolytic anemia, thrombocytopenic purpura, pancytopenia, hyperprolactinemia, galactorrhea, increased libido, excessive weight gain, excessive thirst, hyperpyrexia, insomnia, weakness

PHARMACOKINETICS AND PHARMACODYNAMICS

Onset of action: variable 1–3 h oral; 30–60 min IM
Peak plasma levels: 2–3 h
Plasma half-life: 8–12 h
Bioavailability: 30%–60%
Metabolism: hepatic, several metabolites; little is known regarding potential activity
Excretion: enterohepatic and renal
Protein binding: > 95%
Hepatic impairment: may increase bioavailability and decrease elimination

PROLONGED USE

Antipsychotic drugs may be indicated for maintenance and prophylactic treatment in some disorders (particularly schizophrenia). To lessen the likelihood of adverse reactions related to cumulative drug effects, patients on long-term therapy should be evaluated periodically to determine if dose can be lowered or drug therapy discontinued; short-acting IM preparations are not intended for long-term use. Patients should be examined periodically for the development of tardive dyskinesia or tardive dystonia.

OVERDOSAGE

Possible symptoms include dystonic reactions, hypothermia, tachycardia, tachypnea, cardiac arrhythmia, fever, autonomic reactions, hypotension, somnolence, and coma. There is no specific antidote. Early treatment should include gastric lavage. *Do not attempt to induce emesis.* If a vasoconstrictor is indicated, use norepinephrine (*not epinephrine*). Observe for bladder or intestinal distention. Hemodialysis is not effective. Use conservative symptomatic treatment for CNS depression. Extrapyramidal reactions can produce dysphagia and respiratory dysfunction.

(Continued on next page)

DOSAGE

Adults: Oral route is appropriate for most patients; however, IM injections may be desirable in severely ill patients for the first 24 hours. Oral dosage can be initiated at 25 to 50 mg, three to four times daily. Dosages above 600 mg/d are not likely to be of added benefit. IM 25 to 30 mg three to four times daily. For patients receiving maintenance treatment, attempts should be made to reduce dosage to the lowest effective level after symptoms have been controlled for a reasonable time.

Elderly: Usually one third to half the usual adult dose, and increase more gradually.

Children: Guidelines not established for children younger than 6 years. Children aged 6 to 12 years, 30 to 100 mg/d in divided doses. Children aged 13 to 18 years, low end of adult range.

PATIENT INFORMATION

Patients should be given a list of common side effects and instructed to report extrapyramidal symptoms. Patients should protect themselves from sun exposure. Caution should be used when performing activities requiring mental alertness. Patients should limit alcohol consumption. Given the likelihood that a proportion of patients exposed to antipsychotic drugs will develop tardive dyskinesia, all patients for whom long-term use is contemplated should be given information about this risk. The decision of when to inform patients (or guardian) should take into account the clinical circumstances and the competency of the patient to understand the information provided. The risks of discontinuing treatment must also be described.

AVAILABILITY

Tablets—10 mg in 100s; 25, 50, and 100 mg in 100s and 500s
Concentrate—100 mg/5 mL with fruit flavor in 480 mL
Injection—12.5 mg/mL in 2-mL amps

THIOTHIXENE

(Navane)

Thiothixene is an antipsychotic agent classified as a thioxanthene derivative. It has moderate extrapyramidal and antiemetic effects and minimal sedative, hypotensive, and anticholinergic effects. Thiothixene is structurally similar to the phenothiazines; its potency is similar to the piperazine-type phenothiazines.

SPECIAL PRECAUTIONS

The neurologic syndromes that can occur with use of thiothixene (parkinsonism, dystonia, akathisia, tardive dyskinesia, tardive dystonia) may be confused with other behavioral or neurologic syndromes.

Tardive dyskinesia, a syndrome of involuntary abnormal movements, may develop in patients treated with this drug. In some cases, these movements can be severe or persistent. The elderly are at highest risk, but it can occur at any age. Tardive dystonia unassociated with tardive dyskinesia has also been reported with antipsychotic drug use. The condition is characterized by delayed onset of choreic or dystonic movements and may become irreversible.

A potentially fatal syndrome involving high fever, rigidity, autonomic instability, altered level of consciousness, and elevated creatine phosphokinase referred to as *neuroleptic malignant syndrome* can occur in patients receiving antipsychotic medications.

Avoid or use with caution in patients with a history of bone marrow depression or previous hypersensitivity reaction.

Administer with caution in patients with cardiovascular disease, chronic respiratory disorders, parkinsonism, epilepsy, myasthenia gravis, narrow-angle glaucoma, and those exposed to extreme heat or cold.

Sexual dysfunction, particularly retrograde ejaculation, is seen with some frequency.

In Brief

INDICATIONS

Manifestations of psychotic disorders, mania, severe behavioral disturbances associated with some organic mental syndromes or developmental disorders

CONTRAINDICATIONS

Known hypersensitivity, comatose states or depressed levels of consciousness of unknown cause, presence of large amounts of CNS depressants

INTERACTIONS

Alcohol, narcotics, barbiturates, sedatives, tranquilizers, antihistamines, phenothiazines, atropine or related drugs
Drug/laboratory test interactions: False-positive pregnancy test

ADVERSE EFFECTS

Tachycardia; hypotension; lightheadedness; syncope; drowsiness; restlessness; agitation; insomnia; cerebral edema; CSF abnormalities; pseudoparkinsonism; akathisia; dystonia; rhythmic involuntary movements of tongue, face, mouth, or jaw; leukopenia; leukocytosis; agranulocytosis; eosinophilia; hemolytic anemia; thrombocytopenia; pancytopenia; rash; pruritus; urticaria; photosensitivity; anaphylaxis (rare); lactation; moderate breast enlargement; amenorrhea; dry mouth; blurred vision; nasal congestion; constipation; increased sweating; increased salivation; impotence; hyperpyrexia; anorexia; nausea and vomiting; diarrhea; increased appetite and weight; weakness; polydipsia; peripheral edema

(Continued on next page)

153

THIOTHIXENE (CONTINUED)

SPECIAL GROUPS

Race: Generally effective regardless of race; dosage requirements may vary.

Children: Use with caution. Do not use in children or adolescents whose symptoms suggest Reye syndrome. Tardive dyskinesia can occur in children.

Elderly: The prevalence of tardive dyskinesia is highest in the elderly. Use lower doses, and increase more gradually; observe for hypotensive reactions.

Renal impairment: Administer with caution.

Hepatic impairment: Administer with caution—smaller doses may be required.

Pregnancy: Safety not established. Use only when potential benefit outweighs potential risk.

Breast-feeding: Antipsychotic drugs are excreted in low concentrations in breast milk. Use with caution.

DOSAGE

Adults: Oral route is appropriate for most patients. Initially 2 to 5 mg twice daily. Optimum dose is 20 to 30 mg/d. If necessary, increase to 60 mg/d is often effective. Exceeding 60 mg/d rarely increases beneficial response. Use IM for more rapid control and treatment of severely ill patients and when oral administration is impractical. Give 4 mg 2 to 4 times/daily. Most patients are controlled on 16 to 20 mg/d (maximum 30 mg/d). Institute oral medication as soon as feasible. For patients receiving maintenance treatment, attempts should be made to reduce dosage to lowest effective level after symptoms have been controlled for a reasonable time.

Elderly: Use with caution; administer low end of adult dosage.

Children: Dosage guidelines not established for children younger than 12 years; use with caution. In patients aged 12 to 18 years, administer low end adult dosage.

PHARMACOKINETICS AND PHARMACODYNAMICS

Onset of action: erratic and variable

Peak plasma levels: 1–3 h

Plasma half-life: 34 h

Bioavailability: readily but incompletely absorbed; distribution great because it is lipid soluble with relatively high it apparent volume of distribution

Metabolism: metabolized extensively in the liver; no active metabolites have been identified

Excretion: primary route is hepatic clearance; little unchanged drug excreted

Protein binding: bound significantly to plasma proteins

Hepatic impairment: impaired metabolism may increase availability and decrease elimination.

Elderly: half-life may be extended

PROLONGED USE

Antipsychotic drugs may be indicated for maintenance and prophylactic treatment in some disorders (particularly schizophrenia). To lessen the likelihood of adverse reactions related to cumulative drug effects, patients on long-term therapy should be evaluated periodically to determine if dose can be lowered or drug therapy discontinued; short-acting IM preparations are not intended for long-term use. Patients should be examined periodically for the development of tardive dyskinesia or tardive dystonia.

OVERDOSAGE

Symptoms include muscular twitching, drowsiness, and dizziness. Symptoms of gross overdose may include CNS depression, rigidity, weakness, torticollis, tremor, salivation, dysphagia, hypotension, disturbances of gait, or coma. Treatment is essentially symptomatic and supportive. Early gastric lavage is helpful. Keep patient under careful observation and maintain open airway because involvement of the extrapyramidal system may produce dysphagia and respiratory difficulty in severe overdosage. If hypotension occurs, the standard measures for managing circulatory shock should be used (IV fluids or vasoconstrictors). If a vasoconstrictor is needed, levarterenol or phenylephrine is most suitable; epinephrine is not recommended. If CNS depression is marked, symptomatic treatment is indicated. Extrapyramidal symptoms can be treated with antiparkinsonian drugs. There are no data on use of peritoneal dialysis or hemodialysis, but they are known to be of little value in phenothiazine intoxication.

PATIENT INFORMATION

Patients should be given a list of common side effects and be instructed to report extrapyramidal symptoms. Patients should protect themselves from sun exposure. Caution should be used when performing activities requiring mental alertness. Patients should limit alcohol consumption. Given the likelihood that a proportion of patients exposed to antipsychotic drugs will develop tardive dyskinesia, all patients for whom long-term use is contemplated should be given information about this risk. The decision of when to inform patients (or guardian) should take into account the clinical circumstances and the competency of the patient to understand the information provided. The risks of discontinuing treatment must also be described.

AVAILABILITY

Capsules—1 mg in 100s and UD 100s; 2, 5, and 10 mg in 100s, 500s, 1000s, and UD 100s; 20 mg in 100s, 500s, and UD 100s

Concentrate—5 mg/mL in 30 and 120 mL with or without fruit flavor and with or without dropper

IM solution—2 mg/mL in 2-mL vials

Powder for injection—5 mg/mL (reconstituted) in 2-mL vials

Solution—5 mg/mL in 30 and 120 mL with dropper

Antianxiety Agents: Benzodiazepine Derivatives

Edward M. Sellers

The effective use of benzodiazepines is based on a familiarity with the clinical characteristics of the disorders for which they are effective. The reader should consult the *Diagnostic and Statistical Manual, 4th edition* (DSM IV) of the American Psychiatric Association for the description of anxiety disorders and the diagnostic criteria [1]. From a clinical perspective, it is important to have a series of screening questions to use in clinical practice (Table 6-1).

OVERALL EFFICACY

High-potency benzodiazepines have proven efficacy for the following indications: panic attack, agoraphobia, panic disorder, and generalized anxiety disorders.

A panic attack is a discrete period in which there is the sudden onset of intense apprehension, fearfulness, or terror, often associated with feelings of impending doom. During these attacks, symptoms such as shortness of breath, palpitations, chest pain or discomfort, choking or smothering sensations, and fear of "going crazy" or losing control are present.

Agoraphobia is anxiety about, or avoidance of, places or situations from which escape might be difficult (or embarrassing) or in which help may not be available in the event of having a panic attack or panic-like symptoms.

Panic disorder without agoraphobia is characterized by recurrent unexpected panic attacks about which there is persistent concern. Panic disorder with agoraphobia is characterized by both recurrent unexpected panic attacks and agoraphobia.

Generalized anxiety disorder is characterized by at least 6 months of persistent and excessive anxiety and worry.

Benzodiazepines may be useful for the following indications: agoraphobia without history of panic disorder, specific phobia, social phobia, obsessive-compulsive disorder, posttraumatic stress disorder, acute stress disorder, anxiety disorder due to a general medical condition, and anxiety disorder not otherwise specified.

Agoraphobia without history of panic disorder is characterized by the presence of agoraphobia and panic-like symptoms without a history of unexpected panic attacks.

Social phobia is characterized by clinically significant anxiety provoked by exposure to certain types of social or performance situations, often leading to avoidance behavior. Benzodiazepines are possibly useful.

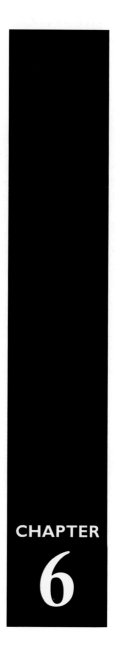

CHAPTER

6

Obsessive-compulsive disorder is characterized by obsessions (which cause marked anxiety or distress) or by compulsions (which serve to neutralize anxiety), or both. Benzodiazepines are possibly useful.

Posttraumatic stress disorder is characterized by the reexperiencing of an extremely traumatic event accompanied by symptoms of increased arousal and by avoidance of stimuli associated with the trauma. Benzodiazepines are possibly useful.

Acute stress disorder is characterized by symptoms similar to those of posttraumatic stress disorder that occur immediately in the aftermath of an extremely traumatic event. Benzodiazepines are possibly useful.

Anxiety disorder due to a general medical condition is characterized by prominent symptoms of anxiety that are judged to be a direct physiologic consequence of a general medical condition.

Anxiety disorder not otherwise specified is included for coding disorders with prominent anxiety or phobic avoidance that do not meet criteria for any of the specific anxiety disorders defined in this section (or anxiety symptoms about which there is inadequate or contradictory information).

Benzodiazepines are not recommended for specific phobia, which is characterized by clinically significant anxiety provoked by exposure to a specific feared object or situation, often leading to avoidance behavior.

Benzodiazepines often are contraindicated for substance-induced anxiety disorder characterized by prominent symptoms of anxiety that are judged to be a direct physiologic consequence of a drug of abuse, a medication, or toxin exposure.

Some clinical trials have reported benzodiazepines to be effective in the treatment of mixed anxiety and depression. In depressed patients, antidepressants, such as the selective serotonin uptake inhibitors (SSRIs), should be the first therapeutic choice.

METABOLISM

To understand the clinical differences among the benzodiazepines, it is important to have an appreciation of their differing patterns of metabolism in humans (Fig. 6-1) [2].

Triazolam, alprazolam, and diazepam are metabolized by cytochrome P450 3A (CYP3A). This cytochrome is important for metabolizing many other drugs, and interactions with these benzodiazepines should be expected with CYP3A substrates (eg, erythromycin, nefazodone, ketoconazole, tricyclic antidepressants, quinidine) [3,4]. Clinically important interactions consisting of sedation have been reported with several of these and other CYP3A-metabolized medications. Undoubtedly, many other interactions occur.

DRUG ABUSE AND DEPENDENCE

Since the late 1960s, benzodiazepines have received frequent attention with regard to their abuse and dependence potential [5]. Many clinicians and researchers consider that there has been excessive concern because the benzodiazepines are so widely used and clearly safer than are antecedent medications, such as the barbiturates [6]. All benzodiazepines produce neuroadaptation as a result of long-term use, even at therapeutic doses [7]. This may result in a drug withdrawal state on cessation of long-term use, which, although mild in most cases, is misunderstood by many to be synonymous with drug dependence. The extrapolation that long-term use defines abuse is also sometimes made. The major overlooked aspect of this issue is that most long-term users of benzodiazepines have a long history of distressing mental disorders (eg, major depression, panic disorder with agoraphobia, personality disorders) [8,9].

Some benzodiazepines are abused by certain subgroups of individuals who are known to be addicted to various illicit and licit drugs (eg, heroin addicts, methadone-treated patients, cocaine users, alcoholics). Such use by addicts and severely dependent individuals does not represent the risk in persons who have never been addicted and who receive the medication for therapeutic reasons. Some evidence exists that diazepam and alprazolam, and possibly lorazepam, are distinguishable from other benzodiazepines, since they are often chosen by drug abusers and they often produce acute effects (which makes them more desirable to such individuals) [7].

Debate continues concerning the appropriateness of using benzodiazepines in patients with past or current alcohol dependence with a current diagnosis of an anxiety disorder [10]. In the absence of a past history of benzodiazepine abuse, the risk of a new primary dependence on benzodiazepines is probably very small. Careful monitoring should detect an evolving pattern of abuse or dependence. Some clinicians prefer to use an SSRI in such patients.

Table 6-1. Screening Questions for Anxiety Disorders

Question	Follow-up	Probable Disorder
Do you have sudden unexpected attacks of anxiety?	Define a panic attack, describe the symptoms	Panic disorder
Do you avoid going to places from which you can't leave easily?	Establish what the patient can no longer do. Give examples: crowds, line-ups	Agoraphobia
Are you uncomfortable doing tasks in front of people?	Establish if there is fear of being criticized or of being thought to look foolish	Social phobia
Are you afraid of insects, heights, or blood?	Check for severity	Simple phobia
Do you find that you keep thinking thoughts you don't want to have?	Determine the nature of the thoughts: harm to others, fear of dirt or contamination	Obsessive-compulsive disorder
Do you have to keep carrying out actions you don't want to?	Determine the nature of the actions: checking, counting, washing	Obsessive-compulsive disorder
Have you been injured, attacked, or abused?	Establish the nature and timing of the trauma	Posttraumatic stress disorder
Do you worry unnecessarily?	Establish if the worry is about family, work, children, or health	Generalized anxiety disorder
Are you depressed, sad, or blue?	Establish whether the mood change has lasted for 2 wk or if the person is thinking of suicide	Mood disorder

Courtesy of Dr. R.P. Swinson, University of Toronto.

DISCONTINUATION AND WITHDRAWAL

The evidence is now overwhelming that physiologic dependence occurs in both high-dosage and low-dosage use. Even long-term therapeutic use (≥ 3 mo) may have detectable withdrawal symptoms. This occurs particularly if dosages are abruptly stopped and in many cases even if they are tapered too quickly [11].

The major clinical problem that arises is the similarity of the withdrawal symptoms of the preexisting anxiety disorder that may reemerge on cessation of treatment. However, there can be both qualitative differences in the nature of the symptoms and differences in the time course of both sets of symptoms. This has been clearly demonstrated in randomized, double-blind, placebo-controlled trials [11].

The occurrence and timing of withdrawal symptoms are clearly related to the particular pharmacologic properties of the benzodiazepine ingested as well as to the dose and duration of use. The onset of withdrawal symptoms relates directly to the elimination rates of the drug or active metabolites [12,13]. In general, ultra–short-acting (eg, triazolam; half-life, 2–5 h), short-acting (eg, oxazepam; half-life, 6 h), and intermediate-acting (eg, lorazepam; half-life, 12–15 h) benzodiazepines may be more likely to produce withdrawal symptoms. With more slowly eliminated drugs, such as diazepam, withdrawal symptoms may occur after 7 days and may last as long as 1 month or more. The likelihood of major withdrawal symptoms is reduced with longer-acting drugs, although seizures have been reported after sudden cessation of high-dose diazepam ingestion [14].

Benzodiazepine withdrawal symptoms resemble those following abrupt withdrawal from high or sometimes therapeutic doses of barbiturates and, to a lesser extent, those from alcohol. Differences exist, however, in the timing, severity, and range of symptoms, which often persist for a long time (up to 8 weeks in some cases). This is partly attributable to the prolonged elimination phase of some agents, such as diazepam. Some symptoms correspond to psychologic symptoms of anxiety, such as tension, difficulty concentrating, fear, fatigue, restlessness, and irritability. Others correspond to somatic anxiety symptoms, such as headache, insomnia, sweating, tremor, anorexia, and dizziness. Some of these symptoms are due to withdrawal, and it is important to note that they do not represent a return to *preexisting* anxiety. Other symptoms (muscle ache, flu-like illness, and sensory disturbances, such as paresthesias, hyperacusis, photophobia, hypersomnia, and metallic taste) are not typical of anxiety. Some of these symptoms (eg, sensory disturbances) can occur in up to 30% of patients [7,11,14].

PREVENTION OF WITHDRAWAL AND MANAGEMENT OF DISCONTINUATION

The regular consumption of benzodiazepines should be kept to as short a period as possible. In addition, the dosage should be kept as low as possible because clinically important problems are more likely to occur with higher dosages.

For any patient who has been taking benzodiazepines regularly for more than 4 to 6 weeks, a gradual reduction in dosage is appropriate, typically over 6 to 12 weeks. However, because many patients do not have any discontinuation symptoms, a trial of more rapid discontinuation and even abrupt cessation can be considered.

EFFICACY AND USE

Benzodiazepines are among the most commonly used medications for symptomatic relief of a wide range of clinical disorders, including anxiety; anxiety associated with depression; treatment of panic disorder with or without agoraphobia: acute alcohol withdrawal; preoperative apprehension and anxiety; as adjunctive therapy in management of partial seizures; muscle relaxation; as an adjunct before endoscopic procedures; for tetanus in infants, and in management of anxiety, tension, agitation, and irritability in older patients [2]. Treatment should be initiated at the lowest dose appropriate for age and prior use of the medication. The elderly should generally be started at drug doses that are half of the dose of younger patients because of the greater sensitivity of the elderly to benzodiazepines [15]. Initial treatment should be for 6 weeks, at which time the overall response to treatment can be assessed and the need for continued treatment determined. In the case of panic disorder, dose adjustment until the patient is free of panic attacks or the side effects are unacceptable is recommended. In such patients, an initial trial of treatment is rarely for less than 6 months [11].

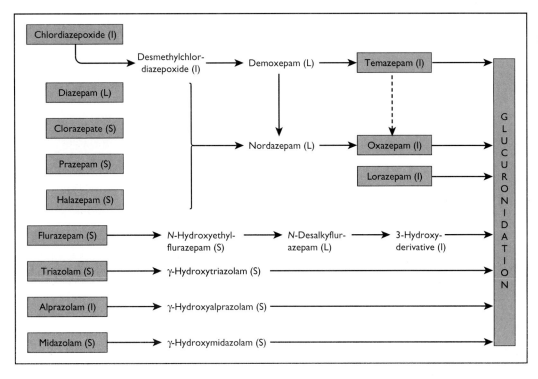

FIGURE 6-1.

Major metabolic relationships between some of the benzodiazepines. Compounds enclosed in *boxes* are marketed in the United States. The approximate half-lives of the compounds are denoted in parentheses: S—< 6 h; I—6–20 h; L—> 20 h. (*Adapted from* Baldessarini [2]; with permission.)

For efficacy in anxiety disorders such as generalized anxiety, most studies have been rather short considering the chronicity of anxiety disorders; hence, efficacy is most clear for treatment over 4 to 12 weeks. As more clinical experience has been gained with each benzodiazepine and longer trials have been conducted, longer-term efficacy has been demonstrated. Therefore, although treatment should be confined to the shortest duration possible, longer-term treatment may be needed and can be effective. A substantial proportion of long-term users (*ie*, > 12 mo) are over 60 years old and many are women. This has raised particular concern about the patterns of benzodiazepine prescribing to the elderly and women.

Initial doses of benzodiazepines may be accompanied by prominent sedation [2]. Patients should be cautioned about this and should not drive or place themselves in situations of risk until the nature of their response is known. Some tolerance to the sedating effects occurs over a few weeks. Benzodiazepines can be discontinued abruptly when they have been used for short duration for acute symptomatic relief or an anxiety disorder for no longer than 4 weeks. For patients receiving the medication for a longer period, the medication should be tapered at a rate acceptable to and tolerated by the patient. The duration of tapering is affected by the dose of medication the patient has received, the duration of use, the patient's determination to stop using the drug, and the chronicity and severity of the underlying psychopathology. For patients with panic disorder who have received medication for long period (*eg*, > 1 y) and higher dose of medication, tapering should take up to 12 weeks or longer [11]. Other patients taking medications for several months may be able to taper over 4 to 6 weeks. The occasional patient may want to stop abruptly. This is not recommended unless the patient is on low doses and has done this successfully in the past.

The purpose of discontinuation is to determine if the patient still requires medication. The symptoms that appear during the trial of discontinuation may be the reappearance of the symptoms of the original disorder, withdrawal symptoms, or a combination. Withdrawal symptoms disappear within a maximum of 10 to 14 days.

All patients receiving benzodiazepines should be cautioned that alcohol may potentiate the sedation caused by benzodiazepines [16].

MODE OF ACTION

Most actions of benzodiazepines are due to the improvement of central neural inhibition by the neurotransmitter γ-aminobutyric acid (GABA) by enhancement of chloride entry into cells. The extent of such entry is elegantly regulated by a macromolecular receptor complex consisting of subunits that are variable in their amino acid sequence. These primary structural changes alter the properties of the receptor. The subunit types seem to vary in different parts of the brain and in the nature of the response they may stimulate. They also may vary in the extent to which they can bind GABA and benzodiazepines and therefore the potency of a given medication. These differences in molecular and neuroanatomic distribution of GABA receptors are the basis for some clinical selectivity of benzodiazepines.

The drugs themselves also may differ in affinity and the extent of receptor occupancy that is needed to produce the same intensity of response. Whereas some benzodiazepines appear to be full agonist and produce sedation (*eg*, triazolam) with low receptor occupancy, others are more similar to partial agonists and produce less sedation (*eg*, clonazepam) but better anticonvulsant action. Some clinical differences among the benzodiazepines occur because of differences in the rate of absorption. In general, the more rapid the absorption, the greater the acute sedation and the greater the risk of abuse [2].

The effects of benzodiazepines can be reversed by the administration of antagonists that compete for these binding sites (*eg*, flumazenil).

REFERENCES

1. Diagnostic & Statistical Manual of Mental Disorders, 4th edition. American Psychiatric Association, Washington, DC: 1994.

2. Baldessarini RJ: Drugs and the treatment of psychiatric disorders. In *Goodman and Gilman's The Pharmacological Basis of Therapeutics*, edn 8. Edited by Gilman AG, Rall TW. New York: Pergamon Press, 1990:387–445.

3. Greene DS, Salazar DE, Dockens RC, *et al.*: Coadministration of nefazodone and benzodiazepines: III. A pharmacokinetic interaction study with alprazolam. *J Clin Psychopharmacol* 1995, 15:399–408.

4. Yasui N, Otani K, Kaneko S, *et al.*: A kinetic and dynamic study of oral alprazolam with and without erythromycin in humans: *in vivo* evidence for the involvement of CYP3A4 in alprazolam metabolism. *Clin Pharmacol Ther* 1996, 59:514–519.

5. Woods JH, Katz JL, Winger G: Benzodiazepines: use, abuse and consequences. *Pharmacological Rev* 1992, 44:151–342.

6. Salzman C: The APA Task Force Report on Benzodiazepine Dependence, Toxicity and Abuse. *Am J Psychiatry* 1991, 148:151–152.

7. Sellers EM, Ciraulo DA, DuPont RL, *et al.*: Alprazolam and benzodiazepine withdrawal. *J Clin Psychiatry* 1993, 54(suppl):64–75.

8. Romach MK, Busto UE, Sobell LC, *et al.*: Long-term alprazolam use. Abuse, dependence or treatment? *Psychopharmacol Bull* 1991; 27:391–395.

9. Rickels K, Case WG, Schweizer E, *et al.*: Long-term benzodiazepine users three years after participation in a discontinuation program. *Am J Psychiatry* 1991, 148:757–761.

10. Ciraulo DA, Barnhill JG, Ciraulo AM, *et al.*: Alterations in pharmacodynamics of anxiolytics in abstinent alcoholic men: subjective responses, abuse liability, and electroencephalographic effects of alprazolam, diazepam, and buspirone. *J Clin Pharmacol* 1997, 37:64–73.

11. Ballenger J, Pecknoid J, Rickels K, Sellers EM: Medication discontinuation in panic disorder. *J Clin Psychiatry* 1993, 54(suppl): 15–21.

12. Kales A, Manfredi RL, Vgontzas AN, *et al.*: Rebound insomnia after only brief and intermittent use of rapidly eliminated benzodiazepines. *Clin Pharmacol Ther* 1991, 49:468–476.

13. Jonas JM: Idiosyncratic side effects of short half-life benzodiazepine hypnotics. Fact or fancy. *Hum Psychopharmacol Clin Exp* 1992, 7:206–216.

14. Noyes R, Garvey MJ, Cook B, Suelzer M: Controlled discontinuation of benzodiazepine treatment for patients with panic disorder. *Am J Psychiatry* 1991, 148:517–523.

15. Greenblatt DJ, Harmatz JS, Shapiro L, *et al.*: Sensitivity to triazolam in the elderly. *N Engl J Med* 1991, 324:1691–1698.

16. Linnoila M, Stapleton JM, Lister R, *et al.*: Effects of single doses of alprazolam and diazepam, alone and in combination with ethanol, on psychomotor and cognitive performance and on autonomic nervous system reactivity in health volunteers. *Eur J Clin Pharmacol* 1990, 39:21–28.

ALPRAZOLAM

(Xanax, Alplax, Apu-Alpraz, Novo-Alprazol, Nu-Alpraz, Tafil, Xanor)

Alprazolam is a benzodiazepine agent classified as an antianxiety drug; its exact mechanism of action is unknown, although its mechanisms of action seem similar to all other benzodiazepines. Alprazolam primarily is prescribed for panic disorder with and without agoraphobia and for generalized anxiety disorder. Some patients use the medication as a sedative hypnotic. Although there has been some concern that alprazolam may be associated with more problems than other benzodiazepines (eg, dependence or abuse), the evidence to support this is not strong. When a drug is widely prescribed, more frequent reports of adverse effects are normal simply because of the greater market exposure. Early clinical trials suggested some antidepressant-like properties of alprazolam. These observations have not held up in patients with depression without anxiety symptoms.

SPECIAL PRECAUTIONS

Withdrawal symptoms can occur with abrupt discontinuance. Although the severity and incidence of withdrawal phenomena appear to be related to dose and duration of treatment, withdrawal symptoms (including seizures) have been reported after only brief therapy with alprazolam at doses within the recommended range for treatment of anxiety.

Psychologic dependence is a risk. The risk may be increased with longer-term use and is increased in patients with a history of alcohol or drug abuse. Alprazolam is a controlled substance under the Controlled Substance Act by the Drug Enforcement Administration and has been assigned to schedule IV.

Alprazolam is not of value in the treatment of psychotic patients and should not be used in place of appropriate treatment for psychosis.

If combined with other psychotropic agents or anticonvulsant drugs, careful consideration should be given to the pharmacology of the agents, particularly with compounds that might potentiate the action of alprazolam.

It is recommended that the dose be limited to the smallest effective dose to preclude development of ataxia or oversedation.

Episodes of hypomania and mania have been reported in association with use of alprazolam in patients with depression.

Precautions should be observed when treating patients with pulmonary function; there have been reports of death in patients with severe pulmonary disease shortly after initiation of treatment with alprazolam.

Because of their CNS-depressant effects, patients should be warned against engaging in hazardous occupations or activities requiring complete mental alertness. For the same reason, patients should be warned about simultaneous ingestion of alcohol and other CNS-depressant drugs during treatment.

Paradoxic reactions, such as excitement, stimulation, and acute rage, have been reported in psychiatric patients and hyperactive, aggressive children. Suicidal tendencies may be present, and protective measures may be necessary.

In Brief

INDICATIONS
FDA-approved: Anxiety disorders including panic disorder with and without agoraphobia, short-term relief of symptoms of anxiety, anxiety associated with depression
Off-label: Agoraphobia with social phobia; depression; premenstrual syndrome

CONTRAINDICATIONS
Drug hypersensitivity, acute narrow-angle glaucoma

INTERACTIONS
Psychotropic medications, anticonvulsants, antihistamines, ethanol, imipramine, desipramine, cimetidine, oral contraceptives

ADVERSE EFFECTS
Drowsiness, lightheadedness, depression, headache, confusion, insomnia, nervousness, syncope, dizziness, akathisia, tiredness or sleepiness, dry mouth, constipation, diarrhea, nausea or vomiting, increased salivation, tachycardia, palpitations, hypotension, blurred vision, rigidity, tremor, dermatitis or allergy, nasal congestion, weight gain or loss

PHARMACOKINETICS AND PHARMACODYNAMICS
Onset of action: intermediate; no information found on specific time range
Peak plasma levels: 1–2 h
Plasma half-life: 12–15 h; half-life may be prolonged with coadministration of oral contraceptives to healthy women and in obese patients
Bioavailability: readily absorbed; distribution may vary in elderly patients
Metabolism: hepatic biotransformation; predominant metabolites are α-hydroxyl-alprazolam and a benzophenon; biologic activity of α-hydroxyl-alprazolam about half that of alprazolam; plasma levels of metabolites low, thus precluding precise pharmacokinetic description
Excretion: alprazolam and its metabolites excreted primarily in urine
Protein binding: about 80% plasma protein bound
Renal impairment: changes in absorption, distribution, metabolism, and excretion reported
Hepatic impairment: changes in absorption, distribution, metabolism, and excretion reported in patients with impaired hepatic function and alcoholism; ability of alprazolam to induce human hepatic enzyme systems has not been determined; in patients with alcoholic liver disease, half-life prolonged

PROLONGED USE
When used at high doses for long intervals, alprazolam can cause severe emotional and physical dependence; ability of patients to discontinue therapy after long-term treatment has not been reliably determined.

(Continued on next page)

ALPRAZOLAM (CONTINUED)

SPECIAL GROUPS

Children: Safety and efficacy in children younger than 18 years have not been established.

Elderly: May be especially sensitive to the effects of alprazolam; only the smallest effective dose should be used.

Renal impairment: Observe usual precautions in treating patients with impaired renal function. Alprazolam has a weak uricosuric effect. Although other medications with weak uricosuric effect have been reported to cause acute renal failure, there have been no reported instances of acute renal failure attributable to therapy with alprazolam.

Hepatic impairment: Use with caution and at reduced doses in patients with advanced liver disease.

Pregnancy: Children born to mothers receiving alprazolam are at risk for withdrawal symptoms from the drug during the postnatal period. Also, neonatal flaccidity and respiratory problems have been reported. The drug has no established use in labor or delivery.

Breast-feeding: Contraindicated.

DOSAGE

Adults: Alprazolam given sublingually is absorbed as rapidly as after oral administration. Individualize dosages. Cautiously increase dosage to avoid adverse effects. Reduce dosages gradually when terminating therapy or decreasing daily dosage. Decrease daily dosages no more than 0.5 mg every 3 days. *Anxiety disorders*—Initial dose of 0.25 to 0.5 mg three times daily. Titrate to total dosage of 4 mg/d in divided doses. If side effects occur with starting dose, decrease dosage. *Panic disorder*—Initial dose of 0.5 mg three times daily. Depending on response, increase dosage at intervals of 3 to 4 days in increments of no more than 1 mg/d. Successful treatment has required dosages over 4 mg/d; in controlled studies, dosages in range of 1 to 10 mg/d were used.

Elderly and debilitated patients: Use with caution and at reduced dosages in debilitated patients and patients with chronic liver disease. Administer 0.25 mg two or three times daily. Gradually increase if needed and tolerated.

OVERDOSAGE

Symptoms include somnolence, confusion, impaired coordination, diminished reflexes, and coma. Death has been reported in association with overdoses of alprazolam. In addition, fatalities have been reported in patients who have overdosed with a combination of alprazolam and alcohol; alcohol levels have been lower than those usually associated with alcohol-induced fatality. Respiration, pulse rate, and blood pressure should be monitored. General supportive measures should be followed along with immediate gastric lavage. IV fluids should be given and an adequate airway maintained. If hypotension occurs, use vasopressors. Dialysis is of limited value. Flumazenil, a specific antagonist, is indicated for complete or partial reversal of sedative effects. Flumazenil is intended as an adjunct to and not as a substitute for proper management of overdosage. Patients should be monitored for resedation and respiratory depression. *The prescriber should be aware of risk of seizure in association with flumazenil treatment, particularly in long-term alprazolam users and in tricyclic antidepressant overdosage.*

PATIENT INFORMATION

Patients should be advised not to increase the dosage without consulting the physician. Patients should not stop taking the drug or decrease the dosage without consulting the physician. Patients should be warned not to consume alcohol, take other CNS-depressant medication, or perform hazardous tasks. Patients should inform physician if they are pregnant or plan to become pregnant. Patients should be informed that alprazolam can produce psychologic and physical dependence.

AVAILABILITY

Tablets—0.25 and 0.5 mg in 100s, 500s, UD 100s, Visipak 100s, and unit-of-issue 30s and 90s; 1 mg in 30s, 90s, 100s, 500s, and UD 100s; 2 mg in 100s, 500s, UD 100s, and Visipak 100s

CHLORDIAZEPOXIDE

(Librium, Lipoxide)

Chlordiazepoxide is a benzodiazepine classified as an antianxiety agent with sedative, appetite-stimulating, and weak analgesic actions; the precise mechanism of action is unknown. This benzodiazepine was the first marketed in North America. Its efficacy has been shown in a wide range of conditions, including anxiety disorders, alcohol withdrawal, and seizures. Unfortunately, newer agents have not often been compared with this medication; hence, whether newer agents are superior is not known. Chlordiazepoxide is available from a variety of suppliers and is quite inexpensive.

In Brief

INDICATIONS

Anxiety disorders, including panic disorder with or without agoraphobia, short-term relief of symptoms of anxiety, symptoms of acute alcohol withdrawal, preoperative apprehension and anxiety

CONTRAINDICATIONS

Known hypersensitivity

INTERACTIONS

Alcohol, barbiturates, sedatives, anticonvulsants, antipsychotic drugs.
Drug/laboratory test interactions: Increased 17-hydroxycorticosteroids and 17-ketosteroids; increased alkaline phosphatase, bilirubin, serum transaminase, and porphobilinogen; decreased prothrombin time in patients taking coumarin

(Continued on next page)

SPECIAL PRECAUTIONS

Chlordiazepoxide is classified by the Drug Enforcement Administration as a schedule IV controlled substance. Withdrawal symptoms similar in character to those noted with barbiturates and alcohol have occurred. After extended therapy, abrupt discontinuance should generally be avoided and a gradual dose-tapering schedule followed. Addiction-prone individuals should be under careful surveillance when receiving chlordiazepoxide.

In general, concomitant administration of chlordiazepoxide and other psychotropic agents is not recommended. If combination therapy is indicated, careful considerations should be given to the pharmacology of all agents.

Paradoxic reactions, such as excitement, stimulation, and acute rage, have been reported in psychiatric patients and hyperactive, aggressive children. It should be borne in mind that suicidal tendencies may be present, and protective measures may be necessary.

Although clinical studies have not established a cause-and-effect relationship, physicians should be aware that variable effects on blood coagulation have been reported in patients receiving oral anticoagulants and chlordiazepoxide.

Injectable chlordiazepoxide is indicated primarily in acute states; patients receiving this form of therapy should be kept under observation, preferably in bed, for up to 3 hours.

Because of their CNS-depressant effects, patients should be warned against engaging in hazardous occupations or activities requiring complete mental alertness. For the same reason, patients should be warned against simultaneous ingestion of alcohol and other CNS-depressant drugs during treatment.

Particular care should be exercised when prescribing benzodiazepines to those with a history of addiction to other drugs, including alcohol.

Benzodiazepines are not of value in the treatment of psychotic patients and should not be used in place of appropriate treatment for psychosis.

Precautions should be observed when treating patients with pulmonary dysfunction; there have been reports of death in patients with severe pulmonary disease shortly after initiation of treatment with benzodiazepines.

SPECIAL GROUPS

Children: Because clinical experience in children younger than 6 years is limited, oral chlordiazepoxide is not recommended in such children. The parenteral dose form is not recommended in children younger than 12 years.

Elderly: Use with caution and at reduced dosages; drowsiness, ataxia, and confusion are more commonly seen in the elderly.

Renal impairment: Usual precautions in treatment of patients with impaired renal function should be observed.

Hepatic impairment: Usual precautions in treatment of patients with impaired hepatic function should be observed.

Pregnancy: An increased risk of congenital malformations associated with use of chlordiazepoxide during first trimester of pregnancy has been suggested in several studies. The possibility that a woman of childbearing potential may be pregnant at time of therapy should be considered. Patients should be advised that if they become pregnant during therapy or intend to become pregnant, they should communicate with their physicians about the desirability of discontinuing the drug. Children born to mothers receiving benzodiazepines are at risk for withdrawal symptoms from the drug during the postnatal period. Neonatal flaccidity and respiratory problems also have been reported. These problems typically are found when high-dose benzodiazepines have been used or abused. The drug has no established use in labor or delivery.

ADVERSE EFFECTS

Drowsiness, ataxia, confusion, syncope, hypotension, tachycardia, skin eruptions, edema, minor menstrual irregularities, nausea, constipation, extrapyramidal symptoms, blurred vision, increased or decreased libido, pain following IM injection, changes in EEG patterns, blood dyscrasias

PHARMACOKINETICS AND PHARMACODYNAMICS

Onset of action: *Oral*—30–60 min; *IM*—15–30 min; *IV*—3–30 min

Peak plasma levels: 30 min–4 h

Plasma half-life: 5–30 h; active metabolites desmethyl, 10–18 h; demoxepam, 28–63 h; and desoxydemoxepam, 39–10 h

Bioavailability: IM absorption may be slow and erratic

Metabolism: hepatic biotransformation; major active metabolite desmethylchlordiazepoxide; active intermediate metabolites demoxepam, desmethyl, and desoxydemoxepam

Protein binding: 93% bound to plasma proteins

PROLONGED USE

When treatment is long term, periodic blood counts and liver function tests are advised; do not use parenteral dose form except for short-term treatment of acute cases.

OVERDOSAGE

Symptoms include somnolence, confusion, coma, and diminished reflexes. Respiration, pulse, and blood pressure should be monitored. General supportive measures should be followed along with immediate gastric lavage. IV fluids should be administered. Hypotension can be combated with norepinephrine or metaraminol. Dialysis is of limited value. There have been reports of excitation in patients following parenteral overdose; if this occurs, barbiturates should not be used. Flumazenil, an antagonist, is indicated for complete or partial reversal of sedative effects. Before administration, secure airway, ventilation, and IV access. Flumazenil is an adjunct to and not a substitute for proper management of overdose. Monitor patients for resedation, respiratory depression, and other residual effects. *The prescriber should be aware of a risk of seizure in association with flumazenil treatment, particularly in long-term chlordiazepoxide users and in tricyclic antidepressant overdose.*

PATIENT INFORMATION

Patients should be advised not to increase the dosage without consulting the physician. Patients should not stop taking the drug or decrease the dosage without consulting the physician. Patients should be warned not to consume alcohol, take other CNS-depressant medication, or perform hazardous tasks. Patients should be informed that chlordiazepoxide can produce psychologic and physical dependence.

AVAILABILITY

Capsules—5, 10, and 25 mg in 20s, 100s, 500s, 1000s, UD 100s, and reverse number 100s

Tablets—5, 10, and 25 mg in 100s

Powder for injection—100 mg/amp in 5-mL amp with 2-mL amp of IM diluent (contains 1.5% benzyl alcohol, polysorbate 80, 20% propylene glycol, maleic acid, and sodium hydroxide)

(Continued on next page)

CHLORDIAZEPOXIDE
(CONTINUED)

DOSAGE
Adults: *Oral*—Individualize dosage. For mild to moderate anxiety, 5 or 10 mg three or four times daily. For severe anxiety, 20 or 25 mg three or four times daily. For anxiety in patients with debilitating disease, 5 mg two to four times daily. For preoperative apprehension and anxiety on days preceding surgery, 5 to 10 mg three or four times daily. For acute alcohol withdrawal, 50 to 100 mg followed by repeated doses as needed up to 300 mg/d. Parenteral form usually used initially. Reduce to maintenance levels. *Parenteral*—Prepare solution immediately before administration. Discard any unused portion. Reconstitute solutions for IM injection only with special diluent provided. Do not use diluent if it is opalescent or hazy. Solutions made with physiologic saline or sterile water for injection should not be given IM. Give deep IM injection slowly into upper outer quadrant of gluteus muscle. Although this preparation has been given IV without untoward effects, such administration is not recommended because air bubbles form on surface of solution. For IV, add 5 mL sterile physiologic saline or sterile water for injection to contents of 100-mg amp. Agitate gently until thoroughly dissolved. Give injection slowly over 1 min. For acute alcohol withdrawal, 50 to 100 mg IM or IV initially; repeat in 2 to 4 hours if necessary. For acute or severe anxiety, 50 to 100 mg IM or IV initially; then 25 to 50 mg three or four times daily if necessary. For preoperative apprehension and anxiety, 50 to 100 mg IM 1 hour before surgery. Although 300 mg can be given during 6-hour period, do not exceed this dose in any 24-hour period.
Elderly and debilitated patients: Use with caution in debilitated patients and patients with kidney or liver disease. Use lowest dose, 25 to 50 mg IV.
Children: Oral not recommended for children younger than 6 years and parenteral not recommended for children younger than 12 years. *Oral*—Initially 5 mg two to four times daily. Can be increased to 10 mg two or three times daily. A dose of 0.5 mg/kg/d every 6 or 8 hours has also been recommended. *Parenteral*—follow dose for debilitated patients. Dose of 0.5 mg/kg/d every 6 to 8 hours IM has also been recommended.

CLORAZEPATE DIPOTASSIUM

(Tranxene)

Clorazepate dipotassium is a benzodiazepine agent classified as an antianxiety drug with anticonvulsant activities. Clorazepate is a prodrug in the sense that its pharmacologic actions are primarily due to its principal metabolite desmethyldiazepam. This metabolite is produced largely in the stomach by acid hydrolysis after the administration of clorazepate. Even though clorazepate is rapidly metabolized, its metabolite is not and has a half-life in excess of 36 hours. From a pharmacokinetic perspective, the resulting profile is not materially different than after diazepam.

SPECIAL PRECAUTIONS
Clorazeapte is not recommended for use in patients with depressive neuroses or psychotic reactions.

Withdrawal symptoms have occurred following abrupt discontinuance of clorazepate.

Caution should be observed in patients who are considered to have a psychological potential for drug dependence.

In patients in whom a degree of depression accompanies anxiety, suicidal tendencies may be present, and protective measures may be required.

Because of their CNS-depressant effects, patients should be warned against engaging in hazardous occupations or activities requiring complete mental alertness. For the same reason, patients should be warned about simultaneous ingestion of alcohol and other CNS-depressant drugs during treatment.

Particular care should be exercised when prescribing benzodiazepines to those with a history of addiction to other drugs, including alcohol.

If combined with other psychotropic agents or anticonvulsant drugs, careful consideration should be given to the pharmacology of the agents, particularly with compounds that might potentiate the action of benzodiazepines. It is recommended that the dose be limited to the smallest effective dose to preclude development of ataxia or oversedation.

(Continued on next page)

In Brief

INDICATIONS
Anxiety disorders including panic disorder with and without agoraphobia, short-term relief of symptoms of anxiety, symptomatic relief of acute alcohol withdrawal, adjunctive therapy in management of partial seizures

CONTRAINDICATIONS
Known hypersensitivity, acute narrow-angle glaucoma

INTERACTIONS
Hexobarbital, ethyl alcohol, chlorpromazine, barbiturates, narcotics, phenothiazines, MAO inhibitors, antidepressants

ADVERSE EFFECTS
Drowsiness, dizziness, GI complaints, nervousness, blurred vision, dry mouth, headache, mental confusion, insomnia, transient skin rashes, fatigue, ataxia, genitourinary complaints, irritability, diplopia, depression, tremor, slurred speech, decrease in hematocrit, abnormal liver function tests, abnormal kidney function tests, decrease in systolic blood pressure

PHARMACOKINETICS AND PHARMACODYNAMICS
Onset of action: fast; no information found on specific time frame
Peak plasma levels: 30 min–2 h
Plasma half-life: average 2 d (range 30–100 h) for active metabolite desmethyldiazepam (nordiazepam); 5–15 h for active metabolite oxazepam
Bioavailability: rapid; parent drug does not circulate; primary metabolite, nordiazepam, quickly appears in the bloodstream
Metabolism: clorazepate is hydrolyzed in stomach and absorbed as desmethyldiazepam (nordiazepam); metabolized in the liver into other metabolites, including active metabolite oxazepam; parent drug is not metabolized
Excretion: 80% recovered in urine and feces within 10 d; excretion primarily in urine with about 1% excreted per day on day 10
Effect of food: concurrent administration of antacids at therapeutic levels does not significantly influence bioavailability
Protein binding: 98% bound to plasma proteins

SPECIAL PRECAUTIONS *(CONTINUED)*

Precautions should be observed when treating patients with pulmonary dysfunction; there have been reports of death in patients with severe pulmonary disease shortly after initiation of treatment with benzodiazepines.

Paradoxic reactions, such as excitement, stimulation, and acute rage, have been reported in psychiatric patients and hyperactive, aggressive children. Suicidal tendencies may be present, and protective measures may be necessary.

SPECIAL GROUPS

Children: Because of the lack of sufficient clinical experience, clorazepate is not recommended for use as anticonvulsant therapy in patients younger than 9 years.

Elderly: Initial dose should be small and increments made gradually in accordance with the response of the patient to preclude ataxia or excessive sedation.

Renal impairment: The usual precautions in treating patients with impaired renal function should be observed in patients on clorazepate for prolonged periods.

Hepatic impairment: The usual precautions in treating patients with impaired hepatic function should be observed in patients taking clorazepate for prolonged periods.

Pregnancy: An increased risk of congenital malformations during the first trimester of pregnancy has been suggested in several studies. Use during this period should be avoided. The possibility that a woman of childbearing potential may be pregnant at time of institution of therapy should be considered. Patients should be advised that if they become pregnant during therapy or intend to become pregnant, they should communicate with their physician about the desirability of discontinuing the drug. Children born to mothers receiving benzodiazepines are at risk for withdrawal symptoms from the drug during the postnatal period. Neonatal flaccidity and respiratory problems also have been reported. These problems typically are found when high-dose benzodiazepines have been used or abused. The drug has no established use in labor or delivery.

Breast-feeding: The drug should not be given to nursing mothers because it has been reported that the major metabolite, nordiazepam, is excreted in human breast milk.

DOSAGE

Adults: *Symptomatic relief of anxiety*—30 mg/d in divided doses. Adjust gradually within the range of 15 to 60 mg/d. Can also be administered as single daily dose at bedtime; initial dose of 15 mg. After initial dose, patient may require adjustment of subsequent doses. Drowsiness may occur at initiation of treatment and with dosage increments. *Maintenance therapy*—Give 22.5-mg tablet in single daily dose as alternate dosage form for patients stabilized on 7.5 mg three times/d. Do not use to initiate therapy. 11.25-mg tablet can be given as single dose every 24 hours.

Elderly and debilitated patients: Use with caution in debilitated patients and in patients with kidney or liver disease. Initiate treatment at 7.5 to 15 mg/d. Lower doses may be indicated.

PROLONGED USE

Effectiveness of clorazepate in long-term management of anxiety, *ie*, more than 4 mo, has not been assessed by systematic clinical studies; patients taking clorazepate for prolonged periods should have blood counts and liver function tests periodically.

OVERDOSAGE

Overdosage is usually shown by varying degrees of CNS depression ranging from slight sedation to coma. There is no specific antidote. Treatment should consist of gastric evacuation either by induction of emesis or lavage. General supportive care and close observation of patient are indicated. Hypotension may occur. Although reports indicate that individuals have survived overdosages as high as 450–675 mg, these doses are not necessarily indicative of amount of drug absorbed because time interval between ingestion and institution of treatment was not always known.

PATIENT INFORMATION

Patients should be advised not to increase the dosage without consulting the physician. Patients should not stop taking the drug or decrease the dosage without consulting the physician. Patients should be warned not to consume alcohol, take other CNS-depressant mediation, or perform hazardous tasks. Patients should not take any other prescription or nonprescription drugs without the approval of the physician.

AVAILABILITY

Capsules—3.75 mg in 100s, 500s, 1000s, and UD 100s; 7.5 and 15 mg in 100s, 500s, and 1000s

DIAZEPAM
(Valium, Vivol, E Pam, Diazemuls)

Diazepam is a benzodiazepine agent classified as an antianxiety drug with muscle relaxant, anticonvulsant, and sedative effects. This agent has achieved widespread use internationally because of its effectiveness, safety, and global marketing and promotion. It is not distinguishable from other benzodiazepines in terms of its pharmacologic actions. Because the medication enters the brain relatively rapidly and is available in a formulation suitable for injection, it can be used for acute treatment of agitation and for acute procedures, for example, endoscopy, when sedation, relaxation, or amnesia is desirable. Diazepam is metabolized to an active and long-acting metabolite (N-desmethyldiazepam) and oxazepam. Both of these metabolites contribute to the overall sustained pharmacologic effects in anxiety states. Because the medication has been marketed since the mid-1960s, it is available in various countries from various suppliers and can be quite inexpensive compared with more recently marketed benzodiazepines. With respect to abuse liability, there is some evidence that drug abusers, including some alcoholics, abuse diazepam. This is probably the consequence in part of the wide availability of diazepam. Among individuals with a therapeutic need for the medication, there is no evidence of abuse.

SPECIAL PRECAUTIONS

Abrupt withdrawal of diazepam may be associated with seizure activity. If the use of diazepam in patients with seizure disorders results in an increase in frequency or severity of grand mal seizures, there may be need to increase the dose of standard anticonvulsant medication.

Withdrawal symptoms similar in character to those noted with barbiturates and alcohol have occurred following abrupt discontinuance of diazepam. Addiction-prone individuals should be under careful surveillance when receiving diazepam because of the predisposition of such patients to habituation and dependence.

When used IV, specific procedures should be followed to reduce the possibility of venous thrombosis, phlebitis, local irritation, swelling, and vascular impairment.

Extreme care must be used in administering injectable diazepam, particularly by the IV route, to patients with limited pulmonary reserve because of possibility of apnea or cardiac arrest.

Injectable diazepam should not be administered to patients in shock, coma, or acute alcoholic intoxication with depression of vital signs.

If diazepam is to be combined with other psychotropic agents or anticonvulsant drugs, careful consideration should be given to the pharmacology of all agents used.

Because of isolated reports of neutropenia, periodic blood counts are advisable for long-term therapy.

Because of their CNS-depressant effects, patients should be warned against engaging in hazardous occupations or activities requiring complete mental alertness. For the same reason, patients should be warned about simultaneous ingestion of alcohol and other CNS-depressant drugs during treatment.

Psychologic dependence is a risk. The risk may be increased with longer-term use and is increased in patients with a history of alcohol or drug abuse. Benzodiazepines are a controlled substance under the Controlled Substance Act by the Drug Enforcement Administration and have been assigned to schedule IV.

Benzodiazepines are not of value in the treatment of psychotic patients and should not be used in place of appropriate treatment for psychosis.

(Continued on next page)

In Brief

INDICATIONS
FDA-approved: Anxiety disorders including panic disorder with or without agoraphobias, short-term relief of symptoms of anxiety, acute alcohol withdrawal, as adjunct before endoscopic procedures, tetanus in infants
Off-label: Panic attacks

CONTRAINDICATIONS
Known hypersensitivity, acute narrow-angle glaucoma, open-angle glaucoma (unless patient is receiving appropriate therapy)

INTERACTIONS
Cimetidine, oral contraceptives, narcotics, barbiturates, alcohol, sedatives, thiazides and other diuretics, d-tubocurarine, gallamine, ranitidine, isoniazid, fluoxetine, valproic acid, propranolol, propoxyphene, neuromuscular blockers, levodopa, phenytoin, probenecid, scopolamine, theophylline

ADVERSE EFFECTS
Most frequent: drowsiness, fatigue, ataxia, venous thrombosis, phlebitis at site of injection
Less frequent: confusion, depression, dysarthria, headache, hypoactivity, slurred speech, syncope, tremor, vertigo, constipation, nausea, changes in libido, incontinence, urinary retention, bradycardia, cardiovascular collapse, hypotension, blurred vision, diplopia, nystagmus, urticaria, rash, hiccups, changes in salivation, neutropenia, jaundice, acute hyperexcited state, anxiety, hallucinations, increased muscle spasticity, insomnia, rage, sleep disturbances, minor changes in EEG pattern

PHARMACOKINETICS AND PHARMACODYNAMICS
Onset of action: *Oral*—30 min–1 h; *IM*—15–30 min; *IV*—< 15 min
Peak plasma levels: *Oral*—30–60 min; *IM*—30–90 min; *IV*—0.25 h
Plasma half-life: 14–60 h for diazepam; 20–70 h for active metabolite nordiazepam; prolonged in obese patients
Bioavailability: rapidly taken into brain and rapidly distributed throughout body; IM administration can be slow and absorption erratic unless given into deltoid muscle
Metabolism: broken down in liver to active metabolites desmethyldiazepam (nordiazepam), methloxazepam (temazepam), and oxazepam
Excretion: diazepam and metabolites primarily eliminated in the kidneys and excreted in urine in form of oxidized and glucuronide-conjugated metabolites
Effect of food: no anticipated effect; may be taken with food without altering absorption and distribution of drug; concomitant ingestion with antacids, however, may alter rate of absorption
Protein binding: 98% bound to plasma proteins
Renal impairment: clearance of drug depends on renal blood flow
Hepatic impairment: pharmacokinetic disposition of drug altered in patients with chronic liver disease

PROLONGED USE
Effectiveness beyond 4 mo has not been assessed by systematic clinical studies.

SPECIAL PRECAUTIONS (CONTINUED)

Precautions should be observed when treating patients with pulmonary dysfunction; there have been reports of death in patients with severe pulmonary disease shortly after initiation of treatment with benzodiazepines.

Paradoxic reactions, such as excitement, stimulation, and acute rage, have been reported in psychiatric patients and hyperactive, aggressive children. Suicidal tendencies may be present, and protective measures may be necessary.

SPECIAL GROUPS

Children: Oral dose form not recommended for use in children younger than 6 months old. Injectable dose form only recommended for treatment of tetanus and seizure activity; doses as antianxiety agent not available.

Elderly: Use extreme care when administering IV because of the possibility of cardiac arrest.

Renal impairment: Metabolites of diazepam are excreted by the kidneys; to avoid excess accumulation, caution should be exercised in administration to patients with compromised kidney function.

Hepatic impairment: The usual precautions in treating patients with impaired hepatic function should be observed. Because of isolated reports of jaundice, periodic liver function tests are advisable for long-term therapy.

Pregnancy: An increased risk of congenital malformations associated with use of diazepam during first trimester of pregnancy has been suggested in several studies. Avoid use during this period. Measurable amounts of injectable diazepam have been found in maternal and cord blood, indicating placental transfer. Until additional information is available, injectable diazepam is not recommended for obstetric use. Children born to mothers receiving benzodiazepines are at risk for withdrawal symptoms from the drug during the postnatal period. Also, neonatal flaccidity and respiratory problems have been reported. These problems are typically found when high-dose benzodiazepines have been used or abused.

Breast-feeding: Diazepam is excreted in human breast milk. Because neonates metabolize diazepam more slowly than do adults, accumulation of the drug and its metabolites to toxic levels is possible. Long-term diazepam use in nursing mothers reportedly causes infants to become lethargic and lose weight; do not give to nursing mothers.

DOSAGE

Adult: *Oral for management of anxiety disorders and relief of symptoms of anxiety*—Depending on severity of symptoms, 2 to 10 mg two to four times daily. If using slow-release capsule, 1 or 2 (15–30 mg) capsules once daily. *Parenteral for management of anxiety disorders and relief of symptoms of anxiety*—Usual recommended dosage ranges from 2 to 20 mg IM or IV, depending on indication and severity. In acute conditions, injection can be repeated in 1 hour, although interval of 3 to 4 hours is usually satisfactory. If giving IM, inject deeply into muscle. If giving IV, solution should be injected slowly, taking at least 1 minute for each 5 mg (1 mL). Do not use small veins, such as those on dorsum of hand or wrist. Extreme care should be taken to avoid intra-arterial administration or extravasation. Do not mix or dilute with other solutions or drugs in syringe or infusion flask. If it is not feasible to administer directly IV, drug can be injected slowly through infusion tubing as close as possible to the vein insertion. Administer 2 to 5 mg IM or IV; repeat in 3 to 4 hours if necessary. For severe anxiety disorders, 5 to 10 mg IM or IV; repeat in 3 to 4 hours if necessary.

(Continued on next page)

OVERDOSAGE

Symptoms include somnolence, confusion, coma, and diminished reflexes. Respiration, pulse, and blood pressure should be monitored, although in general these effects may be minimal. General supportive measures should be initiated along with IV fluids; maintain an adequate airway. Hypotension can be treated with levarterenol or metaraminol. Dialysis is of limited value. Flumazenil, a specific benzodiazepine-receptor antagonist, is indicated for complete or partial reversal of the sedative effects and may be used in situations when an overdosage is known or suspected. Before administration of flumazenil, necessary measures should be instituted for airway security, ventilation, and IV access. Flumazenil is intended as an adjunct to, not as a substitute for, proper management of diazepam overdose. Patients treated with flumazenil should be monitored for resedation, respiratory depression, and other residual diazepam effects for an appropriate period after treatment. Risk of seizure is associated with flumazenil treatment, particularly in long-term diazepam users.

PATIENT INFORMATION

Patients should be advised not to increase the dosage without consulting the physician. Patients should not stop taking the drug or decrease the dosage without consulting the physician. Patients should be warned not to consume alcohol, take other CNS-depressant medication, or perform hazardous tasks. Patients on long-term therapy may experience withdrawal symptoms on abrupt cessation of therapy. Patients should be advised to carry a Medic Alert identification indicating medication use. Do not take with antacids; however, may be taken with food or water if stomach upset occurs.

AVAILABILITY

Tablets—2 mg in 30s, 100s, 500s, 1000s, 2500s, UD32s, UD 100s, UD 500s, and RN 500s; 5 mg in 15s, 30s, 100s, 500s, 720s, 1000s, 1080s, 2500s, UD 32s, UD 100s, and RN 500s; 10 mg in 15s, 30s, 100s, 500s, 720s, 1000s, 1080s, UD 100s, and RN 500s
Capsules (slow-release)—15 mg in 100s and RX pak 30s
Oral solution—5 mg/5 mL with wintergreen-spice flavor in 500 mL and 5- and 10-mg patient cups; 5 mg/mL in 30 mL with dropper
Injection—5 mg/mL in 2-mL amps, 1-, 2-, and 10-mL vials, 2-mL disposable syringes, and 2-mL Tel-E-Ject

DIAZEPAM (CONTINUED)

DOSAGE (CONTINUED)

Elderly or debilitated patients: Use with extreme caution in patients with debilitating disease, including renal impairment. Individualize doses. In presence of debilitating disease, 2 to 2.5 mg one or two times daily initially; increase gradually as needed and tolerated. If 1 or 2.5 mg is desired dose, tablets should be used. Slow-release capsules recommended for debilitated patients only when it has been determined that 5-mg oral diazepam three times daily is optimum daily dose.

Children: IV or IM administration as antianxiety treatment not available. Because of varied responses, initiate therapy with lowest dose and increase as required. Give 1 to 2.5 mg three or four times daily and increase as needed and tolerated.

HALAZEPAM

(Paxipam)

Halazepam is a benzodiazepine agent classified as an antianxeity drug. This benzodiazepine is a pro-drug comparable to clorazepate. Most of its pharmacologic effects are mediated through its long-acting active metabolite N-desmethyldiazepam.

SPECIAL PRECAUTIONS

Prolonged use of therapeutic doses of halazepam can lead to dependence. Withdrawal syndrome has occurred after as few as 4 to 6 weeks of treatment. When discontinuing therapy in patients who have used halazepam for prolonged periods, the dose should be decreased gradually to avoid the possibility of withdrawal symptoms, especially in patients with a history of seizures or epilepsy.

Halazepam is not intended for use in patients with a primary depressive disorder or psychosis or in patients in whom anxiety is not a prominent feature of psychiatric disorders.

In patients in whom depression accompanies anxiety, suicidal tendencies may be present, and protective measures may be required.

Excitement, stimulation, and acute rage have occurred in psychiatric patients and hyperactive, aggressive children treated with halazepam. If acute hyperexcited states, hallucinations, increased muscle spasticity, insomnia, or sleep disturbances occur, discontinue the drug.

Use halazepam with caution in patients if increased salivation causes respiratory difficulty.

Because of their CNS-depressant effects, patients should be warned against engaging in hazardous occupations or activities requiring complete mental alertness. For the same reason, patients should be warned about simultaneous ingestion of alcohol and other CNS-depressant drugs during treatment.

Particular care should be exercised when prescribing benzodiazepines to those with a history of addiction to other drugs, including alcohol.

Psychologic dependence is a risk. The risk may be increased with longer-term use and is increased in patients with a history of alcohol or drug abuse. Benzodiazepines are a controlled substance under the Controlled Substance Act by the Drug Enforcement Administration and have been assigned to schedule IV.

Combined with other psychotropic agents or anticonvulsant drugs, careful consideration should be given to the pharmacology of the agents, particularly with compounds that might potentiate the action of benzodiazepines. It is recommended that the dose be limited to the smallest effective dose to preclude development of ataxia or oversedation.

Precautions should be observed when treating patients with pulmonary dysfunction; there have been reports of death in patients with severe pulmonary disease shortly after initiation of treatment with benzodiazepines.

(Continued on next page)

In Brief

INDICATIONS
Anxiety disorders including panic disorder with and without agoraphobia, short-term relief of symptoms of anxiety

CONTRAINDICATIONS
Known hypersensitivity, psychoses, acute narrow-angle glaucoma

INTERACTIONS
Cimetidine, oral contraceptives, barbiturates, narcotics, sedatives, alcohol, digoxin, levodopa, neuromuscular blocking agents, phenytoin, disulfiram, fluoxetine, isoniazid, ketoconazole, metoprolol, propoxyphene, propranolol, valproic acid, probenecid, ranitidine, rifampin, scopolamine, theophyllines

ADVERSE EFFECTS
Drowsiness, ataxia, confusion, sedation, sleepiness, depression, lethargy, apathy, fatigue, hypoactivity, lightheadedness, memory impairment, disorientation, restlessness, crying or sobbing, delirium, headache, slurred speech, aphonia, dysarthria, stupor, seizures, coma, syncope, rigidity, tremor, agitation, akathisia, hemiparesis, hypotonia, extrapyramidal symptoms, paradoxic reactions, behavior problems, hysteria, suicidal tendencies, constipation, diarrhea, dry mouth, nausea, anorexia, vomiting, difficulty swallowing, increased salivation, incontinence, changes in libido, urinary retention, menstrual irregularities, bradycardia, tachycardia, hypertension, visual disturbances, nystagmus, urticaria, pruritus, hiccup, muscular disturbance, respiratory disturbances, hepatic dysfunction

PHARMACOKINETICS AND PHARMACODYNAMICS
Onset of action: intermediate to slow; no information on time frame found
Peak plasma levels: 1–3 h for parent drug; 3–6 h for metabolite (norhalazepam)
Plasma half-life: 14 h (range 9–28 h) for parent drug; 30–100 h for metabolite
Metabolism: metabolized in the liver into desmethyldiazepam (nordiazepam) and 3-hydroxyhalazepam
Excretion: excreted through kidneys
Protein binding: 98% bound to plasma protein

PROLONGED USE
Clinical studies have not been evaluated for long-term therapy beyond 4 mo.

SPECIAL GROUPS

Children: Safety and efficacy for children younger than 18 years have not been established.

Elderly: Use with caution; adjust doses to avoid ataxia or excessive sedation.

Renal impairment: Observe usual precautions in the presence of impaired renal function.

Hepatic impairment: Observe usual precautions in the presence of impaired hepatic function.

Pregnancy: Halazepam freely crosses the placenta and may accumulate in fetal circulation. An increased risk of congenital malformations associated with the use of halazepam during the first trimester of pregnancy has been reported. Avoid use during this period. Also consider the possibility that a woman of childbearing potential may be pregnant at time of institution of therapy. Halazepam is not recommended for obstetric use (labor and delivery). Children born to mothers receiving benzodiazepines are at risk for withdrawal symptoms from the drug during the postnatal period. Also, neonatal flaccidity and respiratory problems have been reported. These problems are typically found when high-dose benzodiazepines have been used or abused.

Breast-feeding: Halazepam is excreted in human breast milk; do not give to nursing mothers.

DOSAGE

Adults: Usual dosage is 20 to 40 mg three or four times daily. Optimum dosage usually ranges from 80 to 160 mg daily. If side effects occur with the starting dose, lower the dosage.

Elderly (older than 70 years) and debilitated patients: Use with caution in patients with liver or kidney disease or in debilitated patients. Individualize dosages. Increase dosages cautiously to avoid adverse effects. Administer 20 mg once or twice a day and adjust dosage gradually.

Children: Not recommended for use in children 18 years or younger.

OVERDOSAGE

Symptoms include drowsiness, confusion, somnolence, impaired coordination, diminished reflexes, and lethargy. Symptoms of serious overdosage include ataxia, hypotonia, hypotension, hypnosis, and stages 1 to 3 of coma; death has occurred. To treat, induce vomiting and begin general supportive measures along with immediate gastric lavage or ipecac. Follow with activated charcoal administration and a saline cathartic. Monitor respiration, pulse, and blood pressure. Administer IV fluids and maintain adequate airway. Treat hypotension with norepinephrine or metaraminol. In patients with normal kidney function, forced diuresis with osmotic diuretics, IV fluids, and electrolytes may accelerate elimination of drug. Dialysis is of limited value.

PATIENT INFORMATION

Patients should be advised not to increase the dosage without consulting the physician. Patients should not stop taking the drug or decrease the dosage without consulting the physician. Patients should be warned not to consume alcohol, take other CNS-depressant medication, or perform hazardous tasks.

AVAILABILITY

Tablets—20 and 40 mg in 10s

LORAZEPAM

(Almazine, Ativan, Alzapam, Lorax, Lorsilan)

Lorazepam is a benzodiazepine classified as an antianxiety agent with sedative effects. In clinical practice, the principal uses are for anxiety disorders and for insomnia. Lorazepam is distinguishable from other benzodiazepines (eg, diazepam, chlordiazepoxide) because of its shorter half-life (approximately 14 h) and because its metabolism does not result in active metabolites of clinical importance. In addition, the metabolism is less affected by liver disease and drug interactions than are those of diazepam and chlordiazepoxide. The clinical importance of this is not clear. Because the medication has been marketed since the mid-1960s, it is available in various countries from various suppliers and can be quite inexpensive compared with more recently marketed benzodiazepines. With respect to abuse liability, there is some evidence that drug abusers, including some alcoholics, abuse lorazepam. This is probably the consequence in part of the wide availability of lorazepam. Among individuals with a therapeutic need for the mediation, there is no evidence of abuse.

(Continued on next page)

In Brief

INDICATIONS

Anxiety disorders including panic disorder with and without agoraphobia, short-term relief of symptoms of anxiety, anxiety associated with depressive symptoms; *Parenteral*—for preanesthetic medication, to produce sedation, relieve anxiety, and decrease ability to recall events related to surgery

CONTRAINDICATIONS

Oral—Known hypersensitivity, acute narrow-angle glaucoma; *Parenteral*—Intraarterial injection

INTERACTIONS

Ethyl alcohol, phenothiazines, barbiturates, MAO inhibitors, antidepressants, scopolamine, atropine

ADVERSE EFFECTS

Oral: Dizziness, weakness, unsteadiness, disorientation, depression, nausea, change in appetite, headache, sleep disturbance, agitation, eye function disturbance, small decreases in blood pressure, transient amnesia or memory impairment

Parenteral: Drowsiness, excessive sleepiness, restlessness, confusion, crying or sobbing, delirium, hallucinations, diplopia, blurred vision, pain at IM injection site, redness at IV injection site, hypertension, hypotension, skin rash, nausea, vomiting

LORAZEPAM (CONTINUED)

SPECIAL PRECAUTIONS

Before IV use, specific instructions must be followed precisely.

Not recommended for use in patients with a primary depressive disorder or psychosis.

Physical and psychologic dependence can occur with this drug. Withdrawal symptoms similar in character to those noted with barbiturates and alcohol have occurred following abrupt discontinuance of lorazepam.

In patients in whom GI or cardiovascular disorders coexist with anxiety, lorazepam has not been shown to be of significant benefit in treatment.

Because some patients have developed leukopenia, periodic blood counts are recommended for patients on long-term therapy.

Lorezepam can produce CNS-depressant effects when administered with such medications as barbiturates or alcohol.

Parenteral (IV, IM) injection form is primarily used as adjunct to anesthesia (relief of anxiety).

Particular care should be exercised when prescribing benzodiazepines to those with a history of addiction to other drugs, including alcohol.

Withdrawal symptoms can occur with abrupt discontinuance of benzodiazepines. Although the severity and incidence of withdrawal phenomena appear to be related to dose and duration of treatment, withdrawal symptoms (including seizures) have been reported after only brief therapy with alprazolam at doses within the recommended range for treatment of anxiety.

Benzodiazepines are not of value in the treatment of psychotic patients and should not be used in place of appropriate treatment for psychosis.

If combined with other psychotropic agents or anticonvulsant drugs, careful consideration should be given to the pharmacology of the agents, particularly with compounds that might potentiate the action of benzodiazepines. It is recommended that the dose be limited to the smallest effective dose to preclude development of ataxia or oversedation.

Precautions should be observed when treating patients with pulmonary dysfunction; there have been reports of death in patients with severe pulmonary disease shortly after initiation of treatment with benzodiazepines.

Paradoxic reactions, such as excitement, stimulation, and acute range, have been reported in psychiatric patients and hyperactive, aggressive children. Suicidal tendencies may be present, and protective measures may be necessary.

SPECIAL GROUPS

Children: *Oral*—safety and efficacy in children younger than 12 years not established. *Parenteral*—data insufficient to support efficacy or make dose recommendations in patients younger than 18 years; therefore, such use is not recommended.

Elderly: Use with caution; initial dose should not exceed 2 mg to avoid oversedation. Studies, however, show pharmacokinetics of drug remain unaltered.

Renal impairment: *Oral*—Usual precautions should be observed in patients with renal impairment; *Parenteral*—not recommended for patients with renal failure; this does not preclude use in patients with mild to moderate renal disease.

Hepatic impairment: *Oral*—Usual precautions should be observed in patients with renal impairment; *Parenteral*—not recommended for patients with hepatic failure; this does not preclude use of lorazepam in patients with mild to moderate hepatic disease.

(Continued on next page)

PHARMACOKINETICS AND PHARMACODYNAMICS

Onset of action: intermediate; no information found on specific time frame

Peak plasma levels: *Oral*—1–6 h; *IM*—1–1.5 h

Plasma half-life: 10–20 h

Bioavailability: *Oral*—about 90%; *Parenteral*—rapidly and completely absorbed

Metabolism: lorazepam has simple, 1-step metabolism (inactivation of parent drug) with relatively short half-life and duration of action; metabolite is an inactive glucuronide conjugate

Excretion: eliminated through kidneys and excreted in urine

Protein binding: bound 85% to plasma proteins

Renal impairment: kinetic effects may be prolonged in patients with mild to moderate kidney disease

Hepatic impairment: kinetic effects may be prolonged in patients with mild to moderate liver disease

PROLONGED USE

Oral—Used for long-term management of anxiety disorders. *Parenteral*—Used for surgical procedures.

OVERDOSAGE

Symptoms range from drowsiness to coma. Patients with mild cases have drowsiness, mental confusion, and lethargy. More serious overdosage cases result in ataxia, hypotonia, hypotension, and coma; death rarely occurs. Treatment is mainly supportive until the drug is eliminated from the body. Vital signs and fluid balance should be carefully monitored. Adequate airway should be maintained and assisted respiration used as needed. In patients with normal kidney functioning, forced diuresis with IV fluids and electrolytes may accelerate elimination of drug from the body. In addition, osmotic diuretics, such as mannitol, may be effective as adjunctive measures. In more critical situations, renal dialysis and exchange blood transfusions may be indicated.

PATIENT INFORMATION

Patients should be advised not to increase the dosage without consulting the physician. Patients should not stop taking the drug or decrease the dosage without consulting the physician. Patients should be warned not to consume alcohol, take other CNS-depressant medication, or perform hazardous tasks. To ensure safe, effective use, patients should be informed that lorazepam may produce psychologic and physical dependence.

AVAILABILITY

Tablets—0.5 mg in 30s, 100s, 250s, 500s, 1000s, UD 100s and 32s, and Redipak 250s and 100s; 1 mg in 20s, 30s, 100s, 500s, 1000s, UD 100s and 32s, and Redipak 100s and 250s; 2 mg in 20s, 30s, 100s, 250s, 500s, 1000s, UD 100s, and Redipak 100s and 250s

Concentrated oral solution—2 mg/mL in 30 mL with dropper

Injection—2 mg/mL in 1- and 10-mL vials with PEG 400, propylene glycol, and 2% benzyl alcohol; 4 mg/mL of 1-mL fill in 2-mL Tubex with PEG 400, propylene glycol, and 2% benzyl alcohol

SPECIAL GROUPS (CONTINUED)

Pregnancy: *Oral*—Increased risk of congenital malformations during the first trimester has been suggested; use during this period should almost always be avoided. *Parenteral*—Injectable lorazepam can cause fetal damage when administered to pregnant women. There are insufficient data to support use of injectable lorazepam during labor and delivery, including cesarean section. Children born to mothers receiving benzodiazepines are at risk for withdrawal symptoms from the drug during the postnatal period. Also, neonatal flaccidity and respiratory problems have been reported. These problems are typically found when high-dose benzodiazepines have been used or abused.

Breast-feeding: It is unknown whether oral lorazepam is excreted in human breast milk; as a general rule, nursing should not be undertaken. *Parenteral*—Injectable lorazepam should not be administered to nursing mothers.

DOSAGE

Adults: *Oral*—Individualize dosages. Range of 1 to 10 mg/d in divided doses; take the largest dose before bedtime. For anxiety, initial dosage of 2 to 3 mg/d 2 or 3 times daily. For insomnia-related anxiety or transient situational stress, 2 to 4 mg given at bedtime. *IM*—0.05 mg/kg to a maximum of 4 mg. For optimum effect, administer at least 2 hours before surgery. Inject undiluted deep in the muscle mass. *IV*—Before IV use, lorazepam must be diluted with equal volume of compatible solution (sterile water for injection, sodium chloride injection, or 5% dextrose injection). Inject directly into a vein or the tubing of an existing IV infusion. Do not exceed 2 mg/min. Have equipment to maintain patient airway available. Initial dose is 2 mg total or 0.044 mg/kg (0.02 mg/lb), whichever is smaller. Doses as high as 0.05 mg/kg up to total of 4 mg can be given. For optimum effect, administer 15 to 20 min before procedure.

Elderly and debilitated patients: *Oral*—Use oral with caution in debilitated patients and patients with kidney or liver disease. Parenteral use not recommended for patients with renal or hepatic failure. Initial dose of 1 to 2 mg/d in divided doses; adjust as needed and tolerated. *IM*—Same as adult. *IV*—For patients older than 50 years, do not exceed 2 mg total or 0.044 mg/kg (0.02 mg/lb), whichever is smaller.

Children: *Oral*—Not recommended for children younger than 12 years. For children ages 12 to 18 years, follow adult dosage.

OXAZEPAM

(Serax, Zapex)

Oxazepam is a benzodiazepine classified as an antianxiety drug that exerts prompt action in a variety of disorders associated with anxiety, tension, agitation, and irritability as well as anxiety associated with depression. Because oxazepam is absorbed rather slowly with a peak plasma level at about 2.5 hours, it is not particularly well suited to use as a hypnotic. Oxazepam is distinguishable from other benzodiazepines (eg, diazepam, chlordiazepoxide) because of its short half-life (approximately 6 h) and because its metabolism does not result in active metabolites of clinical importance. In addition, the metabolism is less affected by liver disease and drug interactions than are those of diazepam and chlordiazepoxide. The clinical importance of this is not clear.

SPECIAL PRECAUTIONS

Withdrawal symptoms similar in character to those noted with barbiturates and alcohol have occurred following abrupt discontinuance of oxazepam. The more severe withdrawal symptoms have usually been limited to patients who received doses over an extended period of time. Addiction-prone patients should be under careful surveillance when receiving oxazepam because of the predisposition of these patients to habituation and dependence.

Although hypotension has occurred only rarely, oxazepam should be administered with caution to patients in whom a drop in blood pressure might lead to cardiac complications.

Because of their CNS-depressant effects, patients should be warned against engaging in hazardous occupations or activities requiring complete mental alertness. For the same reason, patients should be warned about simultaneous ingestion of alcohol and other CNS-depressant drugs during treatment.

(Continued on next page)

In Brief

INDICATIONS
Anxiety disorders including panic disorder with and without agoraphobia, short-term relief of symptoms of anxiety, anxiety associated with depression; alcoholics with acute tremulousness, inebriation, or anxiety associated with alcohol withdrawal; management of anxiety, tension, agitation, and irritability in older patients

CONTRAINDICATIONS
Known hypersensitivity, psychoses

INTERACTIONS
Alcohol, narcotics, barbiturates

ADVERSE EFFECTS
Transient mild drowsiness, dizziness, vertigo, headache, mild paradoxic reactions, minor diffuse skin rashes, leukopenia, jaundice (rare), ataxia (rare)

PHARMACOKINETICS AND PHARMACODYNAMICS
Onset of action: intermediate to slow; no information found on specific time frame
Peak plasma levels: about 3 h
Plasma half-life: average of 8.2 h (range 5.7–10.9 h)
Bioavailability:
Metabolism: broken down in the liver to inactive metabolites (inactive glucuronide conjugates)
Excretion: excreted through urine (glucuronide) and feces
Protein binding: 86% bound to plasma proteins
Renal impairment:
Hepatic impairment: fatty metamorphosis of the liver may occur; such accumulations of fat are considered reversible, as there is no liver necrosis or fibrosis; significant drug accumulation does not occur

OXAZEPAM (CONTINUED)

SPECIAL PRECAUTIONS (CONTINUED)

Psychologic dependence is a risk. The risk may be increased with longer-term use and is increased in patients with a history of alcohol or drug abuse. Benzodiazepines are a controlled substance under the Controlled Substance Act by the Drug Enforcement Administration and have been assigned to schedule IV.

Benzodiazepines are not of value in the treatment of psychotic patients and should not be used in place of appropriate treatment for psychosis.

If combined with other psychotropic agents or anticonvulsant drugs, careful consideration should be given to the pharmacology of the agents, particularly with compounds that might potentiate the action of benzodiazepines. It is recommended that the dose be limited to the smallest effective dose to preclude development of ataxia or oversedation.

Precautions should be observed when treating patients with pulmonary dysfunction; there have been reports of death in patients with severe pulmonary disease shortly after initiation of treatment with benzodiazepines.

Paradoxic reactions, such as excitement, stimulation, and acute rage, have been reported in psychiatric patients and hyperactive, aggressive children. Suicidal tendencies may be present, and protective measures may be necessary.

SPECIAL GROUPS

Children: Absolute dosage for children 6 to 12 years of age not established; oxazepam not indicated in children younger than 6 years.

Elderly: Because of the potential for hypotension, administer with particular caution.

Hepatic impairment: Because of short duration of activity, oxazepam may be preferred in patients with liver disease.

Pregnancy: Oxazepam has not been studied adequately to determine whether it may be associated with an increased risk of fetal abnormality. Patients should communicate with the physician if they become pregnant or intend to become pregnant during therapy. Children born to mothers receiving benzodiazepines are at risk for withdrawal symptoms from the drug during the postnatal period. Neonatal flaccidity and respiratory problems also have been reported. These problems typically are found when high-dose benzodiazepines have been used or abused. The drug has no established use in labor or delivery.

PROLONGED USE

Effectiveness of oxazepam for more than 4 mo has not been assessed by systematic clinical studies.

OVERDOSAGE

Because oxazepam is a relatively new therapeutic agent, clinical experience for any overdosage cases has not been documented.

PATIENT INFORMATION

Patients should be advised not to increase the dosage without consulting the physician. Patients should not stop taking the drug or decrease the dosage without consulting the physician. Patients should be warned not to consume alcohol, take other CNS-depressant medication, or perform hazardous tasks.

AVAILABILITY

Capsules—10 mg in 100s, 250s, 500s, 100s, and Redipak 25s and 100s; 15 mg in 100s, 500s, 1000s, UD 100s, and Redipak 25s and 100s; 30 mg in 100s, 250s, 500s, 1000s, UD 100s, and Redipak 25s and 100s

Tablets—15 mg in 100s, 500s, and 1000s

(Continued on next page)

DOSAGE

Adults: Because of the flexibility of oxazepam and the range of emotional disturbances responsive to it, doses should be individualized for maximum beneficial effects.

Elderly: For anxiety tension, irritability, and agitation, initial dosage 10 mg three times daily; if necessary increase cautiously to 15 mg three or four times daily.

Symptoms	Dosage
Mild to moderate anxiety with associated tension, irritability, and aggitation, or related symptoms of functional origin or secondary to organic disease	10–15 mg three or four times/d
Severe anxiety syndromes, agitation, or anxiety associated with depression	15–30 mg three or four times/d
Alcoholic patient with acute inebriation, tremulousness, or anxiety following withdrawal	15–30 mg three or four times/d

PRAZEPAM

(Centrax)

Prazepam is a benzodiazepine classified as an antianxiety agent with depressant effects. Much of the pharmacologic action of prazepam is mediated through its active metabolities.

SPECIAL PRECAUTIONS

Addiction-prone individuals should be under careful surveillance when receiving prazepam because of the predisposition of these patients to habituation and dependence. Withdrawal symptoms have occurred following abrupt discontinuance of prazepam, especially in patients who received excessive doses over an extended period of time.

Not recommended for patients in psychotic states or with psychiatric disorders in which anxiety is not a prominent feature.

In patients in whom a degree of depression accompanies the anxiety, suicidal tendencies may be present, and protective measures may be required.

If combined with other psychotropic agents or anticonvulsant drugs, careful consideration should be given to the pharmacology of all agents.

Because of their CNS-depressant effects, patients should be warned against engaging in hazardous occupations or activities requiring complete mental alertness. For the same reason, patients should be warned about simultaneous ingestion of alcohol and other CNS-depressant drugs during treatment.

Psychologic dependence is a risk. The risk may be increased with longer-term use and is increased in patients with a history of alcohol or drug abuse.

Precautions should be observed when treating patients with pulmonary dysfunction; there have been reports of death in patients with severe pulmonary disease shortly after initiation of treatment with benzodiazepines.

Paradoxic reaction, such as excitement, stimulation, and acute rate, have been reported in psychiatric patients and hyperactive, aggressive children. Suicidal tendencies may be present, and protective measures may be necessary.

In Brief

INDICATIONS
Anxiety disorders including panic disorder with and without agoraphobia, short-term relief of symptoms of anxiety

CONTRAINDICATIONS
Known hypersensitivity; acute narrow-angle glaucoma

INTERACTIONS
Barbiturates, narcotics, phenothiazines, MAO inhibitors, other antidepressants

ADVERSE EFFECTS
Fatigue, dizziness, weakness, drowsiness, lightheadedness, ataxia, headache, confusion, tremor, vivid dreams, slurred speech, palpitations, stimulation, dry mouth, diaphoresis, various GI complaints, pruritus, transient skin rashes, swelling of feet, joint pains, various GU complaints, blurred vision, syncope, slight decreases in blood pressure, increases in body weight

PHARMACOKINETICS AND PHARMACODYNAMICS
Onset of action: slow; specific information on time frame not found
Peak plasma levels: 6 h for major metabolite desmethyldiazepam (norprazepam)
Plasma half-life: 30–100 h for major metabolite
Bioavailabillity: slowly absorbed over prolonged period; rather constant blood levels are maintained on multiple-dose schedules
Metabolism: significant first-pass metabolism results in biotransformation to active metabolites desmethyldiazepam (nordiazepam) and oxazepam
Excretion: prolonged; before elimination from the body, prazepam is metabolized in large part to its active metabolities; eliminated through the kidneys and excreted in urine
Protein binding: 98% bound to plasma proteins
Hepatic impairment: prolonged half-life and metabolism in hepatic-impaired patients; significant accumulation of drug and its metabolites

(Continued on next page)

171

PRAZEPAM (CONTINUED)

SPECIAL GROUPS

Children: Safety and efficacy in patients younger than 18 years have not been established.

Elderly: To preclude ataxia or excessive sedation, use with caution and in small initial doses with gradual increments.

Renal impairment: Usual precautions should be observed in patients with impaired renal function.

Hepatic impairment: Usual precautions should be observed in patients with impaired hepatic function; hepatomegaly and cholestasis have been documented in chronic toxicity studies in rats and dogs.

Pregnancy: Prazepam has not been studied adequately to determine whether it may be associated with an increased risk of fetal abnormality. Patients should be advised to communicate with the physician if they become pregnant or intend to become pregnant during therapy. Children born to mothers receiving benzodiazepines are at risk for withdrawal symptoms from the drug during the postnatal period. Neonatal flaccidity and respiratory problems also have been reported. These problems typically are found when high-dose benzodiazepines have been used or abused. The drug has no established use in labor or delivery.

Breast-feeding: Because of their molecular size, prazepam and its metabolites are probably excreted in human breast milk; therefore, this drug should not be given to nursing mothers.

DOSAGE

Adults: Administer orally in divided doses. Usual daily dose is 30 mg. Doses should be adjusted gradually within the range of 20 to 60 mg daily in accordance with patient response. Can also be administered as single daily dose at bedtime; recommended starting nightly dose is 20 mg. Optimum nightly dose usually ranges from 20 to 40 mg.

Elderly and debilitated patients: Use with caution in debilitated patients and patients with liver or kidney disease. In debilitated patients, it is advisable to initiate treatment at a divided daily dose of 10 to 15 mg.

PROLONGED USE

Effectiveness of prazepam for more than 4 mo has not been assessed by systematic clinical studies.

OVERDOSAGE

Multiple-agent overdose must be borne in mind. Vomiting should be induced if it has not occurred spontaneously. Immediate gastric lavage also is recommended. General supportive care is indicated. Hypotension is unlikely. Flumazenil, a specific antagonist, is indicated for complete or partial reversal of the sedative effects. Flumazenil is intended as an adjunct to and not as a substitute for proper management of overdosage. The prescriber should be aware of a risk of seizure in association with flumazenil treatment.

PATIENT INFORMATION

Patients should be advised not to increase the dosage without consulting the physician. Patients should not stop taking the drug or decrease the dosage without consulting the physician. Patients should be warned not to consume alcohol, take other CNS-depressant medication, or perform hazardous tasks.

AVAILABILITY

Capsules—5, 10, and 20 mg in 100s and 500s
Tablets—5 mg in 100s and 500s; 10 mg in 100s, 500s, and IU 100s

Index

178

Index of Proprietary Names

Index of FDA-Approved Indications

Index of Off-Label Indications

Agitation
divalproex sodium, 73
Agoraphobia
alprazolam, 159
Alcohol withdrawal symptoms
lorazepam, 100
Anxiety
lorazepam, 100
Apnea
neonatal
caffeine, 12
doxapram hydrochloride, 13

Bipolar disorders
clozapine, 129
Borderline personality disorder
divalproex sodium, 73

Catatonia
lorazepam, 100

Depression
alprazolam, 159

Electroconvulsive therapy
caffeine, 12

Insomnia
lorazepam, 100

Mania. *See also* Manic-depressive disorder
carbamazepine, 70
Manic-depressive disorder
carbamazepine, 70–71
divalproex sodium, 73

Nausea
lorazepam, 100

Panic disorder
diazepam, 96, 164
divalproex sodium, 73
Parkinson disease
psychosis in
clozapine, 129

Post-traumatic stress disorders
divalproex sodium, 73
Preanesthetic medication
lorazepam, 100
Premenstrual syndrome
alprazolam, 159
buspirone hydrochloride, 107
Psychosis
clozapine, 129

Schizoaffective disorder
clozapine, 129
Sedation
lorazepam, 100
Social phobia
alprazolam, 159
Status epilepticus
lorazepam, 100

Vomiting
lorazepam, 100